CROSS-CULTURAL TRAINING FOR MENTAL HEALTH PROFESSIONALS

CROSS-CULTURAL TRAINING FOR MENTAL HEALTH PROFESSIONALS

Edited by

HARRIET P. LEFLEY

University of Miami School of Medicine

and

PAUL B. PEDERSEN

Syracuse University

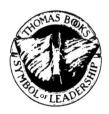

CHARLES C THOMAS • PUBLISHER
Springfield • Illinois • U.S.A.

Published and Distributed Throughout the World by

CHARLES C THOMAS • PUBLISHER

2600 South First Street

Springfield, Illinois 62708-4709

© *1986 by* CHARLES C THOMAS • PUBLISHER

ISBN 0-398-05257-3

Library of Congress Catalog Card Number: 86-5854

With THOMAS BOOKS *careful attention is given to all details of manufacturing and
design. It is the Publisher's desire to present books that are satisfactory as to their physical
qualities and artistic possibilities and appropriate for their particular use.* THOMAS
BOOKS *will be true to those laws of quality that assure a good name and good will.*

Printed in the United States of America
Q-R-3

Library of Congress Cataloging in Publication Data

Cross-cultural training for mental health professionals.

Includes bibliographies and index.
1. Psychiatry, Transcultural--United States.
2. Minorities--Mental health services--United States.
3. Mental health personnel--Education--United States.
I. Lefley, Harriet P. II. Pedersen, Paul, 1936-   .
[DNLM: 1. Community Mental Health Servi-
ces--organization & administration. 2. Cross-Cultural Comparison. 3. Inservice Training--organization &
administration. WA 305 C951]
RC455.4.E8C77   1986   362.2'042   86-5854
ISBN 0-398-05257-3

CONTRIBUTORS

Evalina W. Bestman, Ph.D.

Research Associate Professor, Department of Psychiatry, University of Miami School of Medicine, and Executive Director, New Horizons Community Mental Health Center, Miami, Fl.

Claude Charles, M.A.

Adjunct Assistant Professor, Department of Psychiatry, University of Miami School of Medicine, and Director, Haitian Services, New Horizons Community Mental Health Center, Miami, FL.

Raquel E. Cohen, M.D.

Professor of Psychiatry, University of Miami School of Medicine, and Associate Director, Child and Adolescent Services, University of Miami-Jackson Memorial Medical Center, Mental Health Services Division, Miami, Florida. Past Superintendent, Eric Lindemann Community Mental Health Center, Boston, MA.

Maria De la Roza, M.Ed.

Director of Criminal Justice Program, New Horizons Community Mental Health Center, Miami, FL.

Christine Ho, M.A.

Doctoral Candidate in Clinical Psychology, University of Washington, Seattle, WA.

Gerald Jackson, M.Ed.

Research Associate, Center for the Study of Human Environment, C.U.N.Y. Graduate Center, Visiting Faculty, Cornell University, and President, New Arena Consultants, East Orange, NJ.

William Kurtines, Ph.D.

Professor and Director of Graduate Studies, Department of Psychology, Florida International University, and Adjunct Professor of Psychiatry and Psychology, University of Miami School of Medicine, Miami, FL.

Harriet P. Lefley, Ph.D.

Professor, Department of Psychiatry, University of Miami School of Medicine. Former Director and Principal Investigator, Cross-Cultural Training Institute for Mental Health Professionals, University of Miami School of Medicine, Miami, FL.

Lou Matheson, M.A.

Coordinator, Ethnic Mental Health, Spokane Community Mental Health Center, Spokane, WA

John Papajohn, Ph.D.

Co-Director, Ethnicity and Mental Health Project, Brandeis University, Waltham, MA.

Paul B. Pedersen, Ph.D.

Chairman, Department of Counseling and Guidance, Syracuse University. Former Director and Principal Investigator, Developing Interculturally Skilled Counselors (DISC) Program, University of Hawaii.

Angel Perez-Vidal, Psy.D.

Research Assistant Professor, Coordinator of Clinical Services and Senior Therapist, Miami World Health Organization, Collaborating Center for Research and Training in Mental Health, Alcohol and Drug Dependence, Department of Psychiatry, University of Miami School of Medicine, Miami, FL.

Arturo Rio, Ph.D.

Research Assistant Professor and Research Scientist, Miami World Health Organization Collaborating Center for Research and Training in Mental Health, Alcohol and Drug Dependence, Department of Psychiatry, University of Miami School of Medicine, Miami, FL.

Maria Root, Ph.D.

Clinical Psychologist in private practice, Seattle, WA.

Mercedes C. Sandoval, Ph.D.

Director of Hialeah Center and Professor of Anthropology, Miami-Dade Community College. Former Director of Hispanic Services, New Horizons Community Mental Health Center. Adjunct Assistant Professor, Department of Psychiatry, University of Miami School of Medicine, Miami, FL.

David Santisteban, Ph.D.

Director, Human Systems Institute, and Clinical Psychologist in private practice, Miami, FL.

John P. Spiegel, M.D.

Professor, Florence Heller School, Brandeis University, and Director, Ethnicity and Mental Health Project. Past President, American Psychiatric Association.

Stanley Sue, Ph.D.
Professor of Psychology, University of California, Los Angeles, CA

James N. Sussex, M.D.
Professor and Chairman Emeritus, Department of Psychiatry, University of Miami School of Medicine, and former Director of Mental Health Services, University of Miami-Jackson Memorial Medical Center. Past President, American Board of Psychiatry and Neurology.

Jose Szapocznik, Ph.D.
Research Professor of Psychology and Psychiatry, University of Miami School of Medicine, and Director, Miami World Health Organization Collaborating Center for Research and Training in Mental Health Alcohol and Drug Dependence, Miami, FL.

Hazel H. Weidman, Ph.D.
Professor of Social Anthropology, Department of Psychiatry, University of Miami School of Medicine, and Director, Office of Transcultural Education and Research.

FOREWORD

I FEEL SURE that it is generally regarded as an honor to be asked to write a foreword to a volume like this one. I certainly consider it so. I also choose to believe that it is customary to allow the writer of such an introduction considerable leeway in approaching his task. Surely he is allowed to be as formal or informal as he sees fit, to express his views about the content of the volume and, if he wishes, to reminisce about his personal past and present association with the authors and their work. Having been invited to write the foreword to this volume, I am taking advantage of every one of those implied licenses (whether or not they actually exist!). In any case, I will invoke the privilege of senior citizenship to engage in reminiscence and justify it as placing this volume in "historical perspective."

The publication of this book caps nearly two decades of commitment of the Department of Psychiatry of the University of Miami School of Medicine to the importance of cross-cultural issues in understanding the psychodynamics of psychiatric disorders, in planning and delivering mental health services to a community, and in training people to staff those services. For many years I have been interested in such matters as difference in the experience of shame and guilt in oriental and western cultures. When I was chairman of the Department of Psychiatry of the University of Alabama's medical school in Birmingham, I became fascinated with the field work on family structure and paranoid personality patterns in Burma and Boston that Hazel Weidman had carried out in preparing the dissertation for her doctoral degree at Radcliffe, and I managed to recruit her to the faculty of that school. One of the reasons I came to Miami was the opportunity for pursuing such matters in the context of an especially rich mixture of ethnic and cultural influences. I was able to persuade Dr. Weidman to join me in Miami, and she became the first social scientist in this department. We envisioned developing a program, either within the department or under a separate administrative arrangement, similar to that of the East-West Center at the University of Hawaii.

Many factors have prevented the realization of that dream, but over the years we did manage to develop significant strength in the social sciences within our department. The first major project we undertook was what we called, without noteworthy humility, the Health Ecology Project. This was a four-year study of the health beliefs and practices of five cultural groups (Cubans, Puerto Ricans, Haitians, Bahamian Blacks, and North American Blacks) living in relatively discrete enclaves within a radius of approximately four miles from our medical center. This embraced most of the state-defined mental health catchment area in which the medical center is located, but the population focus was really defined as that served by the Comprehensive Health Care Project, a primary health care service for children and youth, headed by Fred Seligman, M.D., and under the auspices of the Department of Pediatrics. Dr. Weidman recruited a long-time friend, Janice Egeland, Ph.D., who had already established for herself an enviable reputation as a medical sociologist working among the Old-Order Amish in Lancaster County, Pennsylvania. This quartet, comprised of a social anthropologist, a medical sociologist, a pediatrician, and a psychiatrist (yours truly), put together the proposal that resulted in support of this project by the Commonwealth Fund. Under the field supervision of a young anthropologist named Clarissa Scott, who later completed her doctorate and is still a member of our faculty, the staff of this project, only two years into the study, had accumulated so much information and reached so many apparently significant insights about the mental health beliefs, practices, and needs of the people in the community that an application for the development of a community mental health center based on the project findings was submitted, approved and most importantly, funded by NIMH. This community mental health program, for the first seven years of its existence under the auspices of Jackson Memorial Hospital, our department's primary teaching affiliate, ultimately declared its independence. As the New Horizons Community Mental Health Center, under its own multi-ethnic and multi-cultural board of directors, it has continued as a unique undertaking. Under the direction of Evalina Bestman, a clinical psychologist who had already committed herself to the importance of cultural elements in developing appropriate mental health services for the multi-ethnic community for which she was responsible, this program has established an enviable reputation for itself. Dr. Mercedes Sandoval, an anthropologist and internationally known as an expert on Santeria, was one of the original faculty members on the staff of this center. Later, Claude Charles, a Haitian anthropologist, was recruited to strengthen the center's competence in Haitian matters. Dr. Harriet Lefley, a social psychologist specializing in cross-cultural issues, had joined the department in 1973 and from the beginning helped develop this center and played a key role in its research and training activities. Later Dr. Lefley developed the Cross-Cultural Training Institute that is featured in this volume.

At about the same time this program was burgeoning early in the 1970's, another community mental health effort was developing under the auspices of our Department of Psychiatry in Miami's Little Havana, an area of the city with a large portion of its population political refugees from Cuba. Originally called Encuentro, this part of the department ultimately split, one component to become the primary nucleus for another community mental health center in its own catchment area of the county and the other part to remain within the Department of Psychiatry as a separate division, called the Spanish Family Guidance Center, its multidisciplinary staff under the direction of Jose Szapocznik. This program, despite its name, was not officially formed to provide clinical services but focused its entire efforts on health services research relevant to Hispanic populations. In 1982, this division of the department was designated a World Health Organization Collaborating Center for mental health and substance abuse.

In the decade of the 70's a number of other social scientists, particularly medical sociologists and anthropologists, joined the department's Division of Addiction Sciences. Dr. Raquel Cohen, a pioneer in community psychiatry, has been active in working with Cuban refugee youth. As director of Residency Training in Child and Adolescent Psychiatry, she is actively involved in training child psychiatrists in a transcultural perspective. It is not surprising that the cross-cultural emphasis of these consultant, educational and training efforts have resulted in a volume such as this one.

As I approached that magic age when medical schools, notwithstanding Congressman Claude Pepper's valiant effort in behalf of the elderly, regard their departmental chairman as needing to step aside in favor of younger blood, it became apparent to me that our original dream of developing a "North-South Center" for carrying on multi-disciplinary research and training in the multi-ethnic and multi-cultural arena of southern United States, the Caribbean, and Central and South America, was not going to come to fruition. Instead, we decided to create within the department an Office of Transcultural Education and Research, of which Dr. Weidman assumed directorship. Its purpose is to coordinate the efforts of those faculty members in various divisions of the department who are working in areas of cross-cultural importance, and to the extent possible, to do the same thing for the medical school as a whole.

Dr. Lefley has brought together in the contents of this volume the interests of faculty members affiliated with various components of our department. The chapters authored by members of our Miami group reflect their wide experience in dealing with cross-cultural issues in the populations we serve and their commitment to the importance of the transcultural approach to the planning and implementation of health services in general and mental health services in particular. The other authors have been invited to share in this effort because their work has contributed significantly to the field. Together they have produced this volume. I share their hope that it will be as exciting to you as it has been to me and that it will be of practical value in your everyday professional work.

James N. Sussex, M.D.
Professor and Chairman Emeritus, Department of Psychiatry
The University of Miami School of Medicine
Miami, Florida

ACKNOWLEDGMENTS

IN THE FIELD OF manpower development and clinical training of mental health professionals, no single person has done more to help advance our knowlege by stimulating the exchange of ideas and information than Dr. Sam Silverstein, Chief, Center for Clinical Personnel Development, National Institute of Mental Health. Sam Silverstein, in his former position as Chief of Manpower Research and Demonstration at N.I.M.H., was the project officer and prime facilitator of all the training projects described in this book. The authors, and the field as a whole, owe him a deep debt of gratitude.

For the development of this book, Carmen Rivera, M.S.L.S., has been our most valuable asset in logistics, typing, and bibliographic assistance. Carmen also served as research assistant and primary secretarial coordinator of the Cross-Cultural Training Institute described in Part II. Special thanks are due to Luvernice Croskey, M.S.W., Rafael Urrutia, M.S., Ed Ignatoff, M.A., M.S., Herman Dorsett, Ed.D., Clarissa Scott, Ph.D., Herbeline Prier, M.Ed., and Sandra Kelly, M.S.W., for their contributions to process and research.

CONTENTS

PART I: OVERVIEW

PART II: CROSS-CULTURAL TRAINING PROGRAMS

PART III: TRANSCULTURAL SKILLS FOR SPECIAL POPULATIONS

CROSS-CULTURAL TRAINING FOR MENTAL HEALTH PROFESSIONALS

PART I

OVERVIEW

CHAPTER 1

INTRODUCTION TO CROSS-CULTURAL TRAINING

PAUL B. PEDERSEN and HARRIET P. LEFLEY

ADEQUATELY TRAINED mental health professionals will have an awareness of their own cultural biases, knowledge about the research literature relating culture to mental health, and skills to implement the insights resulting from knowledge and awareness in a culturally appropriate format. These three elements of awareness, knowledge and skill provide a sequence of cross cultural training. The goal of cross cultural training is to increase a counselor's intentionality through increasing the person's purposive control over the assumptions which guide his or her behavior, attitudes and insights.

Training can accomplish this basic goal in two ways. First, training can increase awareness of one's own cultural biases and unexamined assumptions which determine, explain and define normal behavior. Second, training can increase the awareness of culturally different alternatives so that counselors can adapt their knowledge and skill to a variety of culturally different populations to enlarge their skill repertoire. In both of these ways training seeks to go beyond the obvious definitions of culture. The most obvious cultural variables are nationality and ethnicity, which have normally defined the boundaries of "cultural" identity. It is increasingly clear, however, that gender, socioeconomic or educational status, life style, job or professional role and a variety of functional roles not only complicate a person's cultural identity, but may even overshadow ethnicity or nationality in defining the person's cultural assumptions. We function both as individuals and as members of cultural clusters. One person's "salient" culture will change from one situation to another over a period of time either as a provider or a consumer of mental health services. Training allows us to both understand the **complexity** of our many faceted culture and the **dynamic** ways in which cultural identities affect our relationships with others.

The mental health professional walks a tightrope. If cultural variables are overemphasized, the provider is guilty of stereotyping the client in one or two of the client's cultural identities. If the cultural variables are underemphasized, the provider is guilty of insensitivity to the dynamic range of influences that intrude on the interview. Mental health has created its own exotic culture crossing national boundaries, dominated by the cultural values of a politically superordinate "majority culture." Mental health services are frequently the vehicles of cultural erosion, from a non-Western point of view. The mental health institutions displace natural support systems such as the family and compete with familial interdependencies which have traditionally provided the foundation of mental health for many non-Western cultures. This process has resulted in profound consequences for less industrialized societies. First, mental health has been strongly influenced by Western dominant cultural values in its formulation and description. Second, social policies in these regions have come to depend on psychological formulations based on pro-Western cultural biases thereby increasing the process of Westernization. Third, those who are most conforming to the dominant system are favored and those who are least conforming to the dominant system are penalized resulting in socialization by force. Fourth, an accurate definition of mental health in a multicultural or culturally differentiated system will require that we first escape from the encapsulated value-assumptions of the dominant culture (Pedersen, 1984).

Wrenn (1962) describes the "culturally encapsulated counselor" as someone who has substituted stereotypes for the real world, disregards cultural variations among clients, and dogmatizes a technique-oriented job definition. A report by the Education and Training Committee of Division 17 (Counseling) of the American Psychological Association (Sue, 1980) identifies minimal cross cultural compentencies for training counselors. There were four criteria for **beliefs and attitudinal** compentencies suggesting that the culturally skilled counselor is (1) aware of and sensitive to his or her own cultural heritage, (2) aware of his or her own values and biases, (3) comfortable with cultural differences in relationships, and (4) knows when to refer clients to members of the client's own culture. With regard to **knowledge** competencies, the culturally skilled counselor will (1) understand the sociology of minority groups, (2) possess adequate cultural knowledge about his or her clients, (3) be competent in generic counseling skills, and (4) be aware of institutional barriers to minority peoples. The **skill** compentencies include the ability to (1) generate a wide variety of verbal/nonverbal counseling responses, (2) send and receive verbal and nonverbal messages accurately and appropriately, and (3) exercise institutional intervention skills to change the system when that might be appropriate.

Although a variety of intercultural training approaches have been developed (Arredondo-Dowd & Gonslaves, 1980; Bryson, Renzaglia, & Danish, 1973; Lewis & Lewis, 1970; Mitchell, 1970) there has been no systematic development of methods, no coordinated articulation of theory, no comparisons of training outcomes, and no universally accepted outcome criteria for the cross cultural training of mental health professionals. Most training approaches can be divided into those that emphasize culturally specific knowledge or skills related to the unique values of a particular culture or group and those emphasizing culturally generalized aspects that would apply in any contrasting culture. While there is a quantity of materials that emphasize the guidelines for working within one or another cultural group (Pedersen, 1981) there are few approaches that successfully generalize from one culture to another. Conceptually and in specific applications, this work is designed to meet that need.

Training Approaches Described in this Book

This book is an attempt to address some of the issues involved in training mental health professionals to deliver services that are culturally sensitive, appropriate, and acceptable to their clients. Although clinical facilities have been nationally mandated to provide culturally responsive services, few professional training programs provide courses on culture and mental health, and today's practitioners often have difficulty understanding and treating patients from culturally contrasting backgrounds. This book addresses the need in terms of methods for developing a transcultural training program. Included are curriculum models and training designs: content areas for specific populations; evaluation strategies; and empirical findings of the impact of cross cultural training on practitioners, their patients, and their institutions. Implications for professional education, clinical practice, and further research directions are indicated.

In Part I, Harriet Lefley demonstrates the need for cross cultural training through an overview of the literature describing the effects of social and cognitive distance between mental health providers and culturally diverse clients in all areas of mental health care. Issues include the interrelations of psychiatric epidemiology and differential diagnosis with cultural differences in symptomatology, normative profiles on screening instruments, cultural perceptions of mental disorders and help-seeking and utilization patterns. Discussed also are a range of treatment issues and the utilization of cultural strengths and adaptive strategies in the therapeutic process.

Three important training programs are discussed in depth in Part II, suggesting the range of models that have been developed to supplement standard clinical education in the United States. The chapter by John Spiegel and John Papajohn describes a training program in ethnicity and mental health which was organized at Brandeis University. Transactional systems theory and cultural value orientation theory were the major conceptual mainstays of the program, applied in two training sites which were also Harvard-affiliated teaching institutions. The chapter by Paul Pedersen emphasizes a broadly defined cross cultural training program in Hawaii for developing interculturally skilled counselors. The chapter by Harriet Lefley describes a series of cross cultural training institutes for mental health professionals at the University of Miami School of Medicine, with an emphasis on continuing education and in-service training for practicing mental health professionals.

In Part III, five chapters discuss background information and skills needed for serving specific ethnic groups, while Part IV focuses on examples of interventions that customize generalized techniques for specific populations. Each of these chapters is written by one or more mental health professionals who have not only worked extensively with the group in question, but are themselves of the same ethnicity and cultural background. Lou Matheson begins Part III by describing the knowledge and special sensitivities needed by a non-Indian provider working with American Indian clients. Blacks and Hispanics are the major ethnic collectivities in the United States today, and there are two chapters which deal in very different ways with each group. Gerald Jackson, long involved in cultural awareness training of mental health professionals and other human services staff, writes of Afrocentric and Eurocentric conceptualization and behavior, embedded in a highly personal account of how he uses an Afrocentric training mode to stay in tune with and lead the audience toward altered insights into the African American experience.

Evalina Bestman, executive director of a large community mental health center, discusses issues germane to training staff in community entry, needs assessment, and utilization of leadership resources in broad-scale interventions affecting mental health in the Black community.

The chapters on Hispanics are similarly diverse, yet equally valuable as training tools. Mercedes Sandoval, an anthropologist and cultural historian for many years organized and directed community mental health services for Hispanics, gives a broad historial and cultural overview of modal value orientations and behavioral patterns which transverse New World Hispanic cultures, illustrating the application of this knowledge in clinical case histories. Clinical psychologist Jose Szapocznik and his associates, long involved in clinical and acculturation research and development of therapeutic modalities for the Cuban population of South Florida, approach their subject from the vantage point of family theory. Their chapter concentrates on a family therapy training model which is specifically geared to the needs of bicultural populations, in this particular case, families of Cuban preadolescents who are in danger of becoming substance abusers.

In other chapters in Part III, Claude Charles writes of the unique mental health problems facing Haitians in the United States today, including an important section on **Vodou** and its relevance as a therapeutic system. The chapter by Root, Ho and Sue on training counselors to work with Asian Americans highlights language barriers, communication styles, and cultural variables involved in determining therapeutic goals, and discusses three levels of training required to work with this population. The authors also discuss the training model used by the National Asian American Training Center in San Francisco, a comprehensive training program for Asian Americans in psychology. In Part IV, in addition to the interventions described by Bestman and by Szapocznik and his associates, Raquel Cohen, a well known community psychiatrist and currently director of a residency training program in child and adolescent psychiatry, presents a comprehensive, well-documented analysis of how to do child psychiatry in cross cultural perspective. Although many of her case examples are from the Latin American population of South Florida, her analysis in reference to psychosocial adaptation and the parental role, key mental health issues and value systems, child development and traditionally family childrearing practice, and the critical questions that must be asked by the sensitive clinician, are highly generalizable as keys for developing optimal diagnostic and therapeutic techniques within a transcultural frame of reference.

The next section of the book looks at the effectiveness of training. Part V discusses evaluation issues and presents a multivariate model with its empirical application to an actual training program. Harriet Lefley presents research findings from the University of Miami's Cross-Cultural Training Institute for Mental Health Professionals to demonstrate the impact of training on trainees, their agencies, and their clients. There is a data-based discussion of affective reactions and identity issues raised by self-cultural awareness, with a special focus on minority providers dealing with value and status conflicts evoked by acknowledging long-felt disparities between their professional education and the needs of their communities.

In the final chapter, Hazel Weidman, architect of multiple anthropologically-based research, service, and training projects in medicine and psychiatry, presents an integrative paradigm which encompasses all of the various cross cultural training models. Viewing mental health service delivery as one component of the orthodox health institutional system, Weidman presents a model that emphasizes value parity and the need for culture brokerage in negotiating dual systems of care.

REFERENCES

Arredondo-Dowd, P., & Gonslaves, J. (1980, June). Preparing culturally effective counselors. *Personnel and Guidance Journal.*

Bryson, S., Renzaglia, G. A., & Danish, S. (1973). Training counselors through simulated racial encounters. *Journal of Non-White Concerns in Personnel and Guidance, 20,* 495-498.

Lewis, M. D., & Lewis, J. A. (1970). Relevant training for relevant roles: A model for educating inner-city counselors. *Counselor Education and Supervision, 10*(1), 31-38.

Mitchell, H. (1970). The black experience in higher education. *The Counseling Psychologist, 2,* 30-36.

Pedersen, P. (1984). Intercultural training of mental health providers. In R. Brislin & D. Landis (Eds.), *Handbook of Intercultural Training* (Volume 2). New York: Pergamon Press.

Pedersen, P. (1981). The cultural inclusiveness of counseling. In P. Pedersen, J. Draguns, W. Lonner, & J. Trimble (Eds.), *Counseling across cultures.* Revised and expanded edition. Honolulu: University Press of Hawaii.

Sue, D. W. (1980). *Cross cultural counseling position paper.* APA Division 17 Executive Committee position paper from the Education and Training Committee, American Psychological Association.

Wrenn, G. C. (1962). The culturally encapsulated counselor. *Harvard Educational Review, 32*(4), 444-449.

CHAPTER 2

WHY CROSS-CULTURAL TRAINING? APPLIED ISSUES IN CULTURE AND MENTAL HEALTH SERVICE DELIVERY

HARRIET P. LEFLEY

THE ULTIMATE objective of any mental health system is to raise levels of mental health for all individuals and communities served. Attainment of this goal involves an accepted conceptual method of defining psychopathology, consensus on appropriate preventive measures, accurate diagnoses of emotional disorder, and, when indicated, selection of effective therapeutic interventions. There is now a substantial body of data indicating that a culture gap between recipient and provider may affect each level of the preventive, diagnostic, and treatment process. Since World War II, at least four disciplines—anthropology, psychiatry, psychology, and sociology—have focused on the interplay of socio-cultural factors and mental health. Many writers in these fields have questioned the transcultural applicability of various definitions of psychopathological categories, their symptomatologies, and their correlative therapies (Al-Issa, 1982; Marsella & White, 1982; Triandis & Draguns, 1980, among others). Within the United States, there is considerable evidence that ethnic co-cultures may differ in their basic perceptions of mental illness and appropriate treatment (Karno & Edgerton, 1969) and that these perceptions may effect utilization of orthodox mental health facilities (Padilla, Ruiz & Alvarez, 1975; S. Sue, 1977). Low utilization rates, of course, can give a misleading epidemiological picture when incidence or prevalence data are drawn from admissions to mental health facilities. They can also be misinterpreted as implying lower levels of psychopathology than actually exist in a

11

particular population (Becerra, Karno, & Escobar, 1982), and can lead to factional disputes about appropriate modes of service delivery (Gaviria & Stern, 1980).

There is now considerable evidence that, lacking normative data on non-psychiatric community populations, the scores of non-White, non-English-speaking patients on diagnostic screening instruments may be of dubious validity, and in some cases, seriously misleading (Gynther, 1979; Penk, et al., 1982).

Under the present system, evaluations of test results are either based primarily on mainstream (typically middle-class Anglo) norms, on code frequencies or profiles of small samples of minority patients (e.g., Cuellar, 1982) or are subjectively "corrected" on the basis of the diagnostician's personal experience and intuitions. On the observational level, misinterpretation of behavioral cues, and differences in symptomatology, may lead to serious diagnostic error (Simon, et al., 1973; Bell & Mehta, 1980). Moreover, the implicit assumption that certain units of behavior invariably go together to make up a global behavioral syndrome has been questioned in cross-cultural research (Guthrie & Bennett, 1971; Lefley, 1976). This is of critical importance since all mental health practitioners, regardless of theoretical persuasion, base their therapeutic strategies on the observation and interpretation of their patients' behavior. Modes of observation are particularly relevant to the influence of ethnic background on the diagnostic process (Katz, Cole, & Lowery, 1979), as well as to the whole issue of evaluating therapies across cultures (Katz, 1981).

With respect to therapy, Triandis and his associates, as well as many others, have stressed the need for understanding the "subjective culture" of patients, i.e., the cognitive, affective, and perceptual modes of their various membership and reference groups, in order to comprehend the referents used in the psychotherapeutic interaction (See Triandis & Draguns, 1980). There is a considerable body of literature, which can only be briefly touched upon here, indicating ways in which psychiatric ethnocentrism may interfere with successful treatment.

While there are many speculations about stressors in minority co-cultures, substantive data on adaptive mechanisms, potentialities, strengths, social support systems, and health factors in socialization are sadly lacking (Hill, 1972; Lindblad-Goldberg & Dukes, 1985; Valle & Vega, 1980). Therapists working with patients of another culture have vacillated between antipodal positions of being overly conscious of racial or ethnic differences or denying these effects altogether. In working with Black patients, for example, some White therapists emphasized racial barriers in transference and countertransference (Schachter & Butts, 1968), while others conceptualized any reference to a segregated experience as "therapeutic resistance" (Waite, 1968, p. 427). Consciousness of cultural variables does not necessarily imply substantive knowledge. Many earlier case reports in the literature that dealt with minority patients appeared to be based on pure speculation, e.g., generalizations about individual ego development "blurred by the phenomenon of color" (Kennedy, 1963, p. 199), or allusions to "modal personality" attributes without empirical documentation (Sclare, 1963). These speculations almost invariably focused on negative rather than positive aspects of the patient's cultural experience.

The larger conceptual considerations of culture and psychopathology have been addressed in a wide range of books and other contributions. Issues such as the cultural variances and invariance of the major psychopathologies, individual and intracultural differences, the etic-emic dilemma, symbolic structuring of concepts of health and illness, mental disorder as deviance, abnormal and adaptive behavior, power relationships and social labelling, stigma and suffering, and the like have been addressed both theoretically and empirically (e.g., Draguns, 1980; Marsella & White, 1982). Presentation and discussion of these issues and sensitization to self-cultural awareness are a fundamental requisite in cross-cultural training of mental health professionals.

Because this book focuses on applied issues, however, the present discussion is restricted to a brief overview of a limited number of studies relating to problematic areas in clinical training and their implications for service delivery. These studies may be conveniently grouped as follows: (a) differences in reported epidemiology of mental disorders among racial/ethnic groups in the United States, including social class and gender variables, (b) potential areas of misdiagnosis that may generate differential statistics, (c) the interaction of (a) and (b) with the disposition of cases and selection of appropriate therapeutic modalities, (d) population variability in service utilization and dropout rates, (e) patient-therapist differences and problems of cultural misunderstanding in evaluation and psychotherapy, (f) culture and psychopharmacology, and (g) population strengths and adaptive strategies that may be enlisted in treatment.

Cultural Differences in Reported Distribution of Psychiatric Disorders

Within the United States, incidence and prevalence figures in minority co-cultures are available primarily for Blacks because of traditional racial classification systems, and to a far lesser extent for Hispanic, American Indian, and Asian groups. For the most part, statistics are based on admissions records of mental health facilities. As Dohrenwend et al. (1980) point out, "It has long been known, however, that such data are biased by a host of selective factors that determine who among those suffering from a particular type of psychiatric disorder actually received treatment. . . Most of those who suffer from clinical psychiatric disorders have not been in treatment with members of the mental health professions and those who have come in to such treatment are frequently not typical of the far larger number of disturbed persons" (p. 2). These authors have further hypothesized that an astonishing three-quarters of adults with clinically significant functional disorders have never been treated by a mental health professional.

An overall low incidence rate for mental illness in any population may, of course, conceal a large number of unknown morbid cases. There may be under utilization of treatment facilities for a variety of reasons related to attitudes, beliefs, socioeconomic variables, alternative healing modalities, or a general alienation from social institutions. Concomitantly, some statisticians have indicated ways in which definitions and distributions of mental disorder may be closely related to institutional racism (Kramer, Rosen, & Willis, 1973).

Because of differential diagnostic, treatment, and utilization factors, authorities have questioned whether a valid picture of mental health in any ethnic group can be obtained by counting patients treated for mental illness, and have called for "true prevalence" studies to determine accurate distributions. Yet one of the first true prevalence studies, the Midtown Manhattan Study (Srole, Langer, Michael, Opler, & Rennie, 1962) was considered seriously flawed, particularly in its implication that the behavior of "Old Americans" (fourth generation) was the standard of mental health. In fact, as Madsen (1969) pointed out, findings must be considered suspect when the percentage of "well" Puerto Ricans was rated as 0.0% for the first generation, with a combined rate of only 3.7% for the first, second, and third generations (pp. 290-291).

One of the major questions with respect to differences in true prevalence studies is whether the reason for cultural variation resides in the culture, the methodology, or the conceptual basis of the instruments used. Consider a major epidemiological study (Dohrenwend, 1975) conducted among five ethnic groups in the Washington Heights section of New York City. Both psychiatric patients and probability samples of adult heads of families were drawn, in roughly equal proportions, from

three "relatively advantaged" groups (White protestants of European an-
cestry, Jews, and Irish) and two "relatively disadvantaged" groups
(Blacks and Puerto Ricans). Two types of interview instruments were
used on a randomly alternated basis, and all interviews were conducted
by psychiatrists. One instrument, the Structured Interview Schedule
(SIS), was a short screening instrument consisting mainly of psychophy-
siological symptoms, together with mild signs of anxiety and depression.
The other instrument, modeled on more traditional clinical interviews
with open-ended questions and probes, was the Psychiatric Status
Schedule or PSS. The results obtained with the SIS showed that the
highest rate of psychiatric impairment was found among Puerto Ricans.
By contrast, Blacks did not differ in rate from the three more advantaged ethnic groups. With the PSS, however, results were strikingly different. Here, Blacks showed the highest rate of psychiatric cases, while
the Puerto Ricans were markedly lower in rate than any of the other
four groups. The contradictory findings appeared to be an artifact of
methodological differences in the two instruments. But as Dohrenwend
(1975) points out, a basic difficulty is that the procedures may be based
on differential, or inadequate, assumptions about the nature of mental
disorders. There is now some attempt to remedy this with DSM III
diagnoses in the current large-scale N.I.M.H. Epidemiological Catchment Area Study (Regier et al., 1984).

Findings of epidemiological studies seem to vary not only in relation
to the instruments used, but also with respect to the geographical area
and the subcultural group studied. While the Midtown Manhattan
study found Puerto Ricans significantly higher in mental health problems than Anglo-Amerians, at about the same time Jaco (1960) was
finding that another Hispanic group — Mexicans-Americans — were significantly lower than "Old American" Anglos in the adjusted incidence
rate for mental illness (taking into account rural-urban differences).
Moreover, they differed in the effects of acculturation; in Manhattan,
mental health increased from the first to the third generation, while in
Texas, it presumably decreased.

Using extremely sophisticated methodology with independent research teams and large N representative samples of the population, the
current Epidemiological Catchment Area Study is also finding urban/
rural and regional differences. With stratification for age, sex, race, and
education, major depressive disorders were found to be twice as frequent in urban areas (Blazer et al., 1985). The ratios of lifetime prevalence for schizophrenia were 2.1% for Blacks versus 1.9% for others in

New Haven, Connecticut, but there were almost no differences between Blacks and others in St. Louis, Missouri and Baltimore, Maryland. Additionally, the rates ranged from only .06 to .08 in the latter sites regardless of race. Overall, lifetime rates for 15 DSM III psychiatric diagnoses showed that "differences between Blacks and others in rates of psychiatric disorders are generally modest and rarely statistically significant" (Robins, et al., 1984, p. 955).

In contrast to these "true prevalence" findings, overall national admission rates to mental hospitals have continued to be disproportionately high for Blacks, both males and females, with rates more than double those of White admissions (Milazzo-Sayre, 1977). The picture has given rise to questions about (a) differential frequency and intensity of stressors, and/or (b) differential diagnostic practices by professionals of contrasting culture. As we shall see, there has also been some concern about sex bias in diagnostic standards.

Social Class Variables

Dohrenwend et al., (1980) have pointed out that although persons from lower socioeconomic groups are more likely to suffer from psychological distress, they are also less likely to have been in treatment with a mental health professional. In almost all investigations conducted in North America and Europe, as well as elsewhere in the world (Segal, 1975), the rates are significantly higher for all types of psychopathology in lower socioeconomic groups, with an average low-high class ratio of 2.59 for North America and Europe, and a similar pattern for psychoses alone (Dohrenwend et al., 1980). In the United States, there is undoubtedly an interaction of social class and minority status, which may account for some of the variance in the Black-White comparison rates. Adebimpe (1984) has stated that apparent differences between Blacks and Whites are largely removed when patients are matched by age, sex, and socioeconomic status. A major psychiatric epidemiological field survey looking at depressive symptomatology in Mexican Americans and Anglos suggests that the distribution of psychiatric symptoms is best predicted by social and economic factors rather than by ethnicity alone (Vega, Warheit, Buhl-Auth, & Meinhardt, 1984). Epidemiological data indicate that the highest prevalence areas for severe mental disorder are poor urban communities; here, mother-father families have the lowest risk, families headed by mother and another adult have varying risk, while loosely organized multi-child mother-alone families have the highest risk (Kellam, Ensminger, & Turner, 1977). Family intactness may be an independent correlate of socioeconomic deprivation. However, these patterns have implications for family therapy, which is largely based on etiological and treatment assumptions derived from the dynamics of two-parent nuclear family structure. Nevertheless, the SES-minority interaction does not appear to be consistent across ethnic groups; viz. the great variability in Puerto Rican and Mexican-American patterns, as well as Asians (Sue & Morishima, 1982) and American Indians (Rhoades et al., 1980).

Sex Differences

In the NIMH Epidemiological Catchment Area Study, significant sex differences were found across geographical sites in several diagnostic categories. Antisocial personality and alcohol abuse/dependence were definitely male predominant, with drug abuse "probably" male predominant. Female predominant diagnoses were major depressive episode, agoraphobia, and simple phobia. It is of interest that agoraphobia was also significantly more prevalent among Blacks (Robins et al, 1984).

The ECA is based on DSM III criteria, however, and recently there has been some concern that our common nosological standard contains implicit sex bias which (a) affects the male-female ratios for specific mental disorders and (b) arbitrarily defines adaptive and maladaptive behavior from a sex-bound societal value system (Kaplan, 1983). Although the task here is not to discuss the separate but interrelated issue of gender in cultural context, the rejoinder by DSM III developers Williams and Spitzer (1983) on reasons for variant epidemiology applies as well to ethnic and cultural differences. The question at issue here is diagnosis of depression, which is found to be twice as common in females as in males in most U.S. and European studies (Weissman & Klerman, 1977). Schwab, Bell, Warheit and Schwab (1979), who confirmed the significantly higher prevalence of depression among females in a major epidemiological survey, suggested that the difference might be due, among other things, to the internalization of aggression by females as opposed to the greater freedom afforded males in acting-out.

Williams and Spizter discussed three categories of theories to account for the unequal sex ratio: (a) theories of how biological and/or cultural factors affect **true prevalence** or expression of a disorder in the two sexes (two separate variables); (b) effects of psychological variables on likelihood of seeking treatment, and therefore being entered into the diagnostic data base; and (c) clinician bias in diagnosis. If we substitute "cultural" for "psychological" under item (b), all apply to the differential diagnosis of depression in White and non-White populations.

Epidemiology, Symptomatology, and Diagnosis

Within the framework of reported cases, almost all studies, regardless of time or locale, have found higher schizophrenia rates for Blacks than for Whites. Studies have ranged from over twice the rate (Malzerg, 1963) to a more modest 65% (Taube, 1971) higher. At the same time, rates for affective disorders, particularly depression, have traditionally been low among Blacks (Bell & Mehta, 1980), Puerto Ricans (Jones, Gray, & Parsons, 1983), and Asians (T-Y Lin, 1983). The picture is unclear for American Indians, although the high suicide rates may certainly be seen as indicative of depression (Ogden, Spector, & Hill, 1970).

Manson and Shore (1981) have been attempting to establish a relationship between ethnopsychiatric data and research diagnostic criteria in identifying depression in an American Indian group. The issue of "masked depression" has been raised many times, with somatization indicated as the major functional equivalent of expressive symptomatology (Kleinman, 1977). Lesse (1981) has reported that depressive episodes masked by hypochondriasis and psychosomatic disorders are relatively uncommon among lower socioeconomic groups in the U.S., in contrast to acting-out behavior as the more common masking process.

The epidemiologic picture, however, is beginning to change. In a major true prevalence survey of almost 2,000 households, Schwab, Bell, Warheit, and Schwab (1979) found that Blacks had significantly higher mean depression scores than Whites. This finding reflected an interaction of race and low socioeconomic status (there was a particularly strong inverse relationship between SES and depression scores). Their explanation of disparity in suicide-homicide rates bears grave consideration.

> For years the prevalence of depression in Blacks was thought to be especially low; in fact, they were believed to be relatively "immune" to depressive illness, as evidenced by their low suicide rates. However, those early studies that also noted the much higher homicide rates among Blacks than Whites did not emphasize the inverse relationship between suicide and homicide in oppressed groups. Psychodynamically, depression is produced in part by internalization of aggression. Thus, when there is evidence of the externalization of aggression, e.g.,

a high homicide rate or war, the frequency of depression is low. From a social psychiatric viewpoint, low suicide and high homicide rates in a group are fundamentals of the psychology of oppression. Recently, however, suicide rates among Blacks have been rising sharply; currently they are higher for non-White females in the United States than at any time in history. Clinically, we have observed that social distance is a factor blocking the sensitivity of White doctors and nurses to their Black patients' emotional distress, such as depression. Consequently, Blacks' depressive conditions are not diagnosed (Schwab et al., 1979, pp. 77-78).

This interpretation is in contrast to earlier psychodynamic explanatory models, many based on Freudian theory, that reinforced stereotypes and thus perpetuated the inappropriate diagnosis/epidemiological cycle. Chief among these was a type of "marginal expectancy" theory originally offered by Prange and Vitols (1961) that suggested that since depression derives from the perception of loss, poor or oppressed people with little to lose are less likely to feel oppressed. Yet rationally, as Weissman and Klerman (1977) have pointed out with respect to women, societal discrimination which generates legal and economic helplessness, low self-esteem, and low aspirations, ultimately leads to clinical depression.

These differentials in diagnosed illness are vitally important to the patient in terms of chemotherapy, other types of treatment offered, length of hospital stay, and prognosis. The schizophrenias are typically more debilitating and chronic disorders than depression. Expectancies regarding functional level and productivity and perceived value of psychotherapy, may well affect hospitalization and other decisions regarding case disposition.

Studies Reversing Diagnosis. Simon, Fliess, Gurland, Stiller and Sharpe (1973) were among the first to question disparate rates for schizophrenia and depression among Blacks on the grounds of diagnostic error. Reclassifying almost 200 patients in nine state hospitals on the basis of rigorous objective criteria, they found that 40% of the Black patients had been misdiagnosed. They suggested that Black depressives were frequently misdiagnosed because they showed significantly higher levels of anxiety and body-related symptoms than Whites, and stated that White clinicians test Blacks for depression by looking for White symptoms. Adebimpe (1984) states that some current figures for depressive illness in Blacks continue to show lower rates than among Whites. One study using the SADS-RDS has indicated a higher rate of current depressive syndromes, but a lower lifetime rate for depression among

Blacks (Vernon & Roberts, 1982). Two studies by Jones, Gray, and Parsons, one on Blacks (1981) and the other on Puerto Ricans (1983), indicated underdiagnosis of manic depressive illness in these populations. With retrospective diagnosis based on DSM III criteria and independent of hospital diagnosis, they diagnosed 11% of the Puerto Rican sample as manic depressive, a rate three times the national admission rate.

In another hospital study of Black and Hispanic patients, Keisling (1981) found a 12:1 ratio of schizophrenic-affective disorders. A careful reassessment of the original diagnoses, using DSM III criteria, showed a 1:1 ratio on the unit studies. Egeland, Hostetter, and Eshleman (1983) have discussed at least three studies in which 50% of the patients previously diagnosed as schizophrenic were actually suffering from bipolar affective illness. In their research, a study of Old Order Amish, 70% of a sample of confirmed bipolar I subjects had earlier diagnoses of schizophrenia. In this landmark study, examples are given of cultural factors involved in the diagnosis of bipolar illness, particularly of Amish concepts of the behavioral correlates of hypomanic symptoms, such as inflated self-esteem, grandiosity, and excessive involvement in activities.

The reported rarity of affective disorders in non-western countries is similarly being contested by current studies. A recent application of DSM III criteria in China to 268 consecutive admissions to a major psychiatric hospital indicated that nearly a quarter had affective disorder (Shan-Ming et al., 1984).

Symptomatology and Cultural Behavioral Norms

Perhaps the most comprehensive study addressing the interaction of ethnicity and psychopathology was conducted in Hawaii by Martin Katz and his associates. In a two-part investigation, the researchers studied almost 300 Hawaii-Japanese, Hawaii-Caucasians, Part-Hawaiians and Hawaii-Filipino psychotic patients both in the hospital and the community. Significant differences in symptomatology were particularly pronounced among Japanese and Caucasians, with depression-anxiety the major discriminant feature. Japanese were low and Caucasians high on this factor. Caucasians were also high in belligerence/negativisim and suspicion/persecution/hallucinations, but low in retardation-withdrawal. Japanese peaked on inappropriate/bizarre behavior. Overall, Caucasians showed a more acting out-affective and Japanese a more withdrawn-schizoid pattern (Katz, Sanborn, & Gudeman, 1969).

These differential profiles were in turn related to the second part of the study, which determined community definitions of mental disorder and the discrepancy between normative and pathological behavior in each ethnic group. The investigators found that the behaviors most associated with mental disorder and most likely to lead to hospitalization in the Hawaii-Japanese community were suspiciousness, anxiety, agitation, and negativism — symptoms also found in patients whom clincians described as severely schizoid. In contrast, the major symptom of mental disorder in the Hawaii-Caucasian community was helplessness, a factor associated with depression. "It seems as if depression has a special or more serious meaning for the Caucasians than for other groups, i.e., their community has less tolerance for it; it is associated with 'severe mental disorder.' It is not, apparently, a prominent concern of the Japanese" (Katz, 1981, p. 166).

These community norms are reflected both in help-seeking behavior (decisions as to whom and when to hospitalize), and in diagnostic practices of clinicians.

Observation of Behavior and Cultural Styles in Diagnosis

A seminal study by Katz, Cole and Lowery (1969) studied two large groups of experienced British and American psychiatrists who viewed a filmed diagnostic interview of a U.S. patient. The investigators found that two-thirds of the Americans diagnosed the case as schizophrenic, whereas **no** British psychiatrist gave this diagnosis. More than half the British psychiatrists gave the diagnosis of affective disorder. Moreover, with level of psychopathology controlled, the Americans saw significantly more apathy, the British significantly more depression, in the same patient. In a later review of the findings, Katz (1981) stated: "One might say that the British were generally less sensitive to the emotions of apathy and hostility in a patient from a different national background. Such important insensitivities or misreadings of emotions are very likely to occur in everyday practice in such interethnic situations" (p. 160).

In the U.S.-U.K. Project, which was set up to ultimately standardize psychiatric diagnoses, the first cross-national investigation compared 250 recently admitted patients in mental hospitals in London and New York. Based on the diagnoses, schizophrenia appeared to be almost twice as common in New York as in London, whereas diagnosis for depressive psychosis was almost four times more frequent in London.

> This work confirms and underlines previous findings that the American diagnosis of schizophrenia is much broader than the British diagnosis. It includes most of what British psychiatrists would call

mania, which is hardly recognized at all by New York psychiatrists. It also encompasses substantial parts of what the British psychiatrists would regard as depressive illness, neurotic illness, and personality disorder (Leff, 1981, p. 32).

The British-U.S. diagnostic disparities are also noted in the Scandinavian countries. American studies typically report a ratio of 8:1 of schizophrenic over bipolar affective disorders, while the English and Scandinavian literature shows a 1:1 ratio (Pope & Lipinski, 1978).

The bipolar-unipolar ratio: 4:1 or 1:1? While most epidemiological studies indicate a ratio of 4:1 for unipolar over bipolar disorders (Krauthammer & Klerman, 1979), a number of studies of non-western or isolated cultures suggest that the actual ratio may be 1:1. In a comprehensive discussion of this question, Egeland, Hostetter, and Eshleman (1983) have suggested that cultural factors lending themselves to symptom masking, treatment styles which favor hospital admissions for depression rather than manic/hypomanic episodes, and cultural tolerance of manic behavior, may blur the true prevalence of bipolar illness. It is noteworthy that studies in three cultures with minimal or proscribed alcohol consumption, in Israel (Gershon & Liebowitz, 1975), Iran (Bazzoui, 1970), and among the Old Order Amish (Egeland & Hostetter, 1983) show a relatively high and remarkably similar proportion of bipolar patients, all approaching the 1:1 ratio. Egeland (1982) comments that comparison of the Israeli phenomenon with data from Sweden prompted Belmaker and van Praag (1980) to observe that apparently every other depressed patient in Jerusalem is bipolar, while in Sweden only every fifth depressed patient is bipolar.

Diagnostic Instruments

The current conflict on intelligence testing has been accompanied by concurrent questioning of the transcultural appropriateness of psychological screening instruments, including those projective techniques that were previously considered "culture fair." Differential response patterns have been related to cultural differences in stimulus perception, response style, and environmental variables, including familarity with the materials used in testing. The major problem is that the norming populations typically have inadequate representation of the ethnic groups on whom the measures are subsequently used.

The literature is replete with contradictory findings on responses of culturally diverse groups to diagnostic instruments. Gynther (1972, 1979) has maintained that Blacks show differential profiles on the

MMPI and considers the normative differences large enough to result in misdiagnosis of a significant proportion of Blacks respondents as psychotic. Gynther's (1972) factor-analytic studies of normal black populations suggested that the observed pattern of black subjects differentially peaking on the psychotic tetrad (Schizophrenia, Paranoia and Hypomania scales) may be a cultural artifact. "Item and factor analyses revealed that these differences represent differences between Blacks and Whites in values, perceptions and expectations rather than differences in level of adjustment" (p. 386). More recent studies continue to show conflicting results with respect to the interaction of culture/ethnicity and MMPI response in different diagnostic groups (Bertlesen, Marks, & May, 1982). Penk et al. (1982), have even found an inverse pattern of Black-White differences among substance abusers as opposed to psychiatric patients. Montgomery and Orozco (1985) found significant deficiencies in scores of Anglo and Mexican-American Ss on 10 of the 13 MMPI scales; however, with acculturation and age statistically controlled, the groups differed only on the L and Mf scales. The authors state that personality differences identified by the L and Mf scales reflect genuine characteristics of Mexican-American culture.

Gynther, Lachar and Dahlstrom (1978) suggest that special norms for minorities may be needed, while Butcher, Braswell and Raney (1983), comparing Black, White and American Indian psychiatric inpatients, interpreted the significantly higher scores of Blacks on scales F, Paranoia, Schizophrenia and Hypomania "as reflecting actual symptomatic differences between the groups rather than supporting the conclusion that the MMPI 'overpathologizes' for Black patients" (p. 587). In contrast, Pollack and Shore (1980), focusing on American Indians alone, found that the MMPI profiles were very similar for Native American patients, despite wide differences in behavioral diagnoses.

Similar contradictions have been found in studies of Mexican-American patients. Research by Fabrega, Swartz and Wallace (1968) indicated that Mexican-American psychotic inpatients were more regressed and evidenced significantly more psychoticism than Anglo inpatients. Cuellar (1982), however, found that mean scores of Mexican-Americans on the Psychotic Inpatient Profile (PIP) were all within one standard deviation of the mean of the standardization sample, and were actually very close to the behaviors manifested in other ethnic groups.

One of the most cogent discussions of cultural influence in projective testing has been provided by Abel (1973), with respect to the use of Rorschach, Thematic Apperception Test, and similar techniques in cultural context. For example, the Bender-Gestalt has been used primarily as a diagnostic tool for organicity, although replications of the individual design figures are also interpreted psychodynamically. The scores are also used to infer maturational level when the test is administered to children. Several cross-cultural comparisons in the latter category have indicated that White children perform significantly "better" than Black children, i.e., have less "error" scores in replication (Abbott & Gunn, 1971; Snyder, Holowenzak, & Hoffman, 1971). The latter authors, comparing Black ghetto and White suburban children, stated categorically that there is "a problem in perceptual-visual maturation for culturally disadvantaged children" (p. 791). Hartlage and Lucas (1976) found differential correlates of the Bender-Gestalt and Beery Visual Motor Integration Test for Black and White children. Rotation of designs on the Bender is interpreted as a sign of organicity. Yet, testing a Caribbean group, Abel (1973) stated: "A design could have been copied sideways, at a different angle from the original, or even in reverse. Rotation is one of the diagnostic signs of disturbance when it is used clinically in America, but for these subjects in the Caribbean, it could not be evaluated as such" (p. 169). House-Tree-Person and other drawing tests which lack richness of detail (e.g., box-like houses) are similar environmentally rather than psychodynamically determined (Abel, 1973) and may be a function of field-dependence/independence and different socialization practices (Britain & Abad, 1974).

The transcultural application of psychiatric rating scales has similarly been questioned, such as the Brief Psychiatric Rating Scale (Rossi & Gabrielli, 1976), as well as the usefulness of first-rank symptoms in diagnosing schizophrenia in a Saudi-Arabian population (Zarrouk, 1978). Decreased diagnostic weights for Schneiderian symptoms have been described in British Black patients of West African and Caribbean origin, as well as Black-American patients (Adebimpe, 1984).

Symptomatology: Variant and Invariant

Despite these differences in diagnostic style, researchers agree that cross-cultural studies have indicated core symptoms of both the schizophrenias and affective disorders. The W.H.O. (World Health Organization, 1979) International Pilot Study of Schizophrenia demonstrated universality of basic symptoms that could be agreed upon regardless of culture in nine different sites. However, despite consensually validated symptomatology, there were some differences in symptom profiles and significant differences in prognosis, which varied according to technological level of the countries studied. This is discussed further in the section on cultural strengths.

Manic-depressive illness has been considered rare in China. However, a recent study by Shan-Ming, Deyi, Zhen, Jingsu and Taylor (1982) reported that of 1,730 consecutive admissions to an acute inpatient psychiatric unit in China, 8.9% satisfied two sets of research diagnostic criteria for mania, a figure significantly higher than any previously reported in China. Further, the authors found that clinical characteristics of a sample were similar to those of western patients. W.H.O. international studies on depression have indicated that standardized methodology is possible with respect to defining core symptoms (Sartorius, Davidian, Fenton et al., 1977). Escobar, Gomez and Tuason (1983), comparing depressive phenomenology in North American and Colombian patients with standardized protocols and measures, found "an impressive similarity in symptoms of depression across cultures, supporting the idea of a universal core depressive syndrome" (p. 47). Nevertheless, somatization and psychomotor components of depression still differentiated their samples. Guilt, irritability, agitation, and suicidal ideation seem more prevalent in industrialized societies, and physical complaints, sexual problems, and withdrawal more characteristic of the developing countries. Marsella (1980) has pointed out, however, that somatic aspects appear frequently regardless of culture, whereas the fact that reports of depressed mood, guilt, and self-depreciation are largely absent in developing countries "suggests that the epistemic framework of a culture must be considered in evaluating psychiatric disorders. 'Depression' apparently assumes completely different meanings and consequences as a function of the culture in which it occurs" (p. 261).

Therapeutic Issues

Utilization of Services

Any discussion of cultural distance between mental health service providers and consumers must agree that the barriers are bilateral. As we have indicated, cultural groups may differ in their perceptions of appropriate and deviant behavior, their thresholds for identification of a particular behavior as pathological, and their willingness to seek help from the orthodox mental health system. Underutilization of psychiatric facilities usually reflects cultural prejudice in both the institution and the community. As we shall see in the section on adaptive strategies, the community may also perceive alternative systems as more effective in dealing with mental health problems.

A recent evaluative overview of the national community mental health centers program (Dowell & Ciarlo, 1983) indicates that, despite much progress, (a) communities still demonstrate little awareness of the existence or location of mental health centers, and (b) admission rates of minorities do not reflect actual service provision, because of extremely high dropout rates relative to White clients. The Seattle Project, a study of nearly 14,000 patients in 17 community mental health centers in the Northwest over a three year period, indicated that about half of all clients from minority ethnic groups (American Indian, Asian-American, Black, and Chicano) failed to return after one session, a significantly higher percentage than the 30% dropout rate for Whites (S. Sue, 1977). An analysis of services indicated that Blacks received "differential treatment and poorer outcomes as measured by premature termination rates" (p. 616). Sue suggested that the emphasis be placed on responsive services rather than on demonstrating inequities.

The same landmark study (Sue & McKinney, 1975) revealed that (a) a disproportionate underutilization of services by Asian Americans, (b) a 52% dropout rate after the first session of those who did use services, and (c) for those remaining, an average of only 2.35 therapy sessions. Yamamoto et al., (1982) have noted that despite 60% underutilization of mental health services by Asian Americans and Pacific Islanders in Los Angeles, a higher percentage of Asian patients were found to be psychotic and chronically ill on the Psychiatric Status Schedule for Asian Americans. Hispanics have traditionally been underutilizers (Becerra, Karno, & Escobar, 1982). Blacks vary, tending to be high users of public mental health facilities (Mollica, Blum, & Redlich, 1980) but to drop out earlier (Bernal, Deegan, & Konjevich, 1983; S. Sue, 1977).

Underutilization and Therapist Ethnicity. Whether different ethnicity of the therapist is an initial barrier to utilization, or emerges as a factor because of lack of cultural knowledge and sensitivity, remains an unresolved question. Although some commentators, for example, have suggested that a major reason for high Hispanic dropout rates is the presence of Anglo therapists, many studies fail to show preference of Hispanics for Hispanic therapists, and at least one study indicated a preference for Anglo therapists (Cortese, 1979). With respect to the Black population, several studies have shown that therapeutic skill is more important than the race of the therapist (Adebimpe, 1984). At this point in history, however, the question is moot, since years of institutional racism in education and admission to training programs have generated an insufficiency of minority mental health professionals to meet the need. Acosta (1980), who solicited the reasons that Black, Mexican, and Anglo-American patients dropped out of treatment, found that the highest ranking reasons for all ethnic groups were negative attitudes toward therapists and the perception that therapy was of no benefit. Baekland and Lundwall (1975) found that therapists' attitudes and behavior, and discrepancies between patients' and therapists' treatment expectations, were major factors in dropout. Acosta, Yamamoto, and Evans (1982) ultimately developed patient and clinician orientation programs to clarify therapeutic roles. The research indicates an apparent need to close a substantial culture gap between patients and therapists, regardless of ethnic specificity.

Culture and Psychotherapy

This is an expanding range of cultural issues that continue to plague patient-therapist interactions. In addition to the basic issue of differential expectancies (Higginbotham, 1977), these include basic communication difficulties and bias in interviewing (Carkhuff & Pierce, 1967); linguistic barriers in evaluating psychopathology (Marcos & Alpert, 1976; D. Sue, 1981); misinterpretation of psychodynamics (Thomas & Sillen, 1972); false "color blindness" of therapists that interferes with authenticity and accurate evaluation (Beaton, 1974); differential self-disclosure by patients (Acosta & Sheehan, 1978); advice that is counter to cultural mores (Abad, Ramos, & Boyce, 1974); and failure to differentiate between adaptive and maladaptive behavior (Smith, 1981). The net result has been differential treatment and outcome, together with massive avoidance behavior on the part of mental health professionals. The research indicates that non-White, non-Anglo patients are less often accepted by psychotherapy, more often assigned to inexperienced therapists, seen for shorter periods of time, and more often receive either supportive or custodial care, or drugs alone (Lefley, 1974).

Some of the major issues involved in counseling and psychotheray with the culturally different involve differential values, expectancies, and conceptions of the self which make many patients unsuitable candidates for traditional psychodynamic therapies. As Mazur (1973) has defined it, psychotherapy works best for people who share the therapist's values regarding personal autonomy, who feel comfortable in an ambiguous relationship, believe in change and the future, and "who value their 'I' " as an issue of overwhelming concern (p. 114). Although many therapists continue to believe that long-term personality restructuring is the treatment choice for all patients, regardless of background, many investigators are beginning to suggest short-term, ahistorical, directive, relational, and problem-focused therapy for low-income minority patients. Psychoanalytic taboos, such as not touching the patient and avoiding therapist self-disclosure, are counterindicated if the patient is to remain willingly in treatment (Lefley, 1985b).

Recent years have seen the emergence of a large number of books specifically dealing with cross-cultural counseling and psychotherapy. Examples are: Acosta, Yamamoto, and Evans (1982); Atkinson, Morten, and Sue (1979); Gaw (1982); LeVine and Padilla (1980); Marsella and Pedersen (1982); McGoldrick, Pearce, and Giordano (1982); Padilla and Padilla (1977); Pedersen, Draguns, Lonner, and Trimble (1981); D. Sue (1981); Walz and Benjamin (1978) and others.

Family Therapy. Because of continuity of family primacy in many traditional groups, development of culturally appropriate treatment approaches has involved an emphasis on family therapy. This is not necessarily related to systems approaches with family units perceived as dysfunctional. Rather, it means total involvement of the family as a natural support and co-therapeutic system. Gaw (1982) has echoed the opinions of many others in emphasizing the importance of therapist-family communications in Asian, Hispanic, and other traditional cultures. In discussing Chinese patients, he states:

> Family involvement in the management of the patient's problems is natural to Chinese Americans. The psychiatrist should not hesitate to conduct family interviews, to give advice to members of the family as to how to handle the patient's problem, and to obtain feedback through periodic family interviews. . .If psychotherapy or psychoanalysis is to be attempted so that the technical requirement of the therapeutic process necessitates minimal or no involvement with family members, the rationale and process of treatment should be carefully explained to both patient and family members (p. 25).

Although family therapy appears to be more consonant with the needs of traditional cultural groups who continue to be highly family-oriented, there are patent pitfalls involved. Significant differences have been found in assessment of relationships between parents and children when these were done by family therapists of the same and different cultural backgrounds. Tseng, McDermott, Ogino, and Ebata (1982) described a cross-cultural research project in which a Japanese family interaction videotape was shown to Japanese and American psychiatrists for assessment of parent-child interactions. Most American psychiatrists perceived the father (who did not directly interact with the mother or daughter, but only with the teenage son), as being passive and noninvolved, while the the Japanese psychiatrists found him both involved and appropriate for his behavior.

Specifics on involvement of different cultural groups in family therapy are given in Falicov (1983) and McGoldrick, Pearce, and Giordano (1982). Of particular interest are normative interaction styles which should be learned by psychotherapists in order to avoid misinterpretation of family dynamics. For example, McGoldrick (1982) has described scapegoating of a selected child, discipline by ridicule and belittling, an emphasis on sin and human badness, and various levels of communication deviance, including double-binding, as rather typical patterns of Irish-American socialization. In contrast, Italian families show "frequent symbiotic-like relationships between parents and children, and Italian families may not achieve the level of differentiation that predominates in the larger culture" (Rotunno & McGoldrick, 1982, p. 357). These authors caution against viewing enmeshment in Italian families as pathogenic. They even suggest that if emotional fusion is lacking, it might suggest a "buried issue" because it would be so culturally anomalous.

Culture and Chemotherapy

Katz (1981) has stated that "Despite more than 25 years of research on the psychotropic drugs and several crossnational clinical trials, it is safe to state that a truly sound study of the efficacy of a drug treatment across diverse cultures has yet to be carried out" (p. 159). Variations in psychotropic dosage have been reported for both the schizophrenias and bipolar affective disorders. T-Y Lin (1983) has reported that "antipsychotic drugs like phenothiazine derivatives can be effective on Chinese patients at about half the dose required by their Western counterparts" (p. 865). Further, he states that in his clinical experience, Chinese manic patients seem to require smaller doses of lithium carbonate per body weight and a lower blood concentration, and that similar findings were obtained in Japan in a large-scale collaborative study (Takahashi, Sakuma, & Itoh, et al., 1975).

Another study, by K-M Lin and Finder (1983), found that effective weight-standardized neuroleptic dose ranges for Asian patients were significantly lower than those for White counterparts matched for age, sex, diagnosis, duration of illness, previous hospitalizations, past neuroleptic exposure, and psychopathology. They also found that extrapyramidal symptoms occurred at a lower dose in Asian patients. Adebimpe (1980), who studied differences in psychopharmacological indices of Blacks and Whites, has suggested that such differences may reflect genetic and race-related variations in drug metabolism. Even though Black-White pharmacologic comparisons are still scarce, some of the research is pointing to interesting clinical implications. A study by Ziegler and Biggs (1977) indicated that Blacks show a more rapid clinical response to anticyclic antidepressants, with a steady state plasma level of nortriptiline 50% higher in Blacks than in Whites. Adebimpe (1984) cites these findings as "suggesting a lower rate of metabolism, the possibility of increased side effects, or treatment failure outside the therapeutic window" (p. 96). Escobar and Tuason (1980) reported on response to antidepressant agents among patients suffering from endogenous depression in the U.S. and Colombia, evaluating the efficacy and safety of the antidepressant trazodone, using imipramine and placebo as comparison drugs. Uniform diagnostic, therapeutic, and evaluative procedures were followed. They found that imipramine was significantly better than placebo in both cultures, while trazodone showed no significant difference. However, Colombian subjects responded better than U.S. subjects regardless of the treatment given. Their findings were given as supporting universality of "core" symptoms, but suggesting that cultural elements "colour" the syndrome (such as higher somatization and sexual disturbance among Colombians). The authors suggest that findings of differential response may have been an artifact of different psychiatric treatment. There are indications that in the U.S. minor clinical gains determined the administration of maximum dosage, and minor side effects resulted in dosage decrements. In Colombia, however, there was a more aggressive escalation of the dosage in spite of anticholinergic side effects, with a trend to reach to maximum dosage by the end of the third week (Escobar & Tuason, 1980, p. 51). The question of culture affecting chemotherapeutic style, as well as patient response, has not typically been addressed in the literature.

An Anglo-Hispanic comparison of depressed patients treated at two New York municipal hospitals, found lower tolerance to medication in Hispanic patients (Marcos & Cancro, 1982). The authors suggest that this may be due to the somatization of the Hispanic groups. They suggested that depressive somatic symptoms are similar to antidepressant side-effects, which are perceived by the patients as signs that the illness is becoming worse. The authors suggested the possibility of biological and psychocultural differences to account for the similar therapeutic response to different medication dosages.

Continuing research on different racial/ethnic groups may indeed yield evidence of different biochemical or morphological parameters. However, as Katz (1982) has pointed out, evaluating a drug treatment cross-culturally involves knowing (1) the psychopathological and social phenomena of the clinical condition being studied and particularly, (2) the quality of change which is expected to occur as a function of treatment (p. 162). The previous work of Katz, Sanborn, Lowery, and Ching (1978), as well as those cited in this chapter, has indicated such significant differences in symptom patterns and behavior, that the measure of outcome in drug therapy would appear to be a function of cultural manifestation, tolerance, and labelling of psychopathological behavior.

Cultural Strengths: Adaptive Strategies and Coping Mechanisms

Much of the research on ethnic groups in the U.S. has been based on what is generally known as the "deficit hypothesis," an assumption that various types of cultural patterns are deficient with respect to U.S. Anglo middle-class norms. In recent years there have been attempts to counteract this with research on strengths in cultural institutions. For example, studies of Afro-American families (Bass, Wyatt, & Powell, 1982; Hill, 1972) have indicated five areas of strength in low-income groups: strong kinship bonds, work orientation, flexible family roles, strong achievement orientation, and strong religious orientation. "In fact, behavior that was seen as pathological in low-income families—women working, the interchangeability of family roles, with children often assuming some parental responsibilities—is now seen as a source of strength and coping when it appears in middle-income families" (Johnson Foundation, 1979, p. 9). Ethnic neighborhoods frequently supply informal networks of support that meet needs and crises of their inhabitants.

Religion and Alternate Healing

Religion, supernatural belief systems, and folk healing have been seen as supportive resources, particularly for populations undergoing socioeconomic and sociocultural stress. The role of the church in Black survival is well established; it has served both as a social and spiritual resource, providing collective human support and a reference point for meaningfulness in life. Therapeutic aspects of the religious experience are so profound that it has been suggested that "the Black church service is a functional community mental health resource for its participants" (Griffith, Young, & Smith, 1984, p. 464).

Some supernatural belief systems have also provided a natural support group needed by individuals with emotional or mental problems. Garrison's (1978) analysis of **Espiritismo** cult houses as therapeutic support systems for schizophrenic Puerto Rican women, and the role of **Santeria** as a mental health care system for Cuban Americans (Sandoval, 1979) are further cases in point.

Religious belief is so powerful in African psychiatric practice, according to Erinosho (1979), that most Nigerian psychiatrists use traditional symbolic rituals and native herbs in healing. One orientation uses rituals that placate diabolical spiritual forces in group psychotherapy without encouraging use of native healers, while a more culture-bound approach not only acknowledges the rituals, but involves native healers as collaborators with western-oriented psychiatrists. In the United States, Ruiz and Lagrod (1976), Delgado (1979), Lefley (1984), and many others have described involvement of folk healers in mental health programs as a means of providing culturally appropriate care for their patients.

The Family

Current years are beginning to see changed attitudes of mental health professionals toward the family. In a recent conference report, the Executive Director of a large Child Guidance center emphasized: "Families are truly support systems and not the enemy. . .The family as a support system must negotiate with many other systems in this society, and a therapist or service professional must consider the impact of these other external systems as well as problems within the family. Perhaps a family dysfunction has its origin, not in the weakness of the family or in an inability to cope, but in the intrusion or intervention of another system. Even ordinarily strong and healthy families cannot always resist the force of external pressures" (Johnson Foundation, 1979, pp. 9-10).

Literature from other countries indicates that in contrast to negative and adversarial attitudes towards families often manifested by western mental health professionals, families in other parts of the world are typically welcomed as participants in patient care (Bell, 1982; Lefley, 1985a). Cross-cultural comparisons are beginning to yield evidence that behavioral patterns observed among families in the United States and United Kingdom are infrequent in other cultural settings (Leff, 1981). For example, high expressed emotion in families of schizophrenics, i.e., excessive criticism and emotional overinvolvement, is apparently minimal in studies done among Mexican-American families (Karno, 1982) and those in Northern India (Day, 1982). There is even some implication that family therapy and family research have yielded iatrogenic interactions because of the expectancies and attitudes of professionals (Terkelsen, 1983). DiNicola (1985), who feels there is a natural synthesis of family therapy and transcultural psychiatry (a better fit than with dynamic "depth" psychology), has pointed out that the expressed emotion researchers "in the more individually-oriented British society emphasize the negative aspects of family involvement, while Third World researchers in Qatar and India highlight instead the positive aspects the family-centeredness and concern, chanelling it into patient care" (p. 99).

Kinship Networks, Support Systems and Stress Reduction

The International Pilot Study of Schizophrenia (World Health Organization, 1979) which studied 1202 patients in nine centers around the world, found diagnostic uniformity but cultural differences in outcome studies conducted two and five years later. The researchers found that the course and history of illness was more benign in developing countries than in technologically advanced societies. Good outcome figures ranged from 58% in Nigeria, to 6% well in Denmark. Leff (1981) has suggested that the two main factors for this differential outcome are (a) the attitudes of the patient's family and (b) the relative ease with which symptomatic patients can be reintegrated into society. Mosher and Keith (1981) have suggested a "low stress-high social support" hypothesis, relating to the possibility of returning to an undemanding but relatively productive role in simple agrarian societies, expectancies that are not too high, and the presence of supportive relatives. Leff (1981) has emphasized that the emotional and financial buffering that occurs in extended kinship networks mitigates the burden of dealing with chronic schizophrenic patients, thereby defusing high expressed emotion and lowering stress for all concerned. Waxler (1979) has suggested that in traditional societies, mental illness is considered brief, easily cured, and nonrecurrent; hence there is less adverse social labelling and better societal and self-expectancies for recovery.

These cross-cultural findings of remission under specific types of conditions have profound implication for psychosocial rehabilitation of the chronic or severely mentally disabled patient in western nations. In particular, a deemphasis of too zealous psychotherapeutic efforts (Linn, Caffey, Klett, Hogarty, & Lamb, 1979), the presence of a supportive family network, a family-professional collaborative relationship, low-stress occupational roles with acceptable levels of productivity, and continuing public education to reduce stigma, seem to be indicated for the long-term mentally ill population.

Coping Mechanisms in Acculturation

Acculturation stress and its resolution seem to be strongly associated with the armamentarium of coping skills available to native and immigrant populations. Native populations, of course, have highly specific problems in determining the extent to which they are willing and able to interface with the larger social system, and the advantages and disadvantages offered by the acculturative process (Manson, 1982).

Apart from the mental health issues involved in selective/nonselective migration, refugee status is presumably more stressful than purposive immigration, since it involves unwilling loss, disenfranchisement, and exposure to trauma both in the home country and in the search for sanctuary. However, specific variables seem to be associated with level of psychosocial adjustment. Among Indochinese refugees, for example, Nicassio (1983) found that Laotians and Vietnamese showed more favorable adjustment and less alienation from American culture than Hmong and Cambodians, "a finding that is consistent with the better English proficiency, higher socioeconomic status and more positive self-perceptions noted in these refugee groups" (p. 349). It is important that mental health workers involved with such groups understand not only something about the respective cultures, but the characteristics and conditions involved in refugee flight.

Another example involves the differential aspects of the Cuban and Haitian migrations to Miami. Recent entrants have been subjected to numerous stressors, including temporary and ongoing incarceration, stigmatization and uncertain acceptance by the local community. Haitians have confronted great ambiguity of legal status and civil rights, and fear of deportation has been an extreme stressor. Mariel refugees find themselves stigmatized by the criminal elements among them who were outsted by the Cuban regime, and significant value differentials with the older Miami compatriots have been reported. However, even among persons similarly classified as entrants, the two populations differ in terms of potential for permanent residency, governmental attitudes, and types and levels of skills available for employment and even for further educational advancement. In each entrant group, both kin and fictive kin networks have provided housing, food, and employment opportunities. For Haitians, many of whom were in hiding and hence not eligible for any type of public welfare, including medical care, the fictive kin community has literally been a mechanism for survival.

A major coping strategy in adjustment to a new environment is the ability to negotiate within the new system without losing the supports of the traditional culture. In contrast to the earlier literature, which seemed to find invariant positive linearity between acculturation and indicators of psychopathology, contemporary literature suggests this is a complex multivariate phenomenon. Acculturation seems to have the potential for becoming a positive learning experience with the addition of new skills and knowledge to the existing base. Among Mexican-American migrants, for example, a recent study found an inverse relationship between acculturation and depressive symptomatology. The authors reported that cultural assimilation appears to lead to acquisition of coping resources (Vega, Warheit, Buhl-Auth, & Meinhardt, 1984).

Yet all too often the process involves cultural loss rather than cultural gain. Particularly among children and young adults, cultural readjustment may involve repudiation of traditional ways, with attendant generational conflict. Research by Szapocznik, Kurtines, and Fernandez (1980) has indicated that both underacculturated and overacculturated youth show lower levels of adjustment than bicultural youth who are at ease in both systems. Based on validation of a biculturalism and cultural involvement scale, the authors have developed Bicultural Effectiveness Training (B.E.T.), which incorporates values clarification and enhancement of communication and negotiation skills in both Hispanic and North American cultures.

Summary

Clinical training has typically been based on universalistic premises regarding distribution, diagnosis, and treatment of mental disorders. An overview of the literature indicates differences in reported epidemiology of mental disorders, both cross-nationally and among racial-ethnic groups in the U.S., which may be related to differential utilization patterns and diagnostic practices. This chapter discusses cultural perceptions of mental disorder, attitudes toward the orthodox mental health system, and availability of alternative healing modalities as factors in service utilization and subsequent effects on epidemiological pattern. Methodological difficulties inherent both in admissions rates and true prevalence studies are compared, together with changing pictures of diagnostic distribution as a consequence of more refined conceptualization and technology. Social class and gender variables are discussed in relation to cultural differences.

The effects of cultural patterning on differential diagnosis are explored both as an element of epidemiology and as a barrier to effective treatment and case disposition. Symptomatology is discussed in relation to cultural norms for appropriate and deviant behavior, observation of behavior, and cultural styles in diagnosis. Cultural differences in responses to diagnostic screening instruments are presented, with questions that have been raised regarding the need for culture-specific normative profiles. All of these issues articulate with global definitions of pychopathology, variant and invariant symptomatology, and the universality of core symptoms of the major disorders.

Treatment issues involve both service utilization and therapeutic process. Underutilization of services of minority patients and high dropout rates may be related to the aforementioned concerns, as well as therapist-patient ethnicity and differential expectations regarding roles, function, and potential outcome in psychotherapy. Basic interactional issues involving communication, interpretation of psychodynamics, self-other perception, understanding of cultural mores and adaptive/maladaptive behavior, are discussed, together with conceptual issues regarding basic therapeutic assumptions and values. Research suggests that cultural differences have generated avoidance behavior on the part of mental health professionals and differential treatment of minority patients.

References are given for new books dealing with culture and psychotherapy, together with specifics on involving families and interpreting interactions in cultural context. As part of the spectrum of therapeutic issues, a new literature on culture and chemotherapy is briefly reviewed, indicating differences in psychopharmacological indices and the possibility of genetic-cultural interaction. Finally, cultural strengths and adaptive strategies that may be enlisted in treatment are discussed. Included are the role of religion, supernatural belief systems and alternative healing modalities; the family; stress-reducing aspects of kinship networks and other social support systems; and coping mechanisms in acculturation.

REFERENCES

Abad, V., Ramos, J., & Boyce, E. (1974). A model for delivery of mental health services to Spanish-speaking minorities. *American Journal of Orthopsychiatry, 44*(4), 584-595.

Abbott, W. L., & Gunn, H. E. (1971). Bender-Gestalt performance by culturally disadvantaged first graders. *Perceptual and Motor Skills, 33,* 247-250.

Abel, T. M. (1973). *Psychological testing in cultural contexts.* New Haven: College & University Press.

Acosta, F. X. (1980). Self-described reasons for premature termination of psychotherapy by Mexican-American, Black-American, and Anglo-American patients. *Psychological Reports, 47,* 435-443.

Acosta, F. X., & Sheehan, J. G. (1978). Self-disclosure in relation to psychotherapist expertise and ethnicity. *American Journal of Community Psychology, 6*(6), 545-553.

Acosta, F. X., Yamamoto, J., & Evans, L. A. (Eds.). (1982). *Effective psychotherapy for low-income and minority patients.* New York: Plenum.

Adebimpe, V. R. (1980). Psychopharmacologic norms in blacks and whites. *American Journal of Psychiatry, 137,* 870.

Adebimpe, V. R. (1984). American blacks and psychiatry. *Transcultural Psychiatric Research Review, 21*(2), 81-111.

Al-Issa, I. (Ed.) (1982). *Culture and psychopathology.* Baltimore: University Park Press.

Atkinson, D. R., Morten, G., & Sue, D. W. (Eds.) (1979). *Counseling American minorities: A cross-cultural perspective.* Dubuque, IA: William C. Brown.

Baekland, F., & Lundwall, R. (1975). Dropping out of treatment: A critical review. *Psychological Bulletin, 82,* 738.

Bass, B. A., Wyatt, G. W. & Powell, G. J. (1982). *The Afro-American family: Assessment, treatment and research issues.* New York: Grune & Stratton.

Bazzoui, W. (1970). Affective disorders in Iraq. *British Journal of Psychiatry, 117,* 195-203.

Beaton, S. R. (1974). The function of "colorblindness." *Perspective in Psychiatric Care, 12,* 80-83.

Becerra, R. M., Karno, M., & Escobar, J. I. (1982). The Hispanic patient: Mental health issues and strategies. In R. M. Becerra, M. Karno, & J. I. Escobar (Eds.), *Mental health and Hispanic Americans: Clinical perspectives* (pp. 1-16). New York: Grune & Stratton.

Bell, J. (1982). The family in the hospital: Experiences in other countries. In H. Harbin (Ed.) *The psychiatric hospital and the family.* New York: Spectrum.

Bell, C. C., & Mehta, H. (1980). The misdiagnosis of black patients with manic-depressive illness. *Journal of the National Medical Association, 72*(2), 141-145.

Belmaker, R. H., & Van Praag, H. M. (Eds.) (1980). *Mania: An evolving concept.* New York: Spectrum.

Bernal, G., Deegan, E., & Konjevich, C. (1983). The EPPI family therapy outcome study. *International Journal of Family Therapy, 5*(1), 3-21.

Bertelsen, A. D., Marks, P. A., & May, G. D. (1982). MMPI and race: A controlled study. *Journal of Consulting & Clinical Psychology, 50,* 316-318.

Blazer, D., George, L. K., Landerman, R., Pennybacker, M. Mellville, M. L., Woodbury, M., Manton, K. G., Jordan, K., & Locke, B. (1985). Psychiatric disorders: A rural/urban comparison. *Archives of General Psychiatry, 42,* 651-656.

Britain, S. D., & Abad, M. (1974). Field-independence: A function of sex and socialization in a Cuban and an American group. *Personality and Social Psychology Bulletin, 1,* 319-320.

Butcher, J. N., Braswell, L., & Raney, D. (1983). A cross-cultural comparison of American Indians, Black and White inpatients on the MMPI and presenting symptoms. *Journal of Consulting & Clinical Psychology, 51,* 587-594.

Carkhuff, R., & Pierce, R. (1967). Differential effects of therapist race and social class upon patient depth of self-exploration in the initial clinical interview. *Journal of Consulting Psychology, 31,* 632-634.

Cortese, M. (1979). Intervention research with Hispanic Americans: A review. *Hispanic Journal of Behavior Sciences, 1*(1), 4-20.

Cuellar, I. (1982). The diagnosis and evaluation of schizophrenic disorders among Mexican-Americans. In R. M. Becerra, M. Karno, and J. I. Escobar (Eds.), *Mental health and Hispanic Americans: Clinical perspectives* (pp. 61-82). New York: Grune & Stratton.

Day, R. (1982). Research on the course and outcome of schizophrenia in traditional cultures: Some potential implications for psychiatry in the developed countries. In National Institute of Mental Health. *Preventive intervention in schizophrenia: Are we ready?*, Goldstein, M. J. (Ed.). (DHHS Pub. No. (ADM) 82-1111). Washington, DC: U.S. Government Printing Office.

Delgado, M. (1979). Therapy Latino style: Implications for psychiatric care. *Perspectives in Psychiatric Care, 17*(3), 107-115.

DiNicola, V. F. (1985). Family therapy and transcultural psychiatry: An emerging synthesis. Part I: The conceptual basis. *Transcultural Psychiatric Research Review, 22,* 81-113.

Dohrenwend, B. P. (1975). Sociocultural and social-psychological factors in the genesis of mental disorders. *Journal of Health and Social Behavior, 16,* 365-392.

Dohrenwend, B. P., Dohrenwend, B. S., Gould, M. S., Link, B., Neugebauer, R., & Wunsch-Hitzig, R. (1980). *Mental illness in the United States.* New York: Praeger.

Dowell, D. A., & Ciarlo, J. A. (1983). Overview of the community mental health centers program from an evaluation perspective. *Community Mental Health Journal, 19,* 95-125.

Draguns, J. G. (1980). Psychological disorders of clinical severity. In H. C. Triandis, J. G. Draguns (Eds.), *Handbook of cross-cultural psychology: Vol. 6. Psychopathology* (pp. 99-174). Boston: Allyn and Bacon.

Egeland, J. A. (1982). *Bipolarity: The iceberg of affective disorders.* Presented at the 135th annual meeting of the American Psychiatric Association, Toronto, Canada, May 15-21.

Egeland, J. A. & Hostetter, A. M. (1983). Amish study I: Affective disorders among the Amish, 1976-1980. *American Journal of Psychiatry, 140*(1), 56-61.

Egeland, J. A., Hostetter, A. M., & Eshleman, S. K. (1983). Amish study III: The impact of cultural factors on diagnosis of bipolar illness. *American Journal of Psychiatry, 140*(1), 67-71.

Erinosho, O. A. (1979). The evaluation of modern psychiatric care in Nigeria. *American Journal of Psychiatry, 136,* 1572-1575.

Escobar, J. I., Gomez, J., & Tuason, V. B. (1983). Depressive phenomenology in North and South American patients. *American Journal of Psychiatry, 140,* 47-51.

Escobar, J. I., & Tuason, V. B. (1980). Antidepressant agents: A cross cultural study. *Psychopharmacology Bulletin, 16*(3), 49-52.

Fabrega, H., Swartz, J. D., & Wallace, C. A. (1968). Ethnic differences in psychopathology with emphasis on a Mexican American group. *Journal of Psychiatric Research, 6,* 121-125.

Falicov, C. J. (1983). *Cultural perspectives in family therapy.* Rockville, MD: Aspen Publications.

Garrison, V. (1978). Support systems of schizophrenic and nonschizophrenic Puerto Rican migrant women in New York City. *Schizophrenia Bulletin, 4*(4), 561-596.

Gaviria, M., & Stern, G. (1980). Problems in designing and implementing culturally relevant mental health services for Latinos in the U.S. *Social Science and Medicine, 14B,* 65-71.

Gaw, A. (Ed.). (1982). *Cross-cultural psychiatry.* Boston: John Wright.

Gershon, E. S., & Liebowitz, J. H. (1975). Sociocultural and demographic correlates of affective disorders in Jerusalem. *Journal of Psychiatric Research, 12,* 37-50.

Griffith, E. E. H., Young, J. L., & Smith, D. L. (1984). An analysis of the therapeutic elements in a Black church service. *Hospital & Community Psychiatry, 35,* 464-469.

Guthrie, G. M., & Bennett, A. B. (1971). Cultural differences in implicit personality theory. *International Journal of Psychology, 6,* 3, 5, 312.

Gynther, M. D. (1972). White norms and Black MMPI's: A prescription for discrimination? *Psychological Bulletin, 78*(5), 386-402.

Gynther, M. D. (1979). Ethnicity and personality: An update. In J. N. Butcher (Ed.), *New developments in the use of the MMPI.* Minneapolis: University of Minnesota Press.

Gynther, M. D., Lachar, D., & Dahlstrom, W. G. (1978). Are special norms for minorities needed? Development of an MMPI F scale for Blacks. *Journal of Consulting & Clinical Psychology, 46,* 1403-1408.

Hartlage, L. C., & Lucas, T. L. (1976). Differentiating correlates of Bender-Gestalt and Beery Visual Motor Integration Test for Black and White children. *Perceptual and Motor Skills, 43,* 1039-1042.

Higginbotham, H. N. (1977). Culture and the role of client expectancy. In R. W. Brislin & M. P. Hamnett (Eds.), *Topics in culture learning* (Vol. 5) (pp. 107-124). Honolulu: East-West Center.

Hill, R. B. (1972). *The strengths of Black families.* New York: Emerson Hall.

Jaco, E. G. (1960). *The social epidemiology of mental disorders: A psychiatric survey of Texas.* New York: Russell Sage Foundation.

Johnson Foundation. A wingspread report. (1979). *Strengthening families through informal support systems.* Racine, WI: Author.

Jones, B. E., Gray, B. A., & Parson, E. B. (1981). Manic-depressive illness among poor urban Blacks. *American Journal of Psychiatry, 138,* 654-657.

Jones, B. E., Gray, B. A., & Parson, E. G. (1983). Manic-depressive illness among poor urban Hispanics. *American Journal of Psychiatry, 140,*(9), 1208-1210.

Kaplan, M. (1983). A woman's view of DSM III. *American Psychologist, 38,* 786-792.

Karno, M. (1982, October). *The experience of schizophrenia in Mexican-American families.* Presented at the meeting of the Society for the Study of Psychiatry and Culture, San Miguel Regla, Mexico.

Karno, M., & Edgerton, R. G. (1969). Perceptions of mental illness in a Mexican-American community. *Archives of General Psychiatry, 20,* 233-238.

Katz, M. M. (1981). Evaluating drug and other therapies across cultures. In A. J. Marsella & P. B. Pedersen (Eds.), *Cross-cultural counseling and psychotherapy* (pp. 159-176). New York: Pergamon.

Katz, M. M., Cole, J. O., & Lowery, H. A. (1969). Studies of the diagnostic process: The influence of symptom perception, past experiences, and ethnic background on diagnostic decisions. *American Journal of Psychiatry, 125,* 109-119.

Katz, M. M., Sanborn, K. O., & Gudeman, H. (1969). Characterizing differences in psychpathology among ethnic groups in Hawaii. In F. Redlich (Ed.), *Social psychiatry.* Baltimore: Williams & Wilkins.

Katz, M. M., Sanborn, K. O., Lowery, H. A., & Ching, J. (1978). Ethnic studies in Hawaii: On psychopathology and social device. In L. C. Wynne, R. L. Cromwell, & S. Matthysse (Eds.), *The nature of schizophrenia: New Approaches to research and treatment.* New York: Wiley.

Keisling, R. (1981). Underdiagnosis of manic-depressive illness in a hospital unit. *American Journal of Psychiatry, 138,* 672-673.

Kellam, S., Ensminger, M., & Turner, R. J. (1977). Family structure and the mental health of children: Concurrent and longitudinal community wide studies. *Archives of General Psychiatry, 34,* 1012-1022.

Kennedy, J. (1963). Problems faced in the analysis of Negro patients. In M. M. Grossack (Ed.), *Mental health and segregation* (pp. 199-221). New York: Springer.

Kleinman, A. (1977). Depression, somatization and the "new cross-cultural psychiatry." *Social Science & Medicine, 11,* 3-9.

Kramer, M., Rosen, B. M., Willis, E. M. (1973). Definitions and distributions of mental disorders in a racist society. In C. V. Willie, B. M. Dramer, & B. S. Brown (Eds.), *Racism and mental health* (pp. 353-459). Pittsburgh: University of Pittsburgh Press.

Krauthammer, C., & Klerman, G. L. (1979). The epidemiology of mania. In Shopsin, B. (Ed.), *Manic illness.* New York: Raven Press.

Leff, J. (1981). *Psychiatry around the globe: A transcultural view.* New York: Marcel Dekker.

Lefley, H. P. (1974, April). *Ethnic patients and Anglo healers: An overview of the problem in mental health care.* Paper presented at the ninth annual meeting of the Southern Anthropological Society, Blacksburg, VA.

Lefley, H. P. (1976). Acculturation, childrearing, and self-esteem in two North American Indian tribes. *Ethos, 4,* 385-401.

Lefley, H. P. (1984). Delivering mental health services across cultures. In P. B. Pedersen, N. Sartorius, & A. M. Marsella (Eds.), *Mental health services: The cultural context.* New York: Sage.

Lefley, H. P. (1985a). Families of the mentally ill in cross-cultural perspective. *Psychosocial Rehabilitation Journal, 8,* 57-75.

Lefley, H. P. (1985b). Mental health training across cultures. In P. Pedersen (Ed.), *Handbook for cross-cultural counseling and therapy.* Westport, CT: Greenwood Press.

Lesse, S. (1981). Masked depression and depressive equivalents. In S. Arieti & H. K. H. Brodie (Eds.), *American handbook of psychiatry* (2nd ed., Vol. 7, pp. 317-329). New York: Basic Books.

LeVine, E. S., & Padilla, A. M. (1980). *Crossing cultures in therapy: Pluralistic counseling for the Hispanic.* Monterrey, CA: Brooks/Cole.

Lin, K-M, & Finder, E. (1983). Neuroleptic dosage for Asians. *American Journal of Psychiatry, 140*(4), 490-491.

Lin, T-Y. (1983). Psychiatry and Chinese culture. *Western Journal of Medicine, 139,* 862-867.

Lindblad-Goldberg, M., & Dukes, J. L. (1985). Social support in Black low-income, single-parent families. *American Journal of Orthopsychiatry, 55,* 42-58.

Linn, M. W., Caffey, E. M., Klett, C. J., Hogarty, G. E., & Lamb, H. R. (1979). Day treatment and psychotropic drugs in the aftercare of schizophrenic patients. *Archives of General Psychiatry, 36,* 1055-1066.

Madsen, W. (1969). Mexican-American and Anglo-Americans: A comparative study of mental health in Texas. In S. C. Plog & R. B. Edherton (Eds.), *Changing perspectives in mental illness.* New York: Holt, Rinehart & Winston.

Malzberg, B. (1963). Mental disorders in the United States. In A. Deutsch & H. Fishman (Eds.), *Encyclopedia of mental health. Vol. 3* (pp. 1051-1066). New York: Franklin Watts.

Manson, S. M. (Ed.) (1982). *New directions in prevention among American Indian and Alaska Native communities.* National Center for American Indian and Alaska Native Mental Health Research. Portland: Oregon Health Sciences University.

Manson, S. M., & Shore, J. H. (1981, December). *Relationship between ethnopsychiatric data and research diagnostic criteria in the identification of depression within a Southwestern Indian tribe.* Paper presented at the annual meeting of the American Anthropological Association, Los Angeles, CA.

Marcos, L. R., & Alpert, M. (1976). Strategies and risks in psychotherapy with bilingual patients. *American Journal of Psychiatry, 133,* 1275-1278.

Marcos, L. R. & Cancro, R. (1982). Pharmacotherapy of Hispanic depressed patients: Clinical observations. *American Journal of Psychotherapy, 36,* 505-512.

Marsella, A. J. (1980). Depressive experiences and disorder across cultures. In H. C. Triandis & J. G. Draguns (Eds.), *Handbook of cross-cultural psychology: Vol. 6. Psychopathology* (pp. 237-289). Boston: Allyn & Bacon.

Marsella, A. J., & Pedersen, P. B. (Eds.). (1981). *Cross-cultural counseling and psychotherapy.* New York: Pergamon.

Marsella, A. J., & White, G. M. (Eds.). (1982). *Cultural conceptions of mental health and therapy.* Dordrecht, Holland: D. Reidel.

Mazur, V. (1973). Family therapy: An approach to the culturally different. *International Journal of Social Psychiatry, 19,* 114-120.

McGoldrick, M. (1982). Irish families. In M. McGoldrick, J. K. Pearce, & J. Giordano, *Ethnicity and family therapy.* New York: Guilford Press.

McGoldrick, M., Pearce, J., & Giordano, J. (Eds.). (1982). *Ethnicity and family therapy.* New York: Guilford Press.

Milazzo-Sayre, L. (1977, November). Admission rates to state and county psychiatric hospitals by age, sex, and race, United States, 1975. N.I.M.H. *Mental Health Statistical Note* No. 140 (DHEW Publication No. (ADM) 78-158).

Mollica, R. F., Blum, J. D., & Redlich, F. (1980). Equity and the psychiatric care of the black patient, 1950-1975. *Journal of Nervous & Mental Disease, 168,* 279.

Montgomery, G. T., & Orozco, S. (1985). Mexican Americans' performance on the MMPI as a function of level of acculturation. *Journal of Clinical Psychology, 41,* 203-212.

Mosher, L. R., & Keith, S. J. (1981). Psychosocial treatment: Individual, groups, family, and community support approaches. *Special Report: Schizophrenia, 1980* (DHHS Publication No. (ADM) 81-1064). Washington, DC: U.S. Government Printing Office.

Nicassio, P. M. (1983). Psychosocial correlates of alienation. *Journal of Cross-Cultural Psychology, 14,* 337-351.

Ogden, M., Spector, M. I., & Hill, C. A. (1970). Suicides and homicides among Indians. *Public Health Reports, 85*(1), 75-80.

Padilla, A. M., Ruiz, R. A., & Alvarez, R. (1975). Community mental health services for the Spanish-speaking/surnamed population. *American Psychologist, 30,* 892-905.

Padilla, E. R., & Padilla, A. M. (Eds.). (1977). *Transcultural psychiatry: An Hispanic perspective* (Spanish Speaking Mental Health Research Center, Monograph No. 4). Los Angeles: Spanish Speaking Mental Health Research Center.

Pedersen, P. B., Draguns, J. G., Lonner, W. J., & Trimble, J. (Eds.). (1981). *Counseling across cultures* (2nd ed.). Honolulu: The University Press of Hawaii.

Penk, W. E., et al. (1982). MMPI differences of Black and White male polydrug users seeking treatment. *Journal of Consulting & Clinical Psychology, 50,* 463-465.

Pollack, D., & Shore, J. (1980). Validity of the MMPI with Native Americans. *American Journal of Psychiatry, 137,* 946-950.

Pope, H., & Lipinski, J. (1978). Diagnosis in schizophrenia and manic depressive illness. *Archives of General Psychiatry, 35,* 811-827.

Prange, H., & Vitols, M. M. (1961). Cultural aspects of the relatively low incidence of depression in Southern Negroes. *International Journal of Social Psychiatry, 8,* 104-112.

Regier, D. A., Myers, J. K., Kramer, M., Robins, L. N., Blazer, D. G., Hough, R. L., Eaton, W. W., & Locke, B. Z. (1984). The NIMH Epidemiologic Catchment Area Program. *Archives of General Psychiatry, 41,* 934-941.

Rhoades, E. R., Marshall, M., Attneave, C., Echohawk, M., Bjorck, J., & Beiser, M. (1980). Mental health problems of American Indians seen in outpatient facilities of the Indian Health Service, 1975. *Public Health Reports, 95,* 329-335.

Robins, L. N., Helzer, J. E., Weissman, M., Orvaschel, H., Gruenberg, E., Burke, J. D., & Regier, D. A. (1984). Lifetime prevalence of specific psychiatric disorders in three sites. *Archives of General Psychiatry, 41,* 949-958.

Rossi, R., & Gabrielli, F. (1976). The use of rating scales for studying diagnosis models: Evidence of dubiousness in the principles of classification (French). *Encephale, 2*(2), 283-286.

Rotunno, M., & McGoldrick, M. (1982). Italian families. In M. McGoldrick, J. K. Pearce, & J. Giordano, *Ethnicity and family therapy.* New York: Guilford Press.

Ruiz, P., & Langrod, J. (1976). The role of folkhealers in community mental health services. *Community Mental Health Journal, 12*(4), 392-398.

Sandoval, M. (1979). Santeria as a mental health care system: An historical overview. *Social Science & Medicine, 13B*(2), 137-151.

Sartorius, N., Davidian, H., Fenton, F. R. et al. (1977, August). *International agreement on the diagnosis of depression: Implications for treatment.* Paper read at the Sixth World Congress of Psychiatry, Honolulu, Hawaii.

Schachter, J., & Butts, H. (1968). Transference and countertransference in interracial analyses. *Journal of the Psychoanalytic Association, 16*(4), 792-808.

Schwab, J. J., Bell, R. A., Warheit, G. J., & Schwab, R. B. (1979). *Social order and mental health: The Florida Health Study.* New York: Brunner/Mazel.

Sclare, A. B. (1963). Cultural determinants in the neurotic negro. In M. Grossack (Ed.), *Mental health and segregation.* New York: Springer.

Segal, J. (Ed.). (1975). *Research in the service of mental health.* Report of the Research Task Force of the National Institute of Mental Health (DHEW Publication No. (ADM) 75-236). Washington, DC: U.S. Government Printing Office.

Shan-Ming, Y., Deyi, C., Zhen, C. Y., Jingsu, J., & Taylor, M. A. (1982). Prevalence and characteristics of mania in Chinese inpatients: A prospective study. *American Journal of Psychiatry, 139,* 1150-1153.

Shan-Ming, Y., De Zhao, X., Zhen, C. Y., Deyi, C., Daqian, Z., & Taylor, M. A. (1984). The frequency of major psychiatric disorder in Chinese inpatients. *American Journal of Psychiatry, 141,* 690-692.

Simon, R. J., Fliess, J., Gurland, B., Stiller, P., & Sharpe, L. (1973). Depression and schizophrenia in hospitalized Black and White mental patients. *Archives of General Psychiatry, 28,* 509-512.

Smith, E. J. (1981). Cultural and historical perspectives in counseling blacks. In D. W. Sue (Ed.), *Counseling the culturally different.* New York: Wiley.

Snyder, R. T., Holowenzak, S., & Hoffman, N. (1971). A cross-cultural item analysis of Bender-Gestalt protocols administered to ghetto and suburban children. *Perceptual and Motor Skills, 33,* 791-796.

Srole, L., Langer, T. S., Michael, S. T., Opler, M. K., & Rennie, T. A. C. (1962). *Mental health in the metropolis: The Midtown Manhattan Study.* New York: McGraw Hill.

Sue, D. W. (1981). *Counseling the culturally different.* New York: Wiley.

Sue, S. (1977). Community mental health services to minority groups. *American Psychologist, 32,* 616-624.

Sue, S. & McKinney, H. (1975). Asian Americans in the community mental health care system. *American Journal of Orthopsychiatry, 45,* 111-118.

Sue, S., & Morishima, J. K. (1982). *The mental health of Asian Americans: Contemporary issues in identifying and healing mental problems.* San Francisco: Jossey-Bass.

Szapocznik, J., Kurtines, W., & Fernandez, T. (1980). Bicultural involvement and adjustment in Hispanic-American youths. *International Journal of Intercultural Relations, 4,* 353-365.

Takahashi, R., Sakuma, A., & Itoh, K. et al. (1975). Comparison of efficacy of lithium carbonate and chlorpromazine in mania. *Archives of General Psychiatry, 32,* 1310-1318.

Taube, C. (1971). Admission rates to state and county mental hospitals by age, sex, and color, United States, 1969. N.I.M.H. Biometry Branch, Statistical Note 41, 1-7.

Terkelsen, K. G. (1983). Schizophrenia and the family: Adverse effects of family therapy. *Family Process, 22,* 191-200.

Thomas, A., & Sillen, S. (1972). *Racism and psychiatry.* New York: Brunner/Mazel.

Triandis, H. C., & Draguns, J. G. (Eds.). (1980). *Handbook on cross-cultural psychology: Vol. 6. Psychopathology.* Boston: Allyn & Bacon.

Tseng, W-S, McDermott, J. F., Ogino, K., & Ebata, K. (1982). Cross-cultural differences in parent-child assessment: U.S.A. and Japan. *International Journal of Social Psychiatry, 28,* 305-317.

Valle, R., & Vega, W. (1980). *Hispanic natural support systems.* State of California, Department of Mental Health.

Vega, W., Warheit, G., Buhl-Auth, J., & Meinhardt, K. (1984). The prevalence of depressive symptoms among Mexican Americans and Anglos. *American Journal of Epidemiology, 120,* 592-607.

Vernon, S. W., & Roberts, R. E. (1982). Use of SADS-RDC in a tri-ethnic community survey. *Archives of General Psychiatry, 39,* 47-50.

Waite, R. (1968). The Negro patient and clinical theory. *Journal of Consulting Psychology, 32,* 427-433.

Walz, G. M., & Benjamin, L. (Eds.). (1978). *Transcultural counseling: Needs, programs and techniques.* New York: Human Sciences Press.

Waxler, N. E. (1979). Is outcome for schizophrenia better in nonindustrial societies? The case of Sri Lanka. *Journal of Nervous & Mental Disease, 167*(3), 144-158.

Weissman, M. M., & Klerman, G. L. (1977). Sex differences and the epidemiology of depression. *Archives of General Psychiatry, 34,* 98-111.

Williams, J. B. W., & Spitzer, R. L. (1983). The issue of sex bias in DSM III: A critique of "A woman's view of DSM III" by Marcie Kaplan. *American Psychologist, 38,* 793-798.

World Health Organization. (1979). *Schizophrenia: An international follow-up study.* Chichester, England: Wiley.

Yamamoto, J., Lam, J., Choi, W-I, Reece, S., Lo, S., Hahn, D. S., & Fairbanks, L. (1982). The Psychiatric Status Schedule for Asian Americans. *American Journal of Psychiatry, 139,* 1181-1184.

Zarrouk, El-Tayeb A. (1978). The usefulness of first-rank symptoms in the diagnosis of schizophrenia in a Saudi Arabian population. *British Journal of Psychiatry, 132,* 571-573.

Ziegler, V. W., & Biggs, J. T. (1977). Tricyclic plasma levels: Effects of age, race, sex, and smoking. *Journal of the American Medical Association, 238,* 2167.

PART II

CROSS-CULTURAL TRAINING PROGRAMS

INTRODUCTORY REMARKS

THE HISTORICAL development of the need for cultural input in the mental health professions has generated a variety of training efforts. At this point in history, cross-cultural programs are nonstandardized, eclectic, and still quite experimental. They range from one-day workshops at professional meetings to full psychology graduate programs, such as a specialization in cross-cultural counseling offered at Western Washington University. In the main, however, cross-cultural mental health training has no subdisciplinary status and is essentially an area in developmental flux.

Because of the large demand for such training (see **Behavior Today,** February 13, 20, 27, 1984, for a mini-series devoted to this demand), Part II is devoted to a comprehensive description of the rationale and operations of three types of training programs. All were offered at major universities and funded by the National Institute of Mental Health Manpower Training Division.

Despite some commonalities, the three programs reflect a heterogeneity of approach that is probably inevitable in any task of amending existing professional disciplines. They vary in duration, emphasis, and format. Although all curricula are oriented toward mental health professionals, the target trainees are noticeably different in terms of their levels of experience and applications in the field. The programs focus on different ethnic groups, contingent on locale, although all purport to transmit a generalizable transcultural perspective. All try to deal directly with overcoming theoretial barriers to a nonuniversalistic approach to mental health service delivery, but different conceptual models are employed.

The Training Program in Ethnicity and Mental Health at Brandeis University was oriented toward mental health professionals at the advanced levels of clinical training: psychiatric residents, and interns in clinical psychology and psychiatric social work. They focused on

Azorean-Portuguese ethnicity, as well as differences in Irish, Italian, Black, Hispanic, Greek subgroups. The project emphasized hands-on, case-oriented applications of training by participants rotating throughout the mental health system in inpatient, outpatient, and satellite clinical services.

The DISC (Developing Interculturally Skilled Counselors) program at the University of Hawaii trained graduate students in cross-cultural counseling and therapy, and designed brief workshops for inservice training for agencies. Trainees were multi-disciplinary, including public health, communication, and anthropology as well as the core disciplines. Resource persons were primarily from Hawaiian and Asian cultures, although other subgroups were represented. An integral component of the DISC model involved hosting an international conference for each year of the project, and in generating ongoing dissemination materials and information exchange with others in the field.

The University of Miami's Cross-Cultural Training Institute for Mental Health Professionals (CCTI) was oriented toward experienced service-providers working in mental health facilities serving low-income multi-ethnic populations. They focused primarily on Afro-American, Afro-Caribbean (Haitian and Bahamian) and Hispanic (Cuban and Puerto Rican) cultures. CCTI emphasized a community mental health perspective and institutional change in the mental health system. To this end, the program was interested in involving administrators and in teaching community outreach as well as clinical techniques.

The descriptions of these three programs are designed to provide information to facilitate development of further cross-cultural training that will meet specific needs and hopefully avoid pitfalls encountered in pioneer experimental efforts. Overall, the three chapters deal with the following elements: background and rationale for the training; preparatory phase; mode of selecting trainees; curriculum models; evaluation and use of feedback for curriculum change; applications and impact of the program; and participants' personal assessment of training in culture and mental health as a component of their professional education. These descriptions are then followed, in Part III, by the detailed comprehensive evaluation of one of these programs, the Cross-Cultural Training Institute for Mental Health Professionals, in terms of its objective impact on the trainees, their patients, and their institutions.

CHAPTER 3

TRAINING PROGRAM IN ETHNICITY AND MENTAL HEALTH

JOHN P. SPIEGEL and JOHN PAPAJOHN

T HE TRAINING PROGRAM in Ethnicity and Mental Health was devised for an interdisciplinary team of non-indigenous mental health professionals in the later stages of their initial clinical training. The choice of "non-indigenous" personnel was based on the assumption that there were already in existence a number of "indigenous" training programs in which Blacks were being trained to deal with Black populations, Hispanics with Latin-American populations, and Asians with Chinese, Japanese, Koreans, and the newcomers from Southeast Asia. Under an affirmative action idealogy, the needs of the "official" minorities were being addressed — although perhaps not perfectly in all instances — while the needs of the so-called "white ethnics" were being overlooked. In addition, we assumed that it would take a long time before there existed a sufficient number of well-trained Blacks, Hispanics, Asians, Native Americans, etc., to meet the needs of the official minorities wherever they happend to be living. In the meantime, such ethnic populations were receiving mental health services from "mainstream" mental health professionals who lacked the cross-cultural perspectives and the skills to provide culturally relevant services. Accordingly, we visualized our Program as one model of a much-needed corrective in the context of the pluralistic and diverse character of the "unmelted" structure of American society.

The approach governing our design of the Training Program utilized the epistemological and theoretical perspectives that constituted the framework that we intended to teach to the trainees. Transactional systems theory and cultural value orientation theory were the two conceptual mainstays guiding us in considering modes of intervening in the two training sites where our work was to be done. These training sites were both Harvard-affiliated teaching institutions, the Cambridge Hospital and Community Health Center and the Erich Lindemann Mental Health Center. We perceived these sites as being systems characterized by discrete cultures, each having a social role structure where relationships among the staff and other personnel were patterned in a consistent manner that reflected the cultural values of the "system" as well as those of individuals, each with his idiosyncratic personality structure. Thus, culture, social roles, and individual psychological organization constituted the three foci in a transacting system of events that would have to be considered if we were to be effective in organizing a successful program for teaching concepts of disordered behavior related to the ethnic backgrounds of individuals who are receiving mental health services in traditional psychiatric settings.

Our target sample of trainees was to consist of psychiatric residents, clinical psychology interns and psychiatric social work students who were working in the clinical settings of university hospitals, outpatient clinics and community mental health centers. They were selected from the general population of trainees already accepted into these programs because of their high motivation for and interest in cross-cultural work.

We considered it important to introduce these trainees to the cross-cultural and ethnic perspective at a relatively early stage of their professional experiences, before their ideas of how to deliver services had become too fixed in "mainstream" patterns which are constructed, for the most part, for urban, middle-class, acculturated populations.

A formal program of this kind almost always develops out of a background of experience which generates ideas that seem useful for educational purposes. For many years we had been engaged in extensive research with several different ethnic groups on the relationship between subcultural values and perceptions, family interaction styles, and mental illness (Papajohn and Spiegel, 1975). Although our interest in research of this sort continued, when we first submitted a grant proposal to NIMH in 1976 we had arrived at the opinion that the time had come to translate our accumulated knowledge base and skills into a training procedure. Because of this opinion we had spent the previous year testing out the feasibility of such a transmission of knowledge and skill by means of a small pilot project conducted at the Cambridge Hospital and the Cambridge Community Mental Health and Retardation Center, funded by the Marcus Foundation of Chicago. During this pilot year we made ourselves available for consultation on "difficult" ethnic cases in the various components of the Department of Psychiatry and in the Emergency Service. During the course of the experimental year we managed to prove to ourselves and to members of the staff that we had something of value to offer. Enough support emerged to encourage us to plan a program to be submitted to NIMH for funding.

In addition, the pilot year had made us acutely aware of some hazards and obstacles that would have to be taken into consideration in order that such a training program would have a reasonable chance of success in the departments of psychiatry of major medical schools. These obstacles were understandable from a systems point of view, and we summarized them as deriving from three sources.

The first of these sources was implicit forms of resistance to a new theoretical approach, i.e., cultural value orientation theory which, in some of its underlying assumptions, could be construed as inconsistent with psychoanalytic theory. Psychoanalysis constitutes the main theoretical basis on which these "traditional" training programs are structured (in a very real way psychoanalysis serves as the ideological or "cultural" foundation of these training programs). Its tenets are shared by the training directors and have a direct patterning effect on the content of the formal teaching inputs and, too, an indirect effect by mediating the epistemological assumptions on which it is based. Psychoanalytic theory assumes a shared genetic (biological) heritage that characterizes human development wherein individuation becomes the goal of therapy. This is a process of continuing differentiation and reintegration through progressive stages of development. Cultural value orientation theory assumes a shared socio-cultural heritage where individual modes of thinking, feeling, and acting are shaped by common environmental (ecological) experiences and are necessary for effective functioning within that cultural system.

The second obstacle we anticipated required that we accommodate our entrance into these two training institutions to the extant role structure. We needed to be allied with and to be validated by both the senior administrators who could facilitate our entrance into their systems and by the line clinical workers who provided direct services to clients. The latter's support needed to be earned by our demonstrating that we could be useful to them in alleviating their burden in treating difficult, that is, restive, ethnic patients.

The third obstacle to be overcome was covert ethnocentricity. That is, the lack of awareness on the part of mental health professionals of their own "learned" tendencies to value patients who shared characteristics common to themselves: white, educated, attractive, middle class. This denial of cultural bias is the factor that allows professionals to see patients as "untreatable" because they are viewed as lacking intelligence, motivation, and other such characteristics associated with their own social class background.

At this juncture it should be noted that while we were able to meet our training objectives more or less successfully during the three years of the Program, in the end we made very little impact on the overall "culture"—the ideological assumptions—that undergird these teaching centers. Indeed, we were able to engage the system, to effect a balanced role for ourselves that assured the support of both the power structure and the line clinical workers, to carry out our specific teaching and training roles, and to earn the respect of the staffs in both institutions. Nevertheless, when we had completed our assignment little interest was expressed in incorporating this ethnocultural dimension as a permanent component of the training capabilities of the two training sites.

Theoretical Concepts

We have made it clear that we attach a great deal of importance to theory and conceptualization as aids to appropriate service delivery and to training procedures. Clinicians need to internalize a frame of reference that equips them to order cultural variables in a useful way in diagnosis and treatment. Next we shall elaborate the theoretical constructs referred to above which are central to our approach to training.

1. Transactional Field Theory

Most of us have learned to order events in cause and effect terms which reflects the Aristotelian assumptions of linear causality. This position is the essence of the scientific method, and it delimits the range of variables that can be examined at one time. A person's neurotic reaction, for example, may be conceptualized as caused by a disturbed relationship to the mother (lack of physical and psychological nuturance, over-control, and over-involvement). The cause of the dysfunctional behavior can be understood as the relationship between a "dependent variable" (a symptom or problematic behavior) for which a cause and "independent variable" needs to be found. This search is limited, furthermore, to the psychological aspects of the individual. An exception will be found in cases of schizophrenia, where biological or genetic causes are also presumed to be present and may "interact" with psychological stress. Even then the causal relationships are conceptualized in a linear fashion.

Transactional systems theory is based on a very different conceptual assumption: That is, that events constitute a field of transaction processes in which change in one part is related to change in all the other parts (see Figure 3-1). An individual's neurosis can be understood as reflecting a transactional interplay of psychological, cultural, social and biological events. The disturbed behavior, for example a symbiotic bond to the mother, is not explained solely as a fixtion in psychological development, but rather as related concomitantly to cultural conflict, social dislocation, biological events, etc. Events in any one of these domains, then, transact with each other domain to produce a neurotic reaction in the individual. Ordinarily, these events are not included in a differential diagnosis. Although they may be noted in the history-taking, they are not viewed as significant data that need to be utilized in the treatment planning. From a transaction system perspective, the treatment objective is to address the disequilibrium in the field of events impinging on the individual to bring about a new and more functional balance.

Figure 3-1

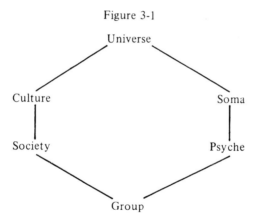

2. Value Orientation Theory and Its Application

In the context of the transactional system approach, culture is the focus to begin the inquiry into families undergoing acculturation since we are dealing with a clash of cultural understandings and norms. For this purpose we need a map. The map we have been using is the theory of variation in cultural value orientations prepared by Florence Kluckhohn. She defines value orientation as follows: **A value orientation is a generalized and organized conception, influencing behavior of time, of nature, of man's place in it, of man's relation to man, and of** the desirable and non-desirable aspects of man-environment and inter-human transactions (Kluckhohn and Strodtbeck, 1961). In addition, value orientations have a directional, a cognitive, and an affective function. These three functions constitute the "program" for selecting between more or less favored choices of alternative behaviors for individuals within a particular culture. Furthermore, communication among individuals in a particular culture is contigent upon the shared value orientations that characterize them.

Kluckhohn postulated five common human problems for which all peoples in all places must find some solution. They are: **Time,** which is the temporal focus of human life; **Activity,** the preferred pattern of action in daily living; the **Relational orientation,** which is the preferred way of relating interpersonally; the **Man/Nature orientation,** which defines the way man relates to the nature or the supernatural environment, however conceptualized; and the **Basic Nature of Man,** concerned with conceptions of innate good and evil in human behavior.

The theory assumes three possible solutions for each of these common human problems, and the variation among and within cultures is based on the rank ordering (pattern of preferences) of these solutions in a dominant-substitute profile of values. It is important to underscore here a central feature of Kluckhohn's theory. Each of the orientations are present in **all** societies; it is the particular rank ordering that differentiates one culture from another. In Table 1 the patterning of preferences for mainstream American lifestyles (American middle class) is compared with profiles characteristic of rural, southern Italian and rural southern Irish families drawn from our work with these migrant groups.

Table 1

COMPARISON OF VALUE ORIENTATION PROFILES

	American Middle Class	Italian	Irish
TIME	Future > Present > Past	Present > Past > Future	Present > Past > Future
ACTIVITY	Doing > Being	Being > Doing	Being > Doing
RELATIONAL	Ind > Coll > Lineal	Coll > Lineal > Ind	Lineal > Coll > Ind
MAN/NATURE	Dom Over > Subj > Harmony	Subj > Harmony > Dom Over	Subj > Harmony > Dom Over

Let us first examine the American middle class value orientation patterns (see Interpretive Key). It becomes readily evident that there is a functional relationship between the value orientation profiles or patterns in the different problem areas or modalities and the adaptational demands of a technologically advanced society like that of the United States. The first-order **future** orientation of a Time area, for example, is a critical one in our society where planning for the future is a necessary condition for effectively carrying on the functions required for maintaining a technologically advanced system. In the Activity area, the first-order **doing** orientation reflects the achievement orientation of this society which is shared by other Western cultures. The opportunities for upward social mobility places demands on individuals to achieve economically and socially. The evaluation of one's individual worth is based on the degree to which one has been able to compete with success. The first-order **individualistic** preference in the Relational area reflects the lifelong thrust toward "individuation" and independence and is consistent with the **doing** orientation in the Activity area. The first-order positioning of the **over nature** preference in the Man-Nature modality is correlated with our assumption that given enough time, money and technology, most problems between man and nature can be solved in the name of "progress." Child-rearing practices in the United States are geared to preparing children for successful functioning in this society. Developmental stages such as weaning, toilet training, are traversed at earlier ages than is the case in other cultures such as rural Italy and rural Ireland from which a significant portion of the American population has emigrated.

VALUE ORIENTATION INTERPRETATIVE KEY

ACTIVITY MODALITY

Doing

Major emphasis is on the kind of activity which results in accomplishments that are measurable by standards conceived to be external to the acting individual, i.e., achievement. EXAMPLE: American middle-class society.

Being

The kind of activity which is a spontaneous expression of what is conceived to be "given" in the human personality — the spontaneous expression of impulses and desires. EXAMPLE: Mexican rural society.

RELATIONAL MODALITY

Individual

Individual autonomy characterizes the relationships of men to each other. Individual goals have primacy over the goals of the group. Reciprocal role relationships are characterized by a recognition of the independence of interrelating individuals. Group goals are attained through the realization of autonomous goals of individual members. EXAMPLE: The American middle-class family.

Collateral

The primacy of the goals of the laterally extended group patterns the relationship of men to each other. Individual autonomous goals are subordinated to the goals of the group. Relationships are ordered on a horizontal, egalitarian dimension. Reciprocal role relationships are characterized by "one for all and all for one" principle. EXAMPLE: The Italian extended family.

Lineal

Group goals again have primacy over individual goals. Relationships, however, on a vertical dimension are patterned by the hierarchically ordered positions that individuals hold in the group. Reciprocal role relationships are characterized by a dominance-submission mode of interrelationship for the position a person holds in the group hierarchy. EXAMPLE: The British upper-classes; the Irish family.

TIME MODALITY

Future

The temporal focus is based on the future. The major emphasis, therefore, is on planning for change at points in time extending away from the present into the future. EXAMPLE: American middle-class society.

Present

The present is the major focus of time. Little attention is paid to the past, and the future is perceived as vague and upredictable. EXAMPLE: rural societies in Latin America and in Italy.

Past

The past is preferred to either the present or the future as the major time focus. Tradition is of central importance in the life of the people. EXAMPLE: traditional Chinese society.

MAN-NATURE MODALITY

Subjugation to Nature

Man is subjugated to the forces of nature and does little to counteract them. EXAMPLE: Spanish rural society.

Harmony with Nature

The sense of wholeness in the individual is based on his continual communion with nature and the supernatural. EXAMPLE: Japanese society; Navaho Indian society.

Mastery over Nature

Natural forces of all kinds are to be overcome and harnessed to man's purpose. EXAMPLE: Americans' emphasis on technology to solve all kinds of problems.

In rural Ireland and rural Italy the first order orientation in the Time area that makes functional sense is the **present**. In rural societies individuals are rooted "existentially" in the present since the future cannot be controlled or predicted and little change is expected. Daily life is modulated by the forces of nature which pattern, also, the economic realities which are encountered. The seasons of the year determine what one does, i.e., planting, harvesting, etc. The planning of activities in accordance with a changing future makes no sense in situations where life goes around in cycles the same way every year.

Irish and Italians are **being** oriented in the Activity dimension. The being orientation places high value on "being oneself," in the sense of spontaneous expression of inner feelings in given situations. Satisfactions are derived from experiencing, here and now, each other, food, and as broad a range of sensual satifactions as possible. While this does not imply an uncontrolled, hedonistic orientation, it is contrasted with the "doing" orientation where immediate pleasure is forfeited for the satisfaction of achievement in the future.

In the relational area the Italians and Irish differ in the rank ordering of the three value orientation preferences. Italians are Coll > Lin > Ind. In both cultures, it should be noted, the individualistic orientation which is the most preferred in American culture is positioned last in the profiles of these two agrarian societies.

The first order collaterality in the Italian pattern reflects the interdependence among family members that is characteristic of Italian family structure. Individuals in this society are socialized for interdependence since the survival of the family is contingent on everyone collaborating with everyone else in common, often agrarian, pursuits. Italians traditionally have never trusted agencies outside the family to protect or to provide for them.

The first order Lineal preference in the Irish value orientation profile represents the essentially matriarchal character of the Irish family. The dominance of the wife and mother derives from a long history of political oppression and economic hardship in Ireland with chronic unemployment relegating the male to a secondary, almost powerless role within the family, despite the wife's attempts to make her husband look good in the eyes of the public.

The **subjugated to nature** first order preference in the Man-Nature area in both Irish and Italian culture is consistent with the **present, being** as well as both the **collateral** and **lineal** orientations in the Rela-

tional area. Man and woman are controlled either by the forces of nature or by a powerful diety. One cannot expect, as in technologically-
advanced societies, to harness the forces of nature to serve man. The
farmer feels helpless and powerless in confronting physical forces beyond his control. This orientation of course generalizes to other areas of
one's life. One is rooted in a present condition with no avenues available
in order to plan for future achievement or upward social mobility. The
alternative is emigration.

The above framework makes it possible to conceptualize the strain
that is experienced by Italian-Americans and Irish-Americans as they
confront the American social system. There is an inconsistency in all
five modalities between the internalized value orientations of the subcul-
ture in which they were socialized with that of the American social system to which they need to adapt. The strain of "acculturation stress"
becomes evident in all domains of adaptation such as occupational, rec-
reational, and social. The clinician who has internalized our frame of
reference can include this cultural understanding in assessing the specific psychological issues that confront his patient. He is not limited to a
psychological theory that is designed to conceptualize developmental
and characterological variables only.

The Program Objectives

We formulated a rather concise training plan which was approved
and accepted by the National Institute of Mental Health on an experimental basis* funded through the Florence Heller Graduate School for
Advanced Studies in Social Welfare at Brandeis University. The program objectives are summarized as follows:

  a. To provide the interdisciplinary staff and students operating clini-
     cal services in community mental health centers with insight into
     the effects of ethnicity on patients and families in treatment.
  b. To differentiate these effects for the different ethnic groups to
     which patients belong.
  c. To provide staff and students with more effective tools for deliver-
     ing services, in respect to:
     • Diagnosis, where distinguishing between subcultural practices
       and psychopathology is a problem;
     • Establishing a therapeutic alliance where social distance or
       ethnocentricity is the problem;

* NIMH Training Grant MH.5-T24-MH14962, Experimental and Special Branch, 1977-1980.

- Assessing psychodynamic formulations where variant or deviant child-rearing customs, marital or parental relations, or extended family transactions are the problem;
- Reorienting therapeutic goals in line with the particular acculturation conflict which the patient and/or the family is undergoing.

The Training Sites

John Spiegel, the Program Director, and John Papajohn, the Associate Program Director, spent a full year exploring potential field settings where the training could take place. In the end, we settled on two Harvard Medical School-affiliated training facilities, the Cambridge/Somerville Community Mental Health Center where the department of psychiatry is based at the Cambridge City Hospital and the Lindemann Community Mental Health Center, an affiliate of the Massachusetts General Hospital department of psychiatry which serves the Harbor Area catchment area.

Our engagement of the Cambridge/Somerville and the Lindemann centers involved several meetings with the respective directors whom we knew personally as well as a protracted twelve-month period of providing consultation to the staff around ethnic cases. Dr. Racquel Cohen, the Lindemann Mental Health Center director, and Dr. Lee Macht, the Cambridge City Hospital chairperson in the department of psychiatry, knew of our research work on ethnic families and were committed to a cultural perspective. Dr. Cohen worked in the area of community psychiatry with Dr. Gerald Caplan at the (Harvard) Laboratory of Community Psychiatry and Dr. Macht's work in community mental health was recognized nationally.

The communities for which the Lindemann Center was responsible included Boston's North End (almost 100 percent Italian-American), East Boston (largely Italian), and the suburbs of Chelsea (30 percent Spanish-speaking, 60 percent old-line Jewish), Revere and Charlestown. At Dr. Cohen's suggestion, our negotiations were confined to the North end and to Chelsea. The reason for beginning in this fashion was the need to determine which ethnic group in which community should be the choice for the "intensive" part of the trainees' experiences. The decision to concentrate on Hispanics in Chelsea was determined by the fact that they were being serviced by the Chelsea Community Counseling Center under the direction of Dr. Matthew Dumont, a psychiatrist dedicated to community psychiatry. He also was familiar with our approach and was supportive of it. While Hispanics comprised only 30 percent of the Chelsea population and only 10 percent of the Center's clientele, the numbers in both instances were rapidly rising. Chelsea also contained some Blacks, some Canadians, Irish and Italians. Most of the Hispanics were Puerto Ricans.

The Cambridge-Somerville Community Mental Health Center comprised a large geographical area that corresponded to the boundaries of these two cities. These are multiethnic, essentially working class communities with a mixture of Irish, Italians, Portuguese, Black, Hispanic, Greek and Haitian subgroups. The neighborhoods are ethnically mixed although North Cambridge is the location of a housing project occupied mainly by Black people, while the neighborhood close to the Cambridge City Hospital has a preponderance of Azorean-Portuguese people. The Greeks and Azorean-Portuguese populations are composed of relatively newly arrived immigrants, who left their homelands after 1965 when the immigration law was changed to allow immigrants from parts of Southern Europe with low quotas to emigrate in larger numbers. The Italians and Irish are the children and grandchildren of the original, first-generation immigrants who established themselves in these communities during the large wave of immigration that occurred at the turn of the century.

We decided to focus on the Azorean-Portuguese population as the group which our trainees might understand in greater depth. The presence of the Egas Moniz Clinic, a health center for Portuguese people nearby, facilitated this effort since it provided a natural site where our trainees could gain experience with Portuguese patients seen in the mental health division.

Program Planning

Two quarter-time Program Coordinators were recruited from the staffs of the two training sites. Both were psychologists who had earned a considerable amount of credibility within their respective organizations and so could serve as mediators for the Training Program. The Cambridge-Somerville Program Coordinator was a Black woman psychologist; her Lindemann counterpart was a male of Hispanic origin who was bilingual. They interpreted and advocated what we intended to do among their colleagues. An advisory committee comprised of senior members of these two training site staffs was created to monitor the Program especially in the difficult phase of getting started. In addition, the Program Directors and the Program Coordinators met with the heads of the different clinical services to acquaint them with Program objectives and contemplated procedures. The directors of training for psychiatry, psychology and social work were also members of the advisory committee. We negotiated with them the criteria for selection of recruits for our Program that would satisfy their own independent training program guidelines. We examined with them the various clinical placements within their mental health centers where the trainees could get the appropriate experiences to satisfy both the hospital training objectives and those of the Ethnicity Training Program as well. We negotiated for blocks of times where the Ethnicity Training Program trainees would be free to attend the formal teaching seminars and clinical conferences that we had designed to be part of the specialized training we were providing. Our effort, in summary, was to integrate our training inputs with those extant forms that constitute the training format in traditional training programs for psychiatry, psychology and social work.

The Training Format

(1) A one-semester course, offered by John Spiegel at the Heller School, "Social Aspects of Mental Health and Illness," was required of all trainees. This was designed to provide the trainees with a macroscopic overview of social psychiatry where issues such as epidemiology in cross-cultural perspective, social class and mental illness, labelling theory, etc. were reviewed.

(2) A one-semester course offered at the Heller School by John Spiegel and John Papajohn entitled "Ethnicity and Mental Health" constituted the second major academic offering. It was in this course that transactional systems theory and cultural value orientation theory with special reference to diagnosis and treatment were reviewed.

(3) A weekly "ethnic clinical teaching conference" was held on alternative weeks at each of the two training sites. Cases seen by the trainees in their respective clinical placements were presented in the traditional mode. John Spiegel and John Papajohn alternated chairing these conferences. Guest consultations with special knowledge of different ethnic groups were invited for special conferences.

(4) Ethnic cases seen by the trainees were supervised individually by John Spiegel and John Papajohn. These were structured in the traditional way with the trainee presenting the case and describing the pro-

cess of treatment with the supervisor providing suggestions and interpretations where appropriate. It was here the trainees could discuss their ideas, questions and doubts about the differential effect of cultural and psychological factors in the clinical process of his or her own individual patient.

(5) In the second year of the Program we instituted an additional seminar entitled, "Ethnocultural Factors in Diagnosis and Treatment." This was a one-semester, weekly, two-hour conference that focused specifically on the application of cultural theory to the clinical process. Formal presentations on different subcultures including Irish, Puerto Rican, Japanese, Haitian, etc. were made by clinicians with special knowledge of these subcultures.

The Recruitment Process

We employed both formal (advertising in professional publications) and informal methods of locating candidates for the NIMH funded traineeships who met our criteria and those of the training directors in the three disciplines. We wanted individuals highly motivated to work with poor ethnic populations who at the same time could meet the criteria for acceptance into the mental health centers' training slots. The mental health center training directors, themselves, were motivated in this recruitment effort by the fact that each could expect to acquire two additional individuals for training in their programs who were funded by the Ethnicity Training Program.

In the end two major sources for recruits for our Program evolved. The first was the mental health center training directors themselves. In reviewing candidates for their own traineeships they introduced the availability of a conjoint program to those who met, in their views, criteria for both programs. In the first year, two psychiatric residents and one of the clinical psychology interns were recruited in this way. The second psychology intern was recruited by word of mouth—a colleague with strong interests in this area introduced to us an associate of his who was in the last stage of completing his doctorate in clinical psychology.

The two psychiatric social work trainees were recruited from the Smith College School of Social Work. There already was in existence a liaison between this school and the department of psychiatric social work at the Cambridge City Hospital. In addition, we had personal contacts with the new administration of this institution that facilitated our collaboration further.

In the second year the recruitment process followed a course similar to the first year with one important exception; we were unable to recruit a psychiatric resident for either the Cambridge City or the Lindemann Mental Health Center sites. We substituted two psychologists in their places: a Ph.D. from the Department of Social Relations at Harvard University and an Ed.D. who wanted to do a post-doctoral internship in clinical psychology at Cambridge City.

As regards ethnic background over the two years, the twelve trainees were almost evenly divided between those whose backgrounds were representative of mainstream American middle-class culture (WASP) and those with an "ethnic" tradition whose parents or grandparents had emigrated from another country. The two psychiatric residents, three psychologists, and one of the psychiatric social workers derived from a mainstream tradition. One psychologist and two of the social workers were Jewish American with very weak ties to Judaism — either second- or third-generation American. One of the psychologists was of Azorean Portuguese parentage and one social worker was born and raised in a slavic country in Eastern Europe. With the exception of the Portuguese American psychologist, all came from predominantly middle-class and professional backgrounds — with strong liberal ideological traditions.

Ethnicity of Cases Seen by Trainees

The ethnicity trainees were rotated through the customary sequence of placements in the mental health center system designed to provide them with a broad range of experience with a variety of different patients. These included the inpatient, outpatient units as well as placements in the satellite clinics where the major portion of patients were ethnic. In Cambridge this was the Egas Moniz Mental Health Clinic serving the Portuguese and in Chelsea the Community Counseling Center serving predominantly the Puerto Rican, low income population. The experiences of our trainees, however, were not uniform as regards the number of ethnic patients that they saw. This was a function of where they were placed, for how long, and was also dictated by the experiences their supervisors (from the mental health centers) determined they needed to have. At the end of the first training year the "ethnicity" trainees were asked to provide a record of the ethnicity, age, and sex of patients they were seeing. This breakdown is provided in Table 2.

Table 2

	Total	Chelsea	Cambridge
Puerto Rican	13	13	0
Irish	13	6	7
Portuguese	12	0	12
Jewish	7	4	3
Italian	6	3	3
Caribbean	3	0	3
Other	24	5	19
Unknown or "American"	14	12	2
	92	43	49

At least 25 of these cases involved more than one family member; hence the total number of persons seen by trainees at this time was actually greater than 92. Some degree of family therapy took place with most of the 25 "family" cases. A correlation of the incidence of family therapy and ethnicity reveals the following:

Table 3

Ethnicity	Number of Cases Involving Family Therapy
Puerto Rican	7
Portuguese	7
Jewish	4
Irish	5
Other	2
	25

Program Evaluation

The Program Evaluator, who was a doctoral student at the Heller School, was present at all the meetings and conferences and continually monitored the progress of the Program over the course of the two training years. He also scheduled an individual conference with each of the trainees twice during their twelve month tenure in each of the two years. He inquired into the trainees' views on the relevance of the training format, the satisfactions and dissatisfactions they derived and their future plans as regards working with ethnic populations.

At the end of the first training year the Program Evaluator's report highlighted the following factors:

1. General Strengths of the Program:

Trainees identified several components of the Program which they considered strong points. Three major strengths were:

  a. The general opportunity to treat ethnic patients in a systematic fashion;

  b. The clinical case conferences, in which specific trainee cases were discussed;

  c. The course held at the Heller School at Brandeis University on ethnicity and mental health.

These components were considered strengths because they served a consciousness-raising function that sensitized trainees to the problems of cross-cultural psychotherapy and the problems of making mental health systems responsive to the needs of ethnic patients. Thus a typical trainee comment was that **before** entering the Program he or she knew that ethnics experienced problems getting appropriate clinical services, but **now** they understood just how serious and complicated the problems really were. They now understood the subtleties and complexities of cross-cultural psychotherapy and the difficulties in altering mental health agencies to respond to needs of ethnics.

These observations are not intended to downplay the acquisition of substantive knowledge on the part of trainees concerning specific ethnic groups and related issues, as this was a significant gain. But, in a general sense, it seems that the primary impact of the Program was in moving trainees from the position of knowing, in an abstract sense, that ethnic patients present unique problems to the clinician to an understanding in a deeper way why this is the case, and what to do about it.

Trainees felt that the experience of treating ethnics—and the first-hand experience of the associated pitfalls—coupled with the critical discussion of their cases in the clinical conferences provided the core of this learning experience. The ethnicity course mentioned above was important for placing their experiences in the context of larger human service delivery systems.

2. General Weaknesses of the Program

Most of the trainees were concerned with what they saw as a lack of communication among various members of the Program staff. In their opinions, poor communication resulted in occasional confusion as to the times and places of meetings, abrupt schedule changes, delays in the receipt of stipend checks, and related matters. They felt that communication among directors and field coordinators was at times confused and strained. They also found it difficult from time to time to contact project directors. They were also aware that directors were often not able to contact them, due to mutually heavy schedules, and that this exacerbated the communication problems. These problems were seen by trainees as administrative problems that needed to be corrected by the directors. Trainees did, however, understand that the newness of the Program was a factor in this problem and made allowances for the need to "debug" any new effort.

The second weakness related to the training process itself. Trainees, and this included all of them, felt that opportunities were provided for them to see ethnic patients and to discuss these patients in a variety of settings. However, the training aspect of the Program was not always effectively put forth. Some trainees apparently wanted a specific, highly delineated model of intervention and were somewhat let down when they learned that such a model was not forthcoming. Others, understanding that one of the intentions of the Program was to experiment with such models, were not clear on what "data" to collect on patients and how to utilize such data.

Related to these concerns was a theme that ran through trainee responses which could be phrased as, "What exactly do I do with the ethnic patients in the counseling situation itself?" For example, they began to understand how to use the value orientation scale to interpret the patient's situation and to make a general treatment plan that was culturally appropriate. However, apart from asking certain specific questions about ethnic background, they were not sure of other clinically-appropriate topics for the therapeutic dialogue, and how this might fit in with whatever treatment approach they were familiar with.

This proved to be a very difficult issue to resolve, given the vagueness with which the trainees described the problem. Nevertheless, it was a real and important issue that needed further consideration. Of particular importance was the development of a way to conceptually merge culturally-relevant approaches with either specific (e.g., analytic, gestalt, cognitive, social learning) therapeutic methodology or an explicitly eclectic model.

A final weakness identified by trainees relates to the issue of inter-organizational communication mentioned above. Trainees wanted the directors and the training coordinators to be more aggressive in their dealings with administrators and supervisors in placement settings. This was of particular concern at the beginning of the year when routines and caseloads were being established. Certain trainees felt that they did not have enough control over the ethnic make-up of their caseloads and that the coordinators and directors could have taken more of a role of advocate in this matter. Also, there were conflicts around the amount of psychological testing expected of psychology interns. One intern felt that, given the demands of the Ethnicity Program and the internship, the requirements around testing placed an excessive demand on an already tight schedule. The issue was how much testing was appropriate, not testing **per se.**

Although there were other individual concerns and problems mentioned by trainees, these discussed here were the ones mentioned by all or most of the trainees.

The main weakness related to the training process itself. They felt that in seeing ethnic patients they were not clear as to how to handle the cultural aspects of the problems that were presented. They had hoped to have learned a specific, highly delineated model of intervention and were somewhat let down when they learned that such a model was not forthcoming. While they understood how to use the value orientation scale to interpret the patient's situation and to make a general treatment plan that was culturally appropriate, they were not sure how to implement it effectively. Specifically they were not sure of how to integrate this cultural perspective with whatever "traditional" treatment approach they were familiar with.

This issue was dealt within the second training year through the introduction of the seminar mentioned earlier in this section entitled "Ethnocultural Factors in Diagnosis and Treatment." The individual presenters in this series discussed specific ethnic groups in relation to the following major parameters: (1) differential diagnosis in which cultural and psychological factors were separated out; (2) establishing a therapeutic alliance; (3) assessment of the presenting problems in the context of the early family socialization process of the patient; (4) refining and monitoring therapeutic intervention accordingly; and, (5) reorientation of therapeutic goals in line with the particular acculturation conflict which the patient and/or the family was undergoing.

A continuing stress report reported by most trainees was that engendered by the concurrent demands of the Ethnicity Program and the mental health center training program. Often the effort to integrate the two segments of their training did not work well and they experienced them as competing for their time and energies. This issue was alleviated somewhat in the second training year through more concentrated work on planning the conjoint program by both the Ethnicity Program Directors and by the Directors of Training in psychiatry, psychology and social work for the two mental health centers. Some strain remained, however, till the end.

In both training years the trainees reported that they found the formal academic courses that were offered as important in broadening their conceptual grasp of the psychological problems of specific ethnic groups. The individual supervision provided by Doctors Spiegel and Papajohn were also reported to be an important teaching experience. The fact that Spiegel was psychoanalytically oriented and Papajohn behaviorally oriented, they felt, enhanced their understanding of the interlacing of psychological and cultural factors in the treatment process.

They also reported gaining an in-depth understanding of both the Portuguese and Puerto Rican groups that were focused on at the Cambridge-Somerville and the Chelsea branch of the Lindemann Community Mental Health Center respectively. Some of the trainees enhanced their understanding through home visits to the families of patients they were treating.

Closing Remarks

John Spiegel interviewed the trainees individually at the end of each of the two training years. Many of the views expressed to the Program Evaluator were shared with him also. The following additional impressions of special relevance to planning future programs will be reported here. One interesting aspect of the Program, which, in some ways is a major strength and at times is a weakness, was the freedom which the Program gave each trainee to carve out his or her own program. Thus, in terms of the trainees' placements, trainees had very different responsibilities and requirements and, hence, very different experiences. Most of the trainees attempted to create a learning situation that best fitted their needs and backgrounds. The problem with this was that some trainees lost time at the beginning of the year as they attempted to "work the system" in order to locate themselves where they wanted to be. A typical problem for trainees involved the various rules about placements that had been created in each organization.

However, the advantage was that, once they got past the bureaucratic hassles, the trainees were to a great extent able to tailor their placements to their own needs.

For example, one trainee was specifically interested in the Portuguese and spent a great deal of time at the Egas Moniz Clinic. Another was interested in family therapy and worked closely with a family therapy training organization. Because trainees actually had a great deal of freedom within the placement aspect of the Program, one cannot say that all of the trainees experienced the "same Program." What they brought with them to supervision and seminars, then, and what they carried away, was a variety of experiences, not one uniform experience. This gave a richness and diversity to the Ethnicity Program that would have been lost if trainees had not been given a great amount of leeway to design a program that provided the kind of educative and growth opportunities they desired.

All the trainees expressed interest in continuing to work with ethnic groups when they finished their training.

Follow-Up

We contacted the trainees two years after the Program was completed. We gathered anecdotal reports from them, principally in the form of letters, as to where they were functioning and whether their training with us was indeed relevant to the work they were doing. The responses were uniformly enthusiastic. While few were working exclusively in settings where ethnic populations were in the majority, all expressed the opinion that it was an invaluable experience in their individual work with clients. Those in private practice said that their conceptualizations of the problems presented to them by their clients was enhanced significantly by a cultural understanding of their cultural backgrounds.

For the year after the Program had been completed John Spiegel and John Papajohn continued an affiliation with the Department of Psychiatry at the Cambridge City Hospital. This involved working as the ethnic consultants on one of the "teams" serving different parts of the community mental health catchment area they were responsible for. This involvement made it possible to assess the impact, if any, we indeed had on one of the two systems we had worked in the previous three years. We came away from this with two main impressions—the first was that we had actually raised the consciousness of the general staff to the point where they would contact us when they had difficulty in either the differential diagnosis of or in treatment planning for an ethnic patient. Secondly, there was no real interest in modifying the traditional training format to include an ethnocultural component in any systematic way.

Conclusion

This overview of the Brandeis-Harvard Training Program represents one model among many others for introducing cross-cultural concepts and techniques to mental health personnel for the more effective and appropriate delivery of services. At the time our Program was proposed (1976), we lacked pre-existing training models upon which we could build our procedure. Since then a variety of models, as represented by this publication, have been experimentally instituted and are just now reaching an increasingly interested audience through the published literature, rather than through word of mouth or preliminary presentations at professional meetings.

As far as we can determine, these models vary along different dimensions, such as: (1) **intensity** — for example, one-to-three consciousness-raising presentations through six-week modules to year-long efforts, such as ours; (2) **ethnic focus** — for eample, one or two ethnic groups versus a broad range and diversity of ethnic populations; (3) **clinical setting** — from academic departments to free-standing service agencies; (4) **discipline** — primarily for psychiatrists, for psychologists, for psychiatric social workers, or some combination (such as ours) of all three; (5) **level of professional experience of trainees** — from pregraduate students through personnel with various degrees of established professional practice willing to be retained and retreaded for this new cultural emphasis; and, (6) **ethnic background of trainees** — from mainly mainstream WASP or Jewish to various minorities seeking to cross over to provide service to other minorities.

All such efforts, to our knowledge, are still in the experimental stages. Their long-term effects, both on trainees and on the institutional settings in which they take place, remain to be evaluated. We who are engaged in such efforts have much to learn from each other. It is our hope that this description of our Program, especially the delineation of its strengths and weaknesses, will contribute to the general pool of knowledge on which the future growth of the field will inevitably depend.

REFERENCES

Kluckhohn, F. & Strodtbeck, F. (1961). *Variations in value orientations.* Evanston, Ill: Row Peterson.

Papajohn, J. & Spiegel, J. P. (1975). *Transactions in families: A modern approach for resolving cultural and generational conflict.* San Francisco: Jossey-Bass.

CHAPTER 4

DEVELOPING INTERCULTURALLY SKILLED COUNSELORS: A PROTOTYPE FOR TRAINING

PAUL B. PEDERSEN

T HE INTERCULTURAL COUNSELOR is facing a modern dilemma where cultural influences of counseling and therapy are
widely recognized as important, but where the dangers of cultural en-
capsulation are more serious now than ever before in history. The National Institute of Mental Health (Fields 1979), the American
Psychological Association (Korman, 1974), and most other professional
mental health organizations have emphasized the urgent ethical responsibility of providers to know their client's cultural values before providing counseling or therapy to them. The Vail Conference (Korman,
1974) emphasized the importance of cross-cultural issues in the levels
and patterns of professional training in psychology. The Dulles Conference in 1978 urged counselors and therapists from minority backgrounds to cooperate in forming a Minority Affairs Office of the
American Psychological Association. As early as 1979 the APA accreditation criteria demanded cultural diversity among faculty and students
in APA approved programs of counseling and clinical psychology.

In spite of the many positive developments in cross-cultural training,
there are numerous indicators that more work is needed. First of all, racial and ethnic minorities are under-represented in clinical and counseling psychology as a profession. Second, this under-representation is
particularly true in applied and academic settings. Third, racial and
ethnic minority persons are most represented in the lower and less influential ranks. Finally, publications and professional presentations
about culturally different perspectives are seriously under-represented

in the primary professional journals as well as in the annual programs of the American Psychological Association (Pedersen & Inouye, 1984).

I. The Rationale for Cross-Cultural Training

Although there is an increased interest in cross-cultural training by counselors and therapists there are still very few comprehensive training programs available. Some universities such as Boston University, Columbia University, The University of Miami, Western Washington University and Syracuse University have begun to develop degree-oriented academic programs at the university level for careers in cross-cultural counseling and therapy. There are more than a dozen excellent textbooks on cross-cultural counseling and each year several hundred new articles are published on cross-cultural variables in counseling (Marsella & White, 1982; Pedersen, Sartorius & Marsella, 1985; Marsella & Pedersen, 1981; Sanders & Pedersen, 1985). Hollis and Wantz (1983) reviewed courses and programs on counseling in 1980 and 1983. In 1980 cross-cultural counseling ranked as the tenth most popular new course and the sixth most popular new course in 1983. By 1983 the number of program emphases in cross-cultural counseling ranked third in a list of twenty new areas of emphasis. By 1983 they identified 44 courses and 61 program emphases on cross-cultural counseling.

Most counselors with an interest in cross-cultural counseling have had to develop their own cross-cultural specialization from courses scattered throughout the curriculum. This dispersion of resources has resulted in several problems. (1) Many of these pre-service courses have emphasized the specialized perspective of one or another ethnic group in relation to the dominant culture. Consequently, there has been less emphasis on the skills required for working in a multi-cultural population where age, gender, lifestyle, socio-economic status **as well** as ethnicity and nationality may determine a person's cultural viewpoint. (2) Many in-service or pre-service courses have emphasized either awareness, knowledge or skill to the exclusion of the other two elements rather than balancing the emphasis of each component with the other two. (3) Many training programs emphasize one disciplinary viewpoint rather than the complimentary viewpoints of different disciplines viewing the same cultural issue. (4) Many training programs emphasize either classroom work or field experience with less involvement of resource persons from cultures being discussed and the cultural problems of field experience. Both the classroom and field work offer perspectives that complement one another in the development of interculturally skilled counselors.

We know that cultural background influences both the way counseling is given and how it is received, but there are extremely few opportunities for counselors to be trained in the specific skills of working with culturally different clients. There is rather a tendency to assume that clients and counselors share the same value assumptions unless there is convincing proof to the contrary. There is an assumption that we all agree on the same meaning for the constructs "healthy and normal" when, in fact, we may merely be reflecting our own political, social or economic values and culturally encapsulated counselors. (Pedersen, 1979, 1981b, 1983, 1985a).

There are several reasons why more cross-cultural training is needed for counselors and therapists. (1) Conventional descriptions of mental health in the textbooks and research literature reflect, to a greater or lesser extent, the cultural bias of a dominant (White, male, urban, young and affluent) cultural stereotype. This bias can easily be counterproductive in translating counseling and therapy to those cultures which do not share a dominant culture perspective. (2) Some cultural groups have developed their own endogenous "self-righting" approaches for promoting mental health without relying on exogenous "outside-the-system" resources. We need to know more about these strategies to supplement conventional counseling and therapy methods. (3) The failure of counseling and therapy in multicultural settings is both emotionally and financially expensive and in some cases appropriate training would prevent failure. (4) The constructs of healthy and normal which guide counselors and therapists are not the same for all cultures and need to be translated to be accurately applied. (5) There is a greater perceived need for reciprocity and interdependence across national, ethnic, and socio-cultural boundaries than previously. Cross-cultural training helps prepare counselors and therapists to understand the socio-political implications of counseling and therapy. (7) Finally, since most therapists come from dominant culture backgrounds and most clients do not share those assumptions, training provides a bridge of understanding from one cultural perspective to the other.

Research on counseling and therapy has failed to develop a comprehensive perspective based on empirical data for several reasons. First, the emphasis has been on abnormal behavior across cultures with less attention to normal behavior from each differing cultural perspective. Second, it is only since the late 1970s that a pancultural core has emerged for the more serious categories of disturbance, such as schizophrenia and affective psychoses (Draguns, 1980). Third, the complexity of re-

search on therapy across cultural lines is difficult to manage and is typically ignored in research on the counseling process (Draguns, 1981).
Fourth, the research which is available has lacked an applied emphasis
related to the practical concerns of program development, service delivery, and techniques of treatment. Fifth, there has been insufficient interdisciplinary collaboration from psychology, psychiatry, and
anthropology among the disciplines most directly related to counseling
and therapy. Sixth, research has emphasized the symptoms as a basic
variable while neglecting the complex interaction of persons, professional perspectives, institutions and community (Pedersen, 1982a).

The literature on how cultural values affect counseling and therapy
vividly describes the need for increased awareness of value assumptions
being made by culturally different clients and counselors. Culturally
biased counseling has resulted in low utilization rates for mental health
services now available and a shortage of coordinated training in cultural
sensitivity for mental health professionals across disciplines (Pedersen,
1981c, 1982b, 1985b).

The DISC Project as a Prototype

In response to the need for a training program to increase an emphasis on cross-cultural variables in the training of counselors and therapists, the National Institute of Mental Health funded a cross-cultural
training project called DISC (Developing Interculturally Skilled Counselors) from 1978 to 1981 in Hawaii. DISC was designed to develop the
previously mentioned priorities for cross-cultural counseling and
therapy. A review of these five DISC components will be useful as an il-
lustration of one attempt to develop the priorities for cross-cultural
training of counselors and therapists.

1. Graduate Seminars: Three graduate level seminars were taught
at the University of Hawaii for three credits each at least three times a
year. The introductory seminar on cross-cultural **awareness** included a
different guest lecture each session by culturally different mental health
service providers in the community. The seminar on cross-cultural psychopathology emphasized **knowledge** of cultural concepts and issues in
the research literature. The seminar on cross-cultural counseling emphasized interviewing **skills** and applications of awareness and knowledge. In addition to the University of Hawaii seminars a series of
DISC-sponsored seminars were also organized at California State University Hayward campus under the direction of Derald Sue, who was at

that time the Evaluator for the DISC project. These seminars combined elements of intercultural awareness, knowledge, and skill.

2. In-Service Training: International and intercultural workshops were designed to provide DISC trainees with practical experience in teaching others what they had learned. Agencies would request an in-service training team from DISC to organize workshops of one-half day to three days or longer in their international/intercultural location, including Samoa, Mexico, Micronesia, the Philippines, Canada, the U.S. mainland, and elsewhere in Hawaii. Some agencies also sent staff members to work with DISC in Hawaii and be trained as cross-cultural trainers. These trainers would then return to their home agency to organize their own training program. The in-service training seminars were useful in developing a network of cross-cultural counselors and therapists, to apply teachings from the pre-service classroom seminars, to disseminate training methods, and to generate additional funds for DISC activities so that DISC trainees could become experienced in teaching others what they had learned. There were 43 workshops conducted over the three years to 1,167 participants for a total time of 275 contact hours in sessions lasting from a half day to several days in length (Sue, 1979, 1981; Brough, 1981).

3. Annual Conference: DISC conferences were scheduled during the summers of 1979, 1980 and 1981 to exchange ideas, data and cross-cultural training methods with recognized leaders in cross-cultural counseling and therapy. Each conference developed its own special focus, with the first year conference emphasizing "Foundations," the second year emphasizing "Theoretical and Conceptual Definitions," and the third year emphasizing the "Research Base" of cross-cultural counseling and therapy. The Annual Conference was designed to become a window both for looking at what other colleagues in related disciplines were doing and for presenting preliminary ideas developed through DISC to the larger community of colleagues. The exchange of ideas in these DISC conferences resulted in three books, numerous articles and other teaching materials that have since been widely distributed (Pedersen, 1981e). A total of 62 international experts in cross-cultural counseling and therapy from the U.S. and other countries presented papers at DISC summer conferences and contributed to the three DISC books which were published.

4. Evaluation: The evaluation design for DISC included an assessment of the on-going activities and procedures of DISC (formative emphasis) as well as an evaluation of the intended outcomes of the program and the long-term impact of DISC on the professional community of counselors and therapists (summative emphasis). Within this conceptual umbrella five distinct evaluation activities were conducted including a daily evaluation of each seminar and classroom activity, separate assessments designed for each workshop, follow up interviews with DISC trainees who had completed the program, and annual exit interviews with all DISC trainees. These data describe DISC as having been very successful by all measures (Brough, 1981; Sue, 1979; Pedersen, 1981d).

Each session of each classroom seminar for the three years of DISC was evaluated on a six point scale with regard to helpfulness, interest, importance and usefulness. Over the three year period the 2,440 evaluations of the Awareness seminar averaged 5.37, the 888 evaluations of the Knowledge seminar averaged 5.68, and the 2,287 evaluations of the Skill seminar averaged 5.32 indicating a uniformly high self-reported evaluation.

5. DISC Trainees: Each year the eight pre-doctoral trainees were selected from nominations by departmental chairpersons at the University of Hawaii. The trainees were selected to represent a balance of gender, cultural background and academic training in fields such as psychology, anthropology, public health, education, communication and social work. Several externally funded pre-doctoral trainees and one externally funded post-doctoral trainee were also included in DISC project activities. Over the period of three years the assignment of responsibilities to DISC trainees became much more specific and structured as we learned how to match a trainer's background to the required tasks and were able to define required tasks more precisely.

In working with the trainees during the three years, several patterns emerged. First, candidates who appeared to be highly qualified in terms of their previous experience and responsibilities were not able to make as much progress in their traineeships as candidates who had less experience but demonstrated facility in interpersonal skills. Second, candidates who were more highly motivated to learn about cross-cultural issues from an interdisciplinary perspective worked out better than candidates who saw themselves more closely tied to a specific field or discipline. Third, candidates who had a lower need for structure worked out better than those who were rigid or had a higher need for structure. Fourth, when trainees were given significant roles where they could share leadership responsibilities in specific areas, they were much more likely to be satisfied than if they felt their own expertise was being overlooked or underutilized. Fifth, the extreme diversity of backgrounds by trainees almost inevitably resulted in some dissention among trainees. Sixth, each group of trainees tended to produce a cluster of three or four students for whom DISC had a higher priority than other aspects of their academic experience. Seventh, some of the trainees who were not intending to become counselors or therapists were able to apply significant skills from DISC to administrative and or educational objectives in terms of their future careers.

III. The Development of a Three-Stage Training Model

Although psychopathology is probably universal, with some special groups having a higher incidence than others, the ways the psychopathology is manifested are different from culture to culture and group to group (King, 1978; Strauss, 1979). There are several modes of therapy that are flexible enough to accommodate a client's world view more inclusively. The interculturally skilled counselor must be trained to integrate the culturally complex alternative perspectives of a client's environment. The DISC training project developed a three-stage cross-cultural training model which emphasized intercultural **awareness** (becoming more intentional in the awareness of one's assumptions), **knowledge** (managing the complex information of cultural perspectives more effectively), and **skill** (balancing the negative and positive variables appropriately in each culturally defined situation).

The goal of cross-cultural training is to increase a counselor's intentionality through increased awareness, knowledge, and skill in the cultural perspectives that control both a consumer's and a provider's behavior. Rather than allow decisions to be made "unintentionally" through disregard or neglect of culturally learned assumptions, cross-cultural training seeks to increase a person's intentional and purposive control over the assumptions that guide their behavior, attitudes, and insights. Training can accomplish this basic goal in two ways. First, training can increase awareness of one's own cultural biases and unexamined assumptions which determine, explain, and define normal behavior. Second, training can increase awareness of culturally different alternatives so that counselors can adapt their knowledge and skill to a variety of culturally different populations, enlarging their skill repertoire.

A report by the Education and Training Committee of Division 17, American Psychological Association, was endorsed identifying minimal cross-cultural compentencies for training counselors in their beliefs/ attitudes, knowledge, and skills (Sue, et al., 1982). There were four

awareness criteria of beliefs and attitudinal competencies: (1) the culturally skilled counseling psychologist is one who has moved from being culturally unaware to being aware and sensitive to his or her own cultural heritage and to valuing and respecting differences; (2) a culturally skilled counseling psychologist is aware of his or her own values and biases and how they may affect minority clients; (3) a culturally skilled counseling psychologist is one who is comfortable with differences that exist between the counselor and client in terms of race and beliefs; and (4) the culturally skilled counseling psychologist is sensitive to circumstances that may dictate referral of the minority client to a member of his or her own race or culture.

There were likewise four criteria of **knowledge** competency; (1) the culturally skilled counseling psychologist will have a good understanding of the sociological system's operation in the United States with respect to its treatment of minorities; (2) the culturally skilled counseling psychologist must possess specific knowledge and information about the particular group he or she is working with; (3) the culturally skilled counseling psychologist must have a clear and explicit knowledge and understanding of the generic characteristics of counseling and therapy; and (4) the culturally skilled counseling psychologist is aware of institutional barriers that prevent minorities from using mental health services.

The **skill** competencies are summarized in three principles: (1) the culturally skilled counseling psychologist must be able to generate a wide variety of verbal and nonverbal responses; (2) the culturally skilled counseling psychologist must be able to send and receive both verbal and nonverbal messages accurately and appropriately; and (3) the culturally skilled counseling psychologist is able to exercise institutional intervention skills on behalf of his or her client when appropriate. These concepts were developed from the baseline of existing data on intercultural training and follow naturally from the limited evidence presently available in an attempt to move beyond rhetorical support for intercultural awareness toward intercultural competence.

The available training approaches can be divided into those that emphasize culturally specific knowledge or skills related to the unique values of a particular culture or group, and those emphasizing culturally generalized aspects that would apply in any contrasting culture. While there is a quantity of materials that emphasize the guidelines for working within one or another cultural group (Pedersen, 1982a, 1984, 1985b), there are few approaches that successfully generalize from one culture to another.

Intercultural skill training approaches must be responsive to the variety of specific contrasting cultures where they are applied. To a large extent the benefit of training will be measured by its relevance to real-life situations in their complexity for their culture. The more action alternatives or strategies counselors possess, the more choices they have for dealing with the environment and the more flexibility they have for responding to culturally complex relationships.

IV. The Triad Model

A Triad Model for cross-cultural training has been developed by Pedersen (1981f, 1982a) that matches a therapist-trainee from one culture with a coached team of two other persons from a contrasting culture, one as a client and the other as an "anticounselor," for videotaping a simulated cross-cultural therapy session. The therapist seeks to build rapport with the culturally different coached client, while the anticounselor seeks to represent the negative elements of counseling from the client's cultural viewpoint. The anticounselor makes explicit the otherwise implicity resistance of culturally different clients. The Triad Model views counseling as a three-way interaction between the counselor, the client, and the anticounselor, where the counselor seeks to establish a temporary, means-oriented coalition with the client against the anticounselor.

Counseling occurs in a force field of push and pull factors in which the counselor seeks to be helpful, the client seeks to reconcile internalized ambiguity and the anticounselor seeks to continue the problem. In the mode of social power theory, counseling occurs in the context of an equilibrium between the counselor seeking coalition with the client against the assistance of a problem. Negotiating a coalition between the client and the counselor describes the task function of counseling in operational terms.

The Triad Model seems to work best when there is positive as well as negative feedback to the counselor from the client and resource persons during or after the simulated interview. For that reason, variations in roles for the client's partner have been developed in the roles of a "procounselor" and an "interpreter" as interchangeable with the anticounselor. The procounselor and interpreter roles are introduced to complement the anticounselor model in more comprehensive cross-cultural training programs. When the client-anticounselor team is highly motivated and feels strongly about the issue under discussion, and when the anticounselor has a high degree of empathy for and acceptance by the client, more relevant insights about intercultural counseling result. The anticounselor needs to provide direct, immediate, and articulate feedback to the trainee, with the client always being free to reject an inauthentic anticounselor. The simulated interview is spontaneous and not scripted. The selection and training of coached client/anticounselor teams are of primary importance. The teams should be as similar as possible, matching ethnicity, socioeconomic status, age, lifestyle, sex role, and other significant variables.

Research with pre-practicum counseling students at the University of Hawaii showed that students trained with the Triad Model achieved significantly higher scores on a multiple-choice test designed to measure counselor effectiveness, had lower levels of discrepancy between real and ideal self-descriptions as counselor, and chose greater numbers of positive adjectives in describing themselves as counselors than students who were not trained with the Triad Model. Students also showed significant gains on Carkhuff measures of empathy, respect, and congruence as well as on the seven-level Gordon scales measuring communication of affective meaning (Pedersen, Holwill & Shapiro, 1978). Bailey (1981) compared a traditional mode of teaching human-relations/intercultural skills with two modes using simulated interviews of two persons, as client and counselor in the first mode, and three persons, with a client, counselor, and an anticounselor in the second mode. She used Ivey's Counselor Effectiveness Scale, A Revised Truax Accurate Empathy scale, the Revised Budner Tolerance of Ambiguity scale as dependent measures. In a three-way analysis of covariance all tests were found significant between the lower scoring traditionally trained group and both high scoring treatment groups. No significant differences were found between the Triad and the dyad training groups on effectiveness, suggesting both approaches were equally effective but similarly superior to the traditional lecture method of intercultural training for counselors.

Hernandez and Kerr (1985) trained three groups of students using (1) a didactic mode, (2) a didactic plus role-play with feedback mode, and (3) a didactic plus triad training mode. After training, videotaped interviews by all students were scored by six professionals on the Global Rating Scale, the Counselor Rating Form-Short and the Cross Cultural Counseling Inventory. "The findings support experiential training and especially the continued use of Pedersen's Triad Model which is geared towards sensitizing and preparing counselors to work more effectively and efficiently with clients from diverse ethnic backgrounds" (p. 14). Niemeyer, Fukuyama, Bingham, Hall, and Mussenden (in press) compared the reactions of 20 counseling students who participated in either the "procounselor" or "anticounselor" conditions of Pedersen's Triad Model. Results indicated that participants in the more confrontive anticounselor version felt more confused and less competent than participants in the procounselor version but no differences in objective ratings of response effectiveness were noted, suggesting a differentiation between perceived expertness and actual effectiveness. Niemeyer et al. (in press) suggest that the more confrontive anticounselor model is better suited to more advanced students who have already developed some confidence for cross-cultural interactions, consistent with other research on the Triad Model (Sue, 1979; Ivey & Authier, 1978).

Derald Sue (1979) field-tested the anticounselor and procounselor training models with 36 counseling students at California State University, Hayward. Sue reported that students felt the anticounselor model was more effective than the procounselor model in achieving self-awareness, developing cultural sensitivity for contrasting cultural values, and for understanding political-social ramifications of cross-cultural counseling. The anticounselor model tended to be most effective for giving participants awareness of their cultural values and biases, obtaining cultural sensitivity to other ethnically defined groups, and helping them understand the political/social ramifications of counseling. The procounselor model was most effective in helping them obtain specific knowledge of the history, experiences, and cultural values of ethnic groups, and helping them develop cross-cultural counseling skills. Students were more comfortable with the procounselor model while the anticounselor model was more anxiety provoking. When asked to rate the most effective model for learning about cross-cultural counseling in the shortest period of time, however, the anticounselor model was seen as far superior. Confrontation by the anticounselor brought out issues of racism, bias, and conflicting values through immediate feedback to the counselor trainees, while the procounselor tended to facilitate acquisition of skills. While the anticounselor showed the mistakes, the procounselor helped remedy a counselor trainee's intercultural style. Ideally, a good training design would incorporate both an anticounselor and a procounselor.

Conclusion

The field of cross-cultural counseling may develop in two different directions. We may either develop a separate field or discipline of "cross cultural specialization" or we can document the importance of cultural perspectives to any and all definitions of competence in counseling and therapy. In either case we need to design better training in cross-cultural counseling and therapy. Such improved approaches would be characterized by several guidelines:

1. The training needs to involve a range of disciplines and professions. The boundaries of field and discipline are sometimes more tenacious than ethnicity or nationality in protecting "cultural" secrets. The selection of trainees, staff, participants, and issues would need to acknowledge a range of disciplinary perspectives related to counseling and therapy.
2. Grass root involvement by cross-cultural agencies in the community will be an important resource. Agencies which can become involved in the training can be approached early so that their specific endorsement of the project will be negotiated and their participation sought out before a proposal for specific training is submitted.
3. There is a demand for clear teaching materials on cross-cultural counseling and therapy. The balanced emphasis on awareness, knowledge, and skill demonstrated its value through the DISC Project and could become the prototype for subsequent educational curricula materials. In addition to written materials, other media could also be developed as educational resources.
4. Other agencies around the world who fund projects related to cross cultural counseling and therapy can be contracted so that a training project can coordinate its efforts with the resources of other agencies. This should be done on an international level to insure the culturally diverse perspective of cooperating institutions.
5. Numerous professional organizations of counselors and therapists have developed policy guidelines that recognize the importance of intercultural issues. The training will develop an active interest in bringing about specific policy changes in professional organizations based on verified data that would support the need for increased facilities to train interculturally skilled counselors and therapists.

When one reviews the field of counseling to discover what is "new" that has not been around for more than a decade it is difficult to identify very many original ideas. Perhaps one contribution of the last ten years to counseling has been a reevaluation of cultural variables. Many arguments can be presented for why we **should** be more responsive to the cultural values of a plural society (Pedersen & Marsella 1982) but the primary argument for cross cultural training is not based on idealism (Lee, 1979). The primary argument for intercultural training is to increase a therapist or counselor's accuracy and measured competence as a professional in all activities and with all populations. The adequately trained professional for the future will need an awareness of cultural bias, knowledge about cultural definitions of mental health and skill to implement these insights responsibly in our own multicultural world society.

REFERENCES

Bailey, F. M. (1981). *Cross-cultural counselor education: The impact of microcounseling paradigms and traditional classroom methods on counselor trainee effectiveness.* Unpublished doctoral dissertation, University of Hawaii, Honolulu.

Barnlund, D. C. *Public and private self in Japan and the United States: Communication styles in two cultures.* Tokyo: Simul Press.

Brough, J. (1981). *Evaluation report from DISC, 1979-1980.* Honolulu, NIMH Final Report (unpublished).

Draguns, J. G. (1980). Psychological disorders of clinical severity. In H. C. Triandis and J. G. Draguns (Eds.), *Handbook of cross-cultural psychology, Volume 6, Psychopathology* (pp. 99-174). Boston: Allyn & Bacon.

Draguns, J. G. (1981). Counseling across cultures: Common themes and distinct approaches. In P. Pedersen, J. G. Draguns, W. Lonner, and J. Trimble (Eds.). *Counseling across cultures; Expanded and revised edition* (pp. 3-21). Honolulu: University Press of Hawaii.

Fields, S. (1979). Mental health and the melting pot. *Innovations, 6*(2), 2-3

Goldstein, A. (1981). *Psychological skill training: The structured learning technique.* New York: Pergamon.

Halleck, S. L. (1971). *The politics of therapy.* New York: Harper & Row.

Hernandez, A. & Kerr, B. (1985). *Evaluating the triad model and traditional cross-cultural training.* Presentation at APA, Los Angeles, California, August.

Hollis, J. W. & Wantz, R. A. (1983). *Counselor preparation 1983-1985: Programs, personnel, trends* (5th edition). Munci, Indiana: Accelerated Development, Inc.

Ivey, A. (1980). *Counseling and psychotherapy: Connections and applications.* New York: Prentice-Hall.

Ivey, A. & Authier, J. (1978). *Microcounseling: Innovations in interviewing training.* Springfield, IL: Charles C Thomas.

Kagan, N. & McQuellon, R. (1981). Interpersonal process recall. In R. Corsini (Ed.), *Innovative psychotherapies* (pp. 443-459). New York: Wiley-Interscience.

King, L. M. (1978). Social and cultural influences on psychopathology. *Annual Review of Psychology, 29,* 405-433.

Korman, M. (1974). National conference on levels and patterns of professional training in psychology: Major themes. *American Psychologist, 29,* 441-449.

Lee, L. (1979). Is social competence independent of cultural context? *American Psychologist, 34,* 795-796.

Marsella, A. & Pedersen, P. (Eds.). (1981). *Cross-cultural counseling and psychotherapy.* Elmsford, NY: Pergamon.

Marsella, A. & White, G. (Eds.). (1982). *Cultural conceptions of mental health and therapy.* Hingham, MA: Reidel.

Neimeyer, G. J., Fukuyama, M. A., Bingham, R. P., Hall, L. E., & Mussenden, M. E. (in press). Training cross-cultural counselors: A comparison of the procounselor and anticounselor model. *Journal of Counseling and Development.*

Pande, S. K. (1968). The mystique of western psychotherapy: An eastern interpretation. *Journal of Nervous and Mental Disorders, 146,* 425-432.

Pedersen, P. (1979). Non-western psychology: The search for alternatives. In T. Marsella, R. Tharp, & C. Cibrowski (Eds.), *Perspectives on cross-cultural psychology* (pp. 77-98). New York: Academic Press.

Pedersen, P. (1981a). Alternative futures for cross-cultural counseling and psychotherapy. In A. Marsella & P. Pedersen (Eds.), *Cross-cultural counseling and psychotherapy* (pp. 312-337). Elmsford, NY: Pergamon.

Pedersen, P. (1981b). Cultural boundaries of education and non-western alternatives. *School Psychology International, 2,* 20-25.

Pedersen, P. (1981c). The cultural inclusiveness of counseling. In P. Pedersen, J. Draguns, W. Lonner, & J. Trimble (Eds.), *Counseling across cultures* (rev. & expanded ed.) (pp. 22-58). Honolulu: University Press of Hawaii.

Pedersen, P. (1981d). *Developing interculturally skilled counselors (DISC).* (Final Report to NIMH). Honolulu: University of Hawaii.

Pedersen, P. (1981e). International conferences: Significant measures of success. *International Journal of Intercultural Relations, 5,* 51-69.

Pedersen, P. (1981f). Triad counseling. In R. Corsini (Ed.), *Innovative psychotherapies* (pp. 840-854). New York: Wiley Interscience.

Pedersen, P. (1982a). Cross-cultural training for counselors and therapists. In E. Marshal & D. Kurtz (Eds.), *Interpersonal helping skills: Models and training methods* (pp. 238-283). New York: Jossey-Bass.

Pedersen, P. (1982b). The intercultural context of counseling. In A. Marsella & G. White (Eds.), *Cultural conceptions of mental health and therapy* (pp. 333-358). Hingham, MA: Reidel.

Pedersen, P. (1983). Asian theories of personality. In R. Corsini & A. Marsella (Eds.), Contemporary theories of personality (rev. ed.) (pp. 537-582). Itasca: Peacock.

Pedersen, P. (1984). Cross-cultural training of mental health professionals. In R. Brislin & D. Landis (Eds.), *Handbook of cross-cultural training: Volume 2. Methodology* (pp. 325-352). Elmsford, NY: Pergamon Press.

Pedersen, P. (1985a). Cross-cultural counseling: U.S. perspectives. In R. Samuda (Ed.), *Cross-cultural counseling: International perspectives* (pp. 71-82). Toronto: C. J. Hogrefe.

Pedersen, P. (1985b). *The handbook of cross-cultural counseling and therapy.* Westport, CT: Greenwood Press.

Pedersen, P., Draguns, J., Lonner, W., & Trimble, J. (Eds.). (1981). *Counseling across cultures* (rev. & expanded ed.). Honolulu: University Press of Hawaii.

Pedersen, P., Holwill, F., & Shapiro, J. (1978). A cross-cultural training procedure for classes in counselor education. *Counselor Education and Supervision, 17*(3), 233-237.

Pedersen, P., & Inouye, K. (1984). The international/intercultural dimension of the APA. *American Psychologist, 39*(5), 560-561.

Pedersen, P., & Marsella, A. (1982). The ethical crises for cross-cultural counseling and therapy. *Journal of Professional Psychology, 13*(4), 492-500.

Pedersen, P., Sartorius, N., & Marsella, A. (Eds.). (1985). *Cross-cultural mental health services.* Beverly Hills, CA: Sage.

Sanders, D., & Pedersen, P. (1985). *Implications of international welfare concerns for the future.* Honolulu: University Press of Hawaii.

Strauss, J. S. (1979). Social and cultural influences in psychopathology. *Annual Review of Psychology, 30,* 397-416.

Sue, D. W. (1979). *Annual evaluation report on developing interculturally skilled counselors.* NIMH training project. Honolulu, Hawaii (unpublished).

Sue, D. W. (1981). *Counseling the culturally different.* New York: Wiley.

Sue, D. W., Bernier, J. E., Durran, A., Feinberg, L., Pedersen, P., Smith, E. J., & Vasquez-Nuttall, E. (1982). Position paper. Cross cultural counseling competencies. *The Counseling Psychologist, 10*(2), 45-52.

Wohl, J. (1981). Intercultural psychotherapy: Issues, questions, and reflections. In P. Pedersen, J. Draguns, W. Lonner, & J. Trimble (Eds.), *Counseling across cultures* (rev. & expanded ed.) (pp. 133-159). Honolulu: University Press of Hawaii.

CHAPTER 5

THE CROSS-CULTURAL TRAINING INSTITUTE FOR MENTAL HEALTH PROFESSIONALS:* REEDUCATING PRACTITIONERS IN CULTURAL AND COMMUNITY PERSPECTIVES

HARRIET P. LEFLEY

THE UNIVERSITY OF MIAMI'S Cross-Cultural Training Institute for Mental Health Professionals (CCTI) began as a training and research project addressing a nationally mandated need for cultural responsiveness in mental health services. Previous chapters in this book have demonstrated the historical emergence of a nationwide network of mental health centers presumably geared toward serving previously unreached populations, and the subsequent inability of the existing system to provide cultural accessibility and acceptability to the target groups. Among these unserved populations, ethnic differences were only one aspect of institutional and conceptual barriers to treatment. Included also were issues relating to poverty, racism, social deprivation, migration, acculturation, and in some cases even illegal alien status. Thus, any approach to resolving cultural differences with clients from diverse groups necessarily involved assessment of a range of human needs, together with integration of case management functions with the purely psychological activities of counseling or psychotherapy. In short, what Schulberg (1977) has called a "community mental health ideology"—involving sociocultural as well as intrapsychic perspectives—was viewed as a necessary component of continuing professional education in culturally appropriate mental health care. This was the theoretical framework underlying the development of the CCTI format.

---

* This project was funded by N.I.M.H. Grant No. 5-T24-MH15429.

An integral component of the conceptual model for the training institute involved development of a comprehensive evaluation. The critical issue in all professional education is, of course, the transfer of training to practice. Any kind of professional training is geared to certain assumptions about time frames and types of learning required to produce a competent practitioner. In the present instance, the time frame was empirically derived from the realities of agency participation and the degree to which busy staff could be released from their functions. Nevertheless, the question remained whether, within the given time-limited curriculum, enough learning would take place so that transfer of training could actually be observed and measured in terms of more skillful performance of practitioners and greater responsiveness of patients. The research project developed for this purpose, and its findings, are presented in the following section on evaluation. In the present chapter, the salient evaluation questions are mentioned briefly in connection with the objectives; however, the major focus is on the conceptualization, history, curriculum development, and implementation of the project.

Developmental History of the Project

The CCTI evolved almost organically from a series of interrelated programs in the Department of Psychiatry of the University of Miami School of Medicine. Integrating research, service, and training initiatives, these programs have provided empirically-derived cultural input into a mental health system delivering multiple services to ethnically diverse clients. The process began over a decade ago when a comprehensive research effort entitled the Health Ecology Project was initiated by social anthropologist Hazel Hitson Weidman with the co-direction of Departmental Chairman James N. Sussex, a psychiatrist. Funded by the Commonwealth Fund of New York, the project investigated, in a federally designated poverty area of Miami, the health systems, beliefs, and behavior of five major ethnic groups: Bahamians, Cubans, Haitians, Puerto Ricans, and Southern U.S. Blacks. In this study of over 500 families (Weidman, 1978), preliminary findings indicated culturally-patterned differences in clustering of symptoms, culture bound syndromes with a large emotional component unrecognized by orthodox medical or mental health professionals (Lefley, 1979b; Weidman, 1979); and differences in conceptions of bodily functioning (Scott, 1974). Alternate healing modalities were widely used, often in conjunction with orthodox medical treatments. However, orthodox mental health treatment was almost never solicited, although sample health calendars and interview information indicated a high degree of emotional stress. Data on cultural variations in the distribution, and conceptualization of mental health problems subsequently became a valuable base for the development of a unique community mental health program designed to serve these populations.

In March 1974, the University of Miami-Jackson Memorial Hospital Community Mental Health Center (now New Horizons CMHC) was funded to serve inner-city Miami, an urban area rich in ethnic diversity, with almost 85% of the population of U.S. Black, Caribbean, Central or South American origin. The CMHC model began with two primary objectives: a) to provide fully accessible, culturally appropriate services which would encompass the full range of presenting complaints, and b) to alleviate environmental stressors by helping residents receive their fair share of adaptive resources. To this end, the program developed six teams of indigenous mental health workers for each of the major groups in the area: Anglo elderly, Bahamian, Cuban, Haitian, Puerto Rican and U.S. Black. A seventh team for black elderly was also added. Each team was led by a social scientist, typically at the Ph.D. level, and all staff, clinical, professional and paraprofessional, were as much as possible, of matching ethnicity to the populations served.

A network of neighborhood clinics was established in each of the ethnic communities. Social scientists and clinicians developed the role of "culture brokers"—a professional role in the health care delivery system first developed by Weidman (1983), involving a bridging, teaching, and training function at the interface of the hospital and community and within the two systems. Culture brokers, as faculty in the Department of Psychiatry, had a combination of academic, applied social scientist, and service provider roles. Hospital linkages facilitated an exchange of transcultural clinical information with a wide range of mental health practitioners.

Within the hospital system, the culture broker's role typically involved consultation and cultural interpretation. In educating mental health and medical staff about culturally appropriate care, the culture broker focused not only on beliefs and practices that may impinge on effective treatment, but also on adaptive strategies, strengths, and supports within the patient's cultural milieu. Concurrently, the culture broker facilitated understanding and utilization of services by the ethnically diverse patients within the context of their belief systems.

Within the community, the teams offered a wide range of decentralized services. Team functions, in addition to traditional chemotherapeutic and psychotherapeutic services, included neighborhood outreach programs; community based consultation and education; direct services in homes, schools, churches board and care homes, etc.; development of supportive networks; programmatic research; and community development. The teams initiated various projects to bring new resources into communities, conducted action research to provide consumer groups with appropriate supportive data for community-requested program, and helped residents learn how to utilize existing resources. Community outreach techniques became an integral aspect of delivery of culturally appropriate services. Program evaluation data subsequently demonstrated the efficacy of these approaches. Empirical data on minority utilization, no-show rates, dropout rates, and client satisfaction demonstrated that, when compared with normative or baseline data from other centers, the model had been successfully applied (Lefley & Bestman, 1984).

In the course of treating our multi-ethnic clientele in the hospital system and the mini-clinics; in ongoing supportive contacts and home visits with families; and in consultation and interventions in the schools, criminal justice system, and other community agencies, a body of information emerged relevant to the application of culturally appropriate care. This information was shared in clinical case conferences, lectures to psychiatric and medical personnel, occasional lectures to interested community groups, papers, and articles (See Bestman & Lefley, 1976; Bestman, Lefley & Scott, 1976; Lefley, 1979a). Additionally, as the research and direct service expertise of the program grew, staff were increasingly called upon as consultants in minority and cross-cultural affairs to a range of agencies and mental health facilities. The CCTI was developed as a mechanism to expand such consultation into a structured learning experience for providers needing cultural input for their staffs.

Rationale and Objectives

The major objective of the three year CCTI was to develop and investigate the effects of a program to provide mental health practitioners with a transcultural perspective and practical skills in serving clients from other cultures, including techniques for outreach and preventive efforts in different ethnic communities. Although the emphasis was on U.S. Black, Caribbean, and Hispanic populations, the training model was expected to be replicable in a variety of settings with a variety of cultural groups. The CCTI was directed toward mental health professionals currently working in clinical facilities serving low-income, ethnically diverse populations. Orientation toward practitioners rather than students was purposive, for two main reasons: the field's need for immediate application, and our need for reciprocal input. The rationale was to increase trainees' personal effectiveness and to provide them with the skills to return to their parent agencies or service networks to train other staff members and key caregivers in the community. In this relatively untapped area, however, we hoped not only to transmit our own insights and techniques developed in working with multi-cultural populations, but to amass insights from the trainees as well. In the investigation of problem areas; the collection of critical incidents of cultural misunderstanding derived from the trainees' own experiences; in exploration of ethnocentrism and the interaction of experiential distance with feelings and values; and in discussion of theoretical orientations and therapeutic techniques applied, modified, questioned, or discarded, we hoped to initiate a bilateral educational process which would open new directions for research and training in this area.

The CCTI thus had the following general goals: a) to provide mental health practitioners with a training experience that would facilitate or improve their work with people of cultures different from their own; b) to develop in trainees a transcultural perspective in the application of mental health skills generally; c) to develop a model for transmitting these transcultural mental health skills to other staff and service providers, and d) to develop and implement a design for evaluating the effects of this training model on cognitive/attitudinal change and therapeutic capability. In the long range, we also hoped to raise theoretical and empirical issues that may be heuristic in furthering new research ideas and/or helping to raise current levels of knowledge in the field. Specific aims of the training workshops were primarily focused on enhancing practical skills of mental health professionals in their therapeutic interactions with clients of other cultures. Involved were the following:

1. Sharpening **diagnostic** skills so as to maximize accurate interpretations of behavior, especially putative behavioral correlates of intrapsychic processes. This includes learning how to assess acceptable and deviant behavior in cultural context-i.e., to separate **normative** and **psychodynamic** properties. (What purpose does the behavior

serve? Is it adaptive/maladaptive in the culture? Is it within the boundaries of "normal"? Does the behavior connote what the practitioner thinks it connotes-whether in manifest or latent interpretation?) Improved diagnostic skills also involve acquisition of knowledge on cultural differences in test responses and normative psychological profiles.

2. Sharpening **therapeutic** skills through bridging the cognitive and social distance between practitioners and the populations they serve. This includes improving **interpretive** skills through providing information that will enable the therapist to better understand the conceptual framework of his client—relevant psycholinguistic referents, and the like. It also includes sharpening **interactional** skills in ways that will decrease patient suspicion and culturally-based resistance and increase the likelihood of cooperation in the therapeutic venture.

3. Sharpening culturally sensitive **administrative** skills that would generate procedures to increase sociocultural accessibility, acceptability, and effectiveness of services to multi-ethnic client populations.

The **measurable objectives** for which the evaluation was designed, included a number of variables anchored to baseline measures. For trainees, we anticipated significant increases in cultural knowledge, comprehension of cultural values, and therapeutic effectiveness, together with decreases in social, affective, and attitudinal distance from persons of other cultures. For clients and agencies, we predicted significant increase in minority utilization, reduction in client dropout rates, and spinoff effects among colleagues and other agency staff. The degree to which these objectives were attained is discussed in the following chapter on Evaluation.

Preparatory Phase

The preparatory phase consisted of two discrete components: (a) conducting a needs assessment and (b) preparing curriculum content.

Prior to the submission of the grant proposal, a letter had been mailed to a random sample of 120 psychiatric hospitals, CMHCs and other mental health facilities describing our intention of developing a CCTI. Attached was a brief questionnaire soliciting interest in participation, nominal reimbursement needs, optimal time frame, ethnic groups of interest to the agency, and the like. The format of the CCTI was developed based on these responses. Time away from work and reimbursement needs are of critical interest to agencies sending practitioners, and these logistical decisions may well determine who attends, benefits from, relays, and implements the training.

Based on the needs assessment, it was determined that eight-day intensive training workshops were the optimal time frame. These would be held four times during the year for approximately 24 participants each, a number considered maximal for the intensive group experiences planned. Because agencies considered this training necessary for high quality culturally appropriate service provision to clients, but varied in their financial ability to send candidates, it was determined that costs would be reimbursable. This permitted selection of participants who were not only highly motivated, but in the best position to utilize and disseminate the information learned.

The second stage of preparation involved curriculum development. During the years prior to the commencement of the CCTI project, the culture broker team leaders of the CMHC had participated in a series of bi-weekly meetings in which they shared knowledge of their respective cultures, discussing significant common and divergent dimensions. Examples of topics under study were cultural history, family structure, and supernatural belief systems as alternate healing modalities. This study group existed in the CMHC structure as a vehicle for augmenting the team leaders' effectiveness in their roles as culture brokers between the ethnic communities and the orthodox mental health care system. The format was as follows: one team leader took responsibility for a prepared presentation while the other leaders prepared themselves for the discussion by reading social science literature on the topic.

In addition, as was customary within the CMHC, both clinicians and team leaders collected "critical incidents" for each local ethnic population. There was also continued recording of cases for which CMHC staff were asked to serve as cultural consultants to other mental health professionals. While this collection of critical incidents and consultation cases was performed in large part to meet the Consultation and Education needs of the CMHC staff (e.g., consultation of specific cases within the Mental Health Institute and Veterans Administration Hospital; Grand Rounds presentations to the Department of Psychiatry faculty; lectures to medical students, nurses, and residents), it served as a useful tool in the development of the curriculum as it pertained to selection of case material for practical illustrations.

A curriculum committee was established as the natural extension of these activities. This working group was entrusted with the design and development of curriculum content and methodology, and subsequent modifications as determined by trainees' group characteristics, evaluations and post-mortems at the closing of each Institute.

The Participants

Trainee Selection and Recruitment

Recruitment was done primarily through dissemination of a brochure to the agencies who had indicated an interest in the needs assessment, together with a selection of clinical facilities located in areas with ethnically diverse clienteles. Target facilities were primarily psychiatric hospitals, CMHCs, and other public and private mental health centers. Because of the importance of cross-cultural training to the field, DHEW (now DHHS) regional offices sent letters supporting the CCTI and encouraging facilities to send their staff. Subsequent distribution of brochures occurred through mailings and distributions at professional meetings and similar events attended by CCTI staff or consultants. Advertising was done only for the final workshop which was self-selective. Initially limited to the Southeast (Region IV), the CCTI subsequently was extended to include interested participants from all over the United States.

Selection of trainees was based on two major criteria. Preference was given to candidates from agencies which (a) served catchment areas with sizeable numbers of Black, Hispanic, or other ethnic populations, and (b) were willing to release at least two participants at the same time, preferably an administrator as well as direct service staff. The latter criterion was critical. Knowing the resistance which one lone change agent is likely to face within an organization, we were interested in training those who were in a position to provide administrative as well as professional support for the sharing of workshop knowledge, spinoff of cross-cultural training efforts, and agency-wide changes. An additional consideration was that, given satisfaction of the above criteria, we wanted to include as many minority participants as feasible. This was based on three factors. First, many individuals feel the need for formal training in their own ethnic history and culture, particularly with respect to different sub-cultural or SES groups. Second, professionals from one minority culture can obviously benefit from cultural information about other minority groups. Finally, it was believed that minority participants would function as motivators and catalysts to get new progress off the ground in their home agencies. It also turned out empirically that minority participants were also extremely helpful as expert consultants, adding their own personal and clinical experiences to the group discussions.

Additional factors in trainee selection included discipline or function, geographic locale, and type of agency, in order to ensure a broad and representative range of service providers and a high level of group process. Roommates were placed together not only on the basis of same sex, but on the basis of different functions as mental health professionals. The housing design—having all trainees stay at the same hotel with roommates preselected for divergent occupational and institutional characteristics—was also part of the training process. The plan was to provide opportunity for optimal after-hours interaction, information exchange, and processing by people representing a variety of professional experiences in the mental health field. Thus, the eight-day workshop would become a total, around the clock experience.

For each Institute, a grid was constructed containing all of the pertinent information of each applicant to facilitate the selection process. A staff team approach was followed in all selection processes resulting in the acceptance of twenty-four trainees and a list of alternates for taking care of last minute cancellations. Names of alternates not utilized became priority candidates for the following Institute.

Trainee and Agency Characteristics

In all, 174 trainees participated in seven workshops (six eight-day sessions and a final four-day session). Participants included 78 males (45%), 96 females (55%), with a median age of 35.6 years. Ethnic distribution as follows: Hispanic, 11%; Black, 35%; Non-Latin White, 52%, Asian/American Indian, 2%.

It is felt that trainees represented a good balance of mental health core disciplines (with the predictable exception of psychiatry). Eighty-one or 47% of the trainees had administrative functions. Of these, 54 or 31% were either exclusively or primarily administrative. The fact that almost one-half had administrative functions was favorable to the likelihood of implementation of the action plans which were an integral component of the workshops.

A total of 97 separate agencies or institutions sent participants to the workshops, and of these 56 (58%) sent administrators. Among the 82 facilities exclusively involved in mental health service delivery, 53 (65%) sent administrators. Twenty-two states were represented, including almost all regions of the United States.

Table 1

CHARACTERISTICS OF TRAINEES BY DISCIPLINE AND OCCUPATIONS

Discipline (by terminal degree)	N (174)	Percent
Clinical Social Work	46	26
Psychology	40	23
Psychiatric Nursing	30	17
Counseling & Guidance	30	17
Psychiatry	2	1
Other*	26	15

Occupations		
Executive Directors	15	9
Other Administrators	25	14
Administrators with Secondary Clinical Role	14	8
Clinicians	72	41
Clinicians with Secondary Administrative Role	27	16
Educators	15	9
Researchers	6	3

*Includes Divinity, Occupational Therapy, Rehabilitation Therapy, Anthropology, Sociology, Human Resources, Corrections, and Business Administration.

Table 2

TYPES OF PARTICIPATING AGENCIES

Types of Agencies	N
Mental Health Service Providers; Hospitals, Clinics, CMHCs, Social Service Agencies With Mental Health Components and Government Bodies Delivering Services	82
Colleges and Universities, Including Museum and University Training Facilities	11
Private Practice	1
State Federal Government Bodies With Administrative Function Only	3
	N = 97

Training Faculty

Trainers for the CCTI represented an unusually rich combination of academicians, clinicans, folk healers, community aides, and various consultants.

The disciplines represented included: clinical, counseling, social, and educational psychology; medical/psychiatric anthropology; clinical social work; nursing; psychiatry; political science; sociology; communications; and cultural history. For the most part, training was administered by mental health professionals and/or social scientists, mostly Black or Hispanic, who were Department of Psychiatry faculty and staff of the University of Miami-Jackson Memorial Community Mental Health Center, now New Horizons CMHC. Although these were the major resources for the didactic lecture materials and group facilitation, the community was drawn upon for: (a) lecturers from local colleges who were experts in various aspects of Black or Hispanic culture; (b) local folk healers; (c) group leaders for community experiences — trained individuals highly familiar with their communities and with open access to neighborhood congregation sites typically closed to outsiders; (d) ministers and church attendants, who interacted with trainee-visitors and responded to their questions; (e) families of clients, who shared their homes and concerns with trainees; (f) ethnic community team personnel, who shared caseload materials and other relevant characteristics; (g) restaurant owners who prepared special ethnic meals (Haitian, Cuban, "soul food," and Bahamian) for the trainees and responded to many questions about eating preferences and cultural interactions; (h) people in the community who interacted with trainees as key informants about their local cultures.

The training took place in multiethnic catchment area IV of Miami, where most of the population is Black (Afro-American and Afro-Caribbean) and/or Spanish-speaking, with heavy representation from the Caribbean and Central and South America. This service area of the New Horizons CMHC also includes the University of Miami-Jackson Memorial Medical Center, focus of a large medical complex and civic center. The Medical Center provided classroom meeting space and trainees visited some of the ambulatory care facilities of the large county-teaching hospital. However, as indicated, much of the training took place in the community — at the various ethnic mini-clinics of the CMHC, in churches, neighborhood restaurants, and in the street experiences described more fully in the curriculum section.

Curriculum

Content and Methods

While our training focus was on transmitting practical knowledge and skills for immediate application in the therapeutic endeavor, one of our primary objectives was to develop a transcultural perspective to enable generalization of skills across a variety of target populations. For this reason, we utilized a categorical approach in applying the knowledge base gained through the CMHC experience with our Miami cultural groups, despite the fact that they may not necessarily have been among those served by all or even most of the trainees. Our premise was that the comparative examination of cognitive systems, value orientations, interpersonal roles, and other cultural dimensions in a transcultural context would facilitate the development of a mode of critical perception which may question the "universality" of some commonly held psychiatric beliefs and enable the trainees to seek alternate interpretations of behavior and more appropriate therapeutic interventions.

The core curriculum was based on four basic training modalities which merged didactic, transactional, experiential, and cultural immersion techniques, as well as goal-oriented planning for future applications.

Didactic materials include overviews of culture and mental health in individual, national, and global perspective. Beginning with culture and self-cultural awareness, trainees were introduced to unconsciously ethnocentric modes of thought and perception which are a function of every enculturation process, and which carry over into the therapeutic enterprise. Materials on culture and mental health gave a developmental overview of the field, with a focus on cultural perceptions of mental illness, epidemiology, symptomatology and diagnosis, communications, and therapeutic transactions. Focusing on culture and mental health in historical perspective, lecture topics included: religion, world view and value systems, family structure and relationships, sex roles, cognitive systems, supernatural beliefs, and alternate healing modalities. Within these contexts, normative behavior, life styles, stressors, coping mechanisms, and support systems were discussed. The interrelationships of ethnic minority status, interracial/intercultural communication and mental health were explored. Lectures also included presentations on community involvement in needs assessment, defining mental health needs, and participation in the planning process for effective service delivery. **Cultural immersion** utilized throughout the CCTI, included systematic participant observation in street and church experiences, visits to ethnic community clinics, and occasionally visits to clients' homes, with group processing of reactions. **Practicum** experiences in the classroom included videotape observation, role-playing and simulation of therapeutic encounters with clients/families of contrasting cultures, utilizing Pedersen's coalition training and similar models. With mandatory **Action Plan development,** participants ended their training by drawing up plans to facilitate transfer of training, with preoperationalized objectives at five levels of predicted attainment. Follow-up and technical assistance strategies, including visits to home agencies by CCTI staff, were also part of the training model.

SAMPLE OF WORKSHOP CURRICULUM COMPONENTS

Culture and Self-Cultural Awareness
Culture and Mental Health/Psychopathology
Group Building
Community Experience: Participant Observation
Church Experience: Religion and Mental Health
Visits with Ethnic Clients in Their Homes
Overview of New World Black/Hispanic Experience
An Approach to Integrating Cultural Experience With Mental Health Service
  Delivery
Family Structure and Relationships
Age and Sex Roles
Support Systems
Ethnic Minority Status
World View and Value Systems
Supernatural Belief Systems
Alternate Healing Practices: Ritual Healing in Operation
Interracial/Intercultural Communication
Visits to Ethnic Community Clinics
Practicum in Interviewing and Counseling Skills
Coalition Training Model
Community Involvement and Outreach
Development of Action Plans

Each institute began formally on a Saturday (after a brief Friday evening get-together) with extensive pretesting and an introductory lecture on culture and self-cultural awareness. This was followed by group-building, an initial curriculum component performed before trainees paired off for the community experience. Logistically, Saturday night offered the best opportunity for community observations, and Sunday for the church visits. Thus, the weekend involved a didactic introduction, followed by cultural immersion. The group-building facilitated subsequent discussion and interaction through trainee introductions, expressions of the interests and problems that brought them to CCTI, expectations, disciplinary interests, and agency concerns. If time permitted, this exchange of information was combined with a simulation game which facilitated processing participants' fantasies regarding what they would gain from the CCTI experience.

Cross-cultural experiences in the community included various types of activities, extending throughout the week. Trainees were given orientations, including demographic data, and guidelines for systematic observation of various structural and interactional variables within these communities. The Saturday night experience typically paired three trainees with a community field guide in a visit to an ethnic neighborhood. There were six to ten community experiences per Institute, varied by ethnicity and type of settlement area. For example, the Black neighborhood experiences focused on different types of inner-city areas; an old Bahamian settlement, and a middle-class Black area in contrast with one dominated by a low-income housing project. Similarly, the Hispanic experiences included Cuban, Puerto Rican, and Mexican migrant neighborhoods, while the Haitian experience showed three different settlement areas in interaction with prior resident populations. The experiences were changed and processed during a wrap up session following the street visits, always relating the observations to clinical practice.

Sunday involved a different type of cultural immersion experience in Cuban, Puerto Rican, Bahamian, Haitian, and Black-American churches. An integrative introduction to religion and mental health focused on the structural supportive role of the church, as well as the cognitive and affective aspects of the religious experience, within these communities. After attendance, again conducted in small groups with leaders, the processing invariably elicited recognition on the part of the trainees of the counseling and supportive functions fulfilled by the church in various ethnic communities, especially if we had been able to arrange a discussion with the pastor following the service. There was also recognition of the compelling and central role both of religious belief and of church affiliation as sources of strength and adaptive coping in the Black community. The importance of outreach and linkages with key religious figures in the community was also highlighted for referral, advisory, and community feedback purposes.

In some early institutes, there were visits with clients in their homes in order to introduce participants to cultural differences in family life-styles, patterns of communication, household density, and psychosocial dynamics. A major objective was to have trainees share the living environment of an inner-city family and become aware of stressors and coping mechanisms used by families in dealing with their social milieu. These visits were ultimately discontinued because the time allotted was too brief for any adequate learning to take place, and sometimes resulted in undue burden on the families. However, the module is still considered a desirable learning experience in the event that adequate time is permitted and resources are available for follow-up work with the families.

The didactic sessions usually began with a lecture on culture and mental health, with an overview of how cultural differences affect the following domains: perceptions of mental disorder; utilization rates; epidemiology; symptomatology and diagnosis in relation to a) observation of behavior and b) responses to screening instruments; communication barriers; patient-therapist interaction; and therapeutic strategies and objectives.

The didactic components of the weekday curriculum, which focused on historical and contemporary perspectives in the New World Black and Hispanic experience and their relationship to mental health service delivery, were interspersed with the learning of practical techniques. An all day practicum involved small group case simulations, with trainees role-playing clients, therapists, and family members, as members of their own and contrast cultures.

Cross-cultural experiences in the classroom utilized Pedersen's (1981) coalition training model, together with a number of exercises in recognizing conceptual boundaries, power relationships, and other variables of importance in therapeutic encounters with clients from another cultural group. In some of these exercises, CMHC staff participated, along with trainees, in bringing particular cases that highlighted cultural differences to the attention of participants. Many trainees cast in the unfamiliar role-simulation of a client or therapist from another culture, or of a third figure giving interpretation or feedback through a cultural filter, reported that for the first time they experienced their own culture-bound values in interpreting someone else's behavior, and were able to empathize at the cultural as well as (and therefore more fully) at the interpersonal level with the other culture role they were simulating.

This was followed by visits to the Community Mental Health Center's ethnic neighborhood clinics, involving discussion and exchange with clinical staff actively serving diverse ethnic caseloads. A long session on supernatural beliefs and alternative healing systems included an overview of the history and functional aspects of **Santeria, Espiritismo,** Root Medicine, and Haitian **Vodou.** Healing systems in operation described the use of alternative healing modalities by some of our own mental health staff, in cases where a client could not otherwise be helped because he believed he had been "rooted," "hexed," or had displeased the spirits. A **Santeria** demonstrated plants and herbs, read the cowrie shells for some of the trainees, and performed cleansing rites for those whose problems became manifest from the readings. Many of the trainees were astonished when the **Santeria** related what seemed to be factual or psychological truths, apparently based on a codified interpretive system (how the shells were thrown) rather than on intuition alone. Some professionals continue to maintain contact with her for ongoing consultation.

Finally, there was a module on community outreach and involvement techniques. This component focused on techniques for community entry, involvement of community leadership in identifying needs, participation on Advisory or Governance Boards and in publicization of services, as well as on recruitment of minority staff. The CMHC's experience in needs assessment, developing community profiles, ethnographies, etc. provided the empirical base for this module. This component also gave rise to the final module, Development of Action Plans, which involved having trainees actually operationalize transfer of training. Action plans were developed along various parameters, most of them involving special agency projects to increase cultural sensitivity. These were set up on a Kiresuk Goal-Attainment Scaling grid at five levels of expected attainment, with a specified time frame for assessment (see Kiresuk & Sherman, 1968).

In addition to the scheduled workshop sessions, trainees sometimes asked for special interest meetings with selected presenters or consultants. All of these requests were honored. Trainees met to discuss "Black language" with the presenter on communication styles. Other presenters who were unable to accommodate all the questions asked similarly agreed to meet with interested persons to pursue sub-topics. Special modules added in the final workshop, some of which are elaborated on in this book, included Child Psychiatry in Cross-Cultural Perspectives, Ethnic Value-Orientations, Bi-Cultural Effectiveness Training, and Attaining the Transcultural Perspective.

Workshop Evaluation: Use of Feedback

Each core component of the curriculum had a printed rationale and objectives. The latter were incorporated in a cognitive test, and were also used by trainees as criteria for daily and overall evaluation of workshops. On a five point Likert scale, each module was rated on four dimensions: (a) interest of topic; (b) quality of presentation; (c) usefulness in own work, and (d) assessment of general importance in training. On the final day, an overall evaluation form was completed requesting feedback on most/least valuable topics and experiences, identification of additional issues that should have been addressed, and suggested changes in workshops. Responses were then categorized and rank-ordered in terms of frequency. These, together with the copious comments on the daily modules, became the basis for ongoing refinement of the curriculum. A third mode of evaluation feedback, which was not pre-planned, was a series of unsolicited letters attesting to the value of the CCTI for the individual trainee, and citing his or her applications of the materials learned.

Almost all trainee suggestions that could be implemented were incorporated in current or forthcoming workshops. There were special sessions on funding sources for minority programs. When time was lacking, luncheon meetings were held with CMHC division Directors on consultation and education, administration, and research and evaluation. There were also meetings on discrete aspects of Cuban and Haitian culture, a special session on American Indians, and several presentations on organizing the elderly into self-help groups.

Long-Range Subjective Evaluation

Although the forthcoming chapter focuses on the long-range objective effects of the training, the continuity of short-term workshop evaluation and long-term evaluation of personal impact is of interest here. Part of the follow-up procedure requested assessment of the impact of the CCTI on participants' thinking and practice. Participants responded to the query from six months to two years following CCTI participation. There were four questions:

In what way has your CCTI experience affected the following areas?
1. Your work as a clinician and/or administrator?
2. Your self-concept as: a) a person; b) a member of your own culture; c) a mental health professional?
3. Your thinking about your own professional education?

4. Your view of what constitutes good mental health care?

Among the clinicians sampled, there was a 63% return rate. However, a substantial number had moved on from their agencies, in accord with the usual mental health turnover, and inquiries were often not forwarded. The actual return rate of available respondents was estimated at 70-75%.

Almost all responses to all items were positive. Six percent reported "no change" in the area of self-concept as a person, and 2% in their view of what constitutes good mental health care. Otherwise, in all other areas, trainees reported a positive change.

Responses were categorized in terms of their dominant themes. Because the richness of content cannot be captured by the quantified categories, brief verbatim samples are given below. The quotations are selected not for adulatory content, but rather for indicating a range of attitudinal and behavioral changes in clinicians, as well as structural changes implemented by administrators as a result of cross-cultural training. Many of the comments indicate a re-shaping of administrative policy with respect to specific types of service provision, as well as a new attitude toward minority issues reflective of personal sensitivity rather than expedient adherence to federal guidelines.

Of great interest also are the large number of responses, only hinted at here, which stated that the trainee had previously considered herself/himself an unprejudiced and culturally sensitive person, and for the first time was exposed to unseen biases in attitude and conceptualization which may have been barriers to effective treatment.

1. Impact On Own Work

A. Impact on Work as Clinician

"I have become more comfortable working with minority clients. I can ask them about their feelings about racial issues in their own personal life. I am more open discussing their feelings about talking with a white therapist. I am somewhat more tolerant of missed appointments and late arrivals now that I understand the cultural context of these behaviors. I am more open to using alternative forms of treatment."

"My therapeutic stance now allows for cultural differences to emerge without being defined as 'pathologically' different."

"More aware of my own 'differentness' to the client. . .more willing to work within someone else's framework, less demanding that they work within mine."

"My work as a clinician has changed as a result of the CCTI training experience of myself and our administrative staff, in that we all provide more linkage/brokerage services to our clients so that exacerbating stresses are reduced, thereby resulting in our clients being in more control of vital resources and rising in their functional level. I also provide more services in the field, including support, brokerages with landlords, transportation to hospitals, and promoting peer support networks in apartment complexes."

"It has taught me to be more aware of all subgroups—people in wheelchairs as well as of other races. . ."

B. Impact on Work as Administrator

"The training has enabled this agency to participate in cross-cultural training with other significant agencies, such as the police department, and the community college. It has also formed the structural basis for presenting community cross-cultural workshops for professional staff."

"[The CCTI] helped in development of decentralized service delivery." (Executive Director who decentralized his CMHC after attending CCTI.)

"Since several top administrators attended CCTI much of the flavor of our present direction in services delivery appears to show some influence from the Miami experience. For example. . .inservice areas where significant concentrations of a particular culture group reside (such as Indochinese refugees) will have a direct influence on staffing patterns. The employ of a worker with the ability to serve as a culture broker would seem quite likely."

"The model posed at CCTI was a particularly helpful one for use since we were able to establish an outpost for our Native American Unit after we returned for CCTI. . .Because of the cutback in funding for FY '83 we seriously have considered closing one or more outposts for fiscal reasons. I am sure that my attendance at CCTI has significantly had an impact on our final decision, which was not to close any outposts and make fiscal cutbacks in other areas. . .I regret that more people have not been exposed to the CCTI model because the learning there was quite powerful and reinforced our own beliefs that decentralization, especially in urban populations that are highly diverse, is a very positive way to offer mental health services." (Executive Director of CMHC).

"As an administrator, I feel responsible for taking the initiative to identify problems and plan for solutions re: mental health service delivery to Blacks. Prior to CCTI, this task I had viewed as necessary to stay within Federal regulations. The percentages of Black clients served and Black staff employed were within an acceptable non-discriminatory range. After CCTI, my perspective changed. I do not think this center will be fulfilling its purpose unless attention is given to the areas of under-served Blacks."

"As an administrator, I am more aware of how to utilize the social network in the minority culture to make services more available and acceptable to minorities."

2. Self-Concept

A. Self-Concept as a Person and Member of Own Culture

"Surprisingly to myself, I became more aware of my own motivations and drives. I believe I learned as much about the influence of my culture on me as I did about other cultures."

"I take more pride in my own culture and background. I feel less alienated from my past."

"The CCTI experience has affected my self concept in terms of my own cultural awareness more than any other specific area. . .It has given me insight into my own belief system, which in turn has aided me in understanding others. In this way, it affected my role as a mental health counselor in a positive way, and in addition, I feel my self-concept as an individual has been enhanced by the experience."

"My self-concept as a person has changed since I realized my liberal 'color blindness' reflected good will but a lot of fear and ignorance too. In the year since CCTI I have come to know some friends and colleagues in a much fuller, honest way and have begun new friendships with culturally diverse people. This is a source of good feelings. . ."

B. Self-Concept as Mental Health Professional

"I have become aware that mental health professionals have their own culture of what is 'good mental health,'—which may be contrary to another culture's concepts."

"In general, my sense of professional competency has increased as a result of having obtained a wider scope and appreciation of cultural diversity. CCTI has sharpened my responding to the needs of the client **where he is**—from his own framework."

"My self-concept as a mental health professional has changed considerably, as I have engaged more activist outreach activities. . .I began to reorient my role concept to that of an experienced mental health professional who does what needs to be done to help clients prosper, rather than a system-oriented clinical psychologist."

3. Thinking About Professional Education

"My professional education. . .did not touch on issues of race or even class distinction as relevant to the counseling process. CCTI was invaluable to me. Continuing education should be part of any professional degree and cross-cultural training without a doubt needs to be included."

"After attending CCTI, it has expanded my scope as a person and as a professional. As a result, I realize my professional education has been valuable but I can now see there is a different need, to understand the external environmental forces better and how they affect. . .the clientele I work with. I intend to get involved with continuing education. . .which will build upon the knowledge obtained by attending this CCTI."

"My own education in social work school was limited to exploring institutional racism, but did not adequately address the need for cross-cultural issues to be considered in planning good sound mental health care. Our current action plan (seminar of Black Culture in America), is allowing other staff to consider these issues and begin to incorporate the ideas into their practice. Without the CCTI training, our hospital staff would never have been confronted with considering these things."

"My professional education had some breadth in that I have been exposed to traditional psychodynamic and new personalistic approaches to treatment by double majoring in Personality and Clinical Psychology, minoring in Experimental Psychology, working with a community psychologist for two years, in a counseling center for five years, and now in a CMHC for four years. CCTI has served to emphasize the need for more knowledge, both theoretical and applied, from the field of cultural anthropology, social services, and community organization. . .Lacking this, our staff try to include cultural issues in our intervention planning at staffings (after CCTI)."

4. What Constitutes Good Mental Health Care

"In order to provide good mental health care, practitioners should be broad in their perceptions, knowledgeable of social forces that affect people's behavior, knowledgeable of the inherent hostility which is reflected in our socialization process toward minority groups. Keeping this generic base in mind, a mental health practitioner needs to not only focus on the individual, but also consider the social context and pull from the community resources other support systems which, if coordinated properly, can offer the client a more comprehensive treatment modality."

"Truly starting where the individual is and then considering him in total — physically, mentally, spiritually, culturally, etc. Then applying treatment that truly meets the client's needs — not necessarily the Rx that the staff knows best or is most comfortable with."

"The CCTI experience enabled me to recognize that good mental health care is not necessarily 'traditional' services. Presently, I realize that environmental intervention and use of natural support systems may have more value in dealing with many clients. I have been able to transfer some of the philosophy of 'cross-cultural training' to rural, lower SES Whites and different age groups."

"Prevention strategies within the community, quality of care issues in agency settings, expertise of the mental health professionals rendering services. . .[CCTI provided] excellent professional education, addressing significant issues in patient care."

"Good mental health care. . .provides an intervention which helps increase a client's functional level. CCTI has helped me understand better that many interventions will fail if they are not developed with an awareness of the cultural acceptability of them as well as the client's functional level. CCTI also helped me realize the impact of basic economics on client functioning. . .[and] pernicious effects of institutional and personal discrimination on our clients. CCTI has reinforced my belief that community/neighborhood care results in better network building."

These responses are not considered solely evaluative of the CCTI program; they are more probably reflective of the changes in values and conceptualization that are a function of the transcultural learning experience in any program, together with the added skill-building that enhances self-confidence as a clinician and service provider. The carryover of this subjective impact into practice is the topic of Chapter 14.

REFERENCES

Bestman, E. W. and Lefley, H. P. (1976). Treatment of Caribbean patients in Miami. Paper presented at the First Annual Meeting of the Association of Caribbean Psychologists, Port-au-Prince, Haiti, August.

Bestman, E. W., Lefley, H. P. and Scott C. S. (1976). Culturally appropriate interventions; Paradigms and pitfalls. Paper presented at the 53rd annual meeting of the American Orthopsychiatric Association, Atlanta, Georgia, March.

Kiresuk, T. J. and Sherman, R. E. (1968). Goal attainment scaling: A general method for evaluating community mental health programs. *Community Mental Health Journal, 4,* 443-453.

Lefley, H. P. (1979a). Prevalence of potential falling-out cases among the Black, Latin and non-Latin white populations of the city of Miami. *Social Science & Medicine, 13B* (2), (April 1979), 113-114.

Lefley, H. P. (1979b). Environmental interventions and therapeutic outcome. *Hospital & Community Psychiatry, 30,* 341-344.

Lefley, H. P. and Bestman, E. W. (1984). Community mental health and minorities: A multi-ethnic approach. In S. Sue and T. Moore (Eds.). *Community mental health in a pluristic society.* New York: Human Sciences Press.

Pedersen, P. B. (1981). Triad counseling. In R. J. Corsini (Ed.), *Handbook of innovative psychotherapies* (pp. 840-854). New York: Wiley.

Schulberg, H. C. (1977). Community mental health and human sciences. *Community Mental Health Review, 2* (6), 1-9.

Scott, C. S. (1974). Health and healing practices among five ethnic groups in Miami, FL. *Public Health Reports, 89* (6), 523-532.

Weidman, H. H. (1978). *Miami Health Ecology Project Report: A statement of ethnicity and health. Vol. 1.* Unpublished report. Miami, FL: University of Miami School of Medicine.

Weidman, H. H. (1979). The trancultural view: Prerequisite to interethnic (intercultural) communication in medicine. *Social Science & Medicine, 13B* (2), 85-87,

Weidman, H. H. (1983). Research, science and training aspects of clinical anthropology: An institutional overview. In D. Shimkin and P. Golde (Eds.) *Anthropology and health services in American Society.* Washington, DC: University Press of America.

PART III

TRANSCULTURAL SKILLS FOR SPECIAL POPULATIONS

CHAPTER 6

IF YOU ARE NOT AN INDIAN, HOW DO YOU TREAT AN INDIAN?

LOU MATHESON

WHILE IT IS NECESSARY to rely on the common humanity between Indian and non-Indian people, in the intimacy of a counseling situation, complexities arise which are not always understood. Somewhere in the relationship between a non-Indian service provider and an Indian service recipient, barriers appear which are not only puzzling, but often mean the total failure of even the most sincere efforts to be helpful. On the part of the Indian client, each failure reinforces the idea of differences and widens the span of misunderstanding between Native American and Euro-American people.

For the purpose of creating positive, growth-enhancing relationships between non-Indian service providers and Indian clientele, three areas of focus are suggested. The first is an inner self-assessment, or self-adjustment. In consulting with, and observing, sensitive non-Indian therapists, it has become clear to the author that successful intervention must begin at a far more personal level than following a prescribed 55 minute script. The essentials of therapy are a basic respect, both human and ideological, and an honesty that is based on an accurate knowledge of self.

The second focus is on becoming knowledgeable about the client. This paper will introduce several examples of the type of knowledge which seems to be important about Indian people. These are generalizations, for the most part, which are not intended to become stereotypes, but to give only some examples of what might be an outsiders' observations of some Indian people.

In the third focus, each of the above elements are related to the process of providing ethnically sensitive psychotherapy and other human services.

Dr. Ignace, a Coeur d'Alene Indian, who is currently chairman of the Board at the Milwaukee Indian Clinic, says "If Indians feel, for any reason, that they are not wanted, they will never come back and never tell why."

1. Stages in Developing Respect

What has been lacking in many instances of "no-return" is a quality for which there is no better word than "respect." Treat an Indian with respect. The term "respect" reflects a deeply inner process. Respect in this context is a quality which one carries with him/her, as constantly as his/her heart or spine. Respect is **not** a **re**-active phenomenon, only stimulated in response to specifically measured behaviors or status. Nor is respect only extended when we judge it to be earned and withdrawn at the whim of a personal affront. Respect in this context refers to a sense that in order for a person to participate in creation, it is essential that the person achieve and nourish a personal and satisfying relationship within self and with all other living forms. This is not a passive, "basking in the sun" event. It is a conscious and active awareness of the ever-changing, fluxing and waning dance between an individual and his/her universe.

For example, even if you place a high value on intellectual verbal skills, you would still be able to feel and express appreciation for the direct simplicity in the language of an Indian client who does not share that value. You might assess his/her verbal behavior as uncommon, but it would not occur to you to label the speaker as inferior. In fact, roughly half of Indian communication is non-verbal. I believe one of the obstacles to the type of constant respect I am speaking of is fear — fear of difference, fear of being disempowered by the unknown.

To overcome the obstacle of fear, I suggest that the first step is having the courage to allow oneself to be vulnerable. "Vulnerability," commonly identified with "weakness" is, paradoxically, the peak of strength and power. At the instant and to the extent one experiences vulnerability, one conquers whatever forces which seem to pose a threat. Once a person gives up fear or hostility or resistance, there is often no longer anything to be afraid of or hostile toward. There are reports of people who, once allowing themselves to be vulnerable to death, for example, find death no longer fearful. And in some instances, they may "magically" find the means to forestall that foreboding angel. Again and again the description of this occurence repeats useful experiences where: "Time stood still." "Everything happened in slow motion." "I don't know how, but somehow I knew exactly the 'right' thing to do." And so forth.

The specific task in identifying the kind of inner universal respect I speak of requires allowing oneself vulnerability to one's own fears, hostilities, and to whatever appears to be in conflict between different cultures. This vulnerability eliminates, or at least lessens the necessity to place a value judgement on every new discovery or old assumption. It is possible to ingest that which appears strange in a different culture, without the fear or the threat that some vague inner attachment will be diminished. It is possible to accept the commonality between you and another person from a different background and that makes the second phase very much easier.

The second phase of gaining respect for another culture can be found in the field of anthropology. "Cultural Relativity" is a way of studying a different culture in which the findings are couched both within the frame of reference set by the culture being studied, and the cultural conditionings which underlie the behaviors of the observer. Relativists make conscious efforts to base each judgement about a person or groups of persons on the host value system rather than from an outsider's own views. At the same time, they respect their own values, being aware of their influence on a person's ability to be objective.

A relativist perspective makes an important difference in our relationships. As Jack O. Wadell (1981) points out in his article about cultural relativity, if I ascribe validity and viability to another system whose basic values and beliefs differ from my own, my attitude toward that system is markedly different than if I take an absolutist ethnocentric approach, assuming that only my own system is valid. It would follow then, that my treatment of the people within each system would also undergo dramatic alterations. The right for an Indian to be different becomes as active and as enriching a component in your relationship as his/her right to be acculturated and similar.

Therefore, the second step I would advocate toward the development of an invariable state of respectfulness is to adopt a relativist approach to Indian cultures and the people emerging from those systems.

The issues which need most to be identified and considered in learning about Indian cultures are those, in my judgement, which are advocated by Bateson (1969). In **Steps To An Ecology of Mind** Bateson proposes that a society is more accurately and usefully assessed by identifying the types of relationships which people form than by drawing conclusions about categories such as religion, economic system, and so forth. Bateson's view is twice as valuable in one's approach to Indian societies, because when you begin thinking relationally, as all things being related, you begin to see things as most Indians do. That is, that almost nothing in life can be taken out of context as not having important impact on everything else.

If you go the step further and accurately define those relationships, many aspects of Indian culture and the behaviors of some Indian people begin to appear natural and predictable. Bateson continues to propose that the common character of a society be seen in terms of the "motifs of relationships between differential sections of the community." In learning to understand or to come to any conclusion about a generalized feature of a Native American Society, Bateson would suggest that you seek to define relationships between husband and wife, parents and children, leaders and common people, and so forth. On the basis of these relationships you may come to acquire a sense of national or cultural character.

Bateson is kind enough to get us started by suggesting a few relationship patterns which he has observed. He calls one relationship pattern **Symmetrical.** This type of relationship occurs when two people or groups of people have the same aspirations and general behavior patterns, but they differ in their basic orientation. For example, you may have two groups who both aspire to accumulate large sums of money but both their motives and economic practices may be very different.

He calls the second relational pattern **Complementary.** A relationship is complementary when the behaviors of each person or group are fundamentally different. Thus, you develop patterns of dependence and succorance, exhibition and admiration, and dominance and submission. He suggests there may be others, as well.

I believe we can observe some instances where the relationship between Indians and Euro-Americans are complementary, but additional problems have created imbalances. For example, if we consider one of our relationship patterns to be the complementarity of dominance and submission, these two poles may become so exaggerated that the relationship totally breaks down until all that is left is antagonism.

A third relationship pattern Bateson defines as **Reciprocity,** when the behaviors within each group are more different among themselves than they are toward other groups. They agree that in exchange for behaviors A, B and C, the other group will provide behaviors X, Y and Z, but not in the same way within their own group among themselves. An example of reciprocity would be the economic or political agreements between two countries.

As I see it, reciprocity is also the dynamic relationship pattern that Indian people try to establish and maintain not only within nearly all internal social structures but with the entire universe. The roles of each person or group in the relationship are fluid, and exchange functions as the circumstances dictate. In this sense, we become complementary. This can be seen clearly in relations between the people and nature. A traditional Indian will never indiscriminately harvest a large amount of herbs and medicines. He/she will select only certain specimens and not without giving some sort of "offering" back to the earth. This can be in the form of tobacco or some sort of jewel or silver. In exchange, the earth will continue to provide for the basic needs of the people. This is only one of thousands of examples of reciprocity.

Once it has been possible to break down some of the internal barriers to clear understanding, such as fear, and to view whatever differences there are in our relationship patterns without biased value judgements, treating an Indian "with honesty" becomes possible. Regardless of how honest we are, how can we begin to treat another person with honesty until we are prepared to deal in truths from both points of view? The approach to truths is paved with information — information which in itself presents matching pieces to a more-or-less objective model.

2. Value System

The information gathering process is one in which a truths-seeker will find better results if the focus is on the movement and activity inherent in the search itself. One must first be aware of one's own inner responses and uncertainties which occur upon each new contact. To willingly float or soar with the currents of discovery leads the adventurer not to the end of his journey, but to the fulfillment of his quest. In other words, it is not helpful to enter into the process of discovery expecting answers and absolutes. A book about Indians should not be read for the purpose of finding a conclusion, but only as a door to increased understanding. The interaction with an individual should not follow the form of a survey. Human contact is to be experienced and absorbed, and, hopefully, to be enjoyed. However, in the course of interfacing, many cruel mistakes have been made which create and re-create the type of polarization which leads to and has led to many of the social, economic and personal conditions which bring Indian people through the doorways of social service and mental health professionals. This is history, not only of 100 years ago, but in the life time of many of us here, maybe just last week.

For instance, one wonders how many Indian school children have been labeled "slow" by teachers who look for aggressive, competitive behavior as a sign of intelligence. One wonders how often an Indian student is expelled from college not because of poor grades, but because "she didn't socialize." This happened at a major university in 1973. The examples are endless, not only in education, but in all sorts of legal and civil rights issues. It is important to accept the reality of these events. It is important to accept them without guilt and without anger, but to remember them as a phase of exploring, as Bateson would say, "the basis upon which a relationship may be formed."

Based on the above theories, I would like to share some information relative to Indian people which may be valuable in providing quality services. In this effort it is essential to bear in mind that I as an individual, am influenced in my observations by my personal, as well as my cultural orientations. The generalities presented do not represent each member of Indian culture as a whole nor of all differentiated social units. Most of what I am sharing with you is based upon my own personal experiences and the words of wisdom from older and wiser individuals I have had the fortune to meet.

Of primary value within Indian culture is relationships, especially harmonious relationships. Such harmonious relationships occur within a nuclear and extended family, between self and important others, one's relationship with trees, animals, ancestors, and relationships as far reaching as the stars. It even appears as though an Indian person reaffirms humanity through the intensity and variety of relationships. Tribal systems are generally "receptive." Therefore, an observer finds Indian societies developing the means to form relationships and creating processes to accept even behaviors which are different from the norm. Thus, you find examples such as the Hopi and their relationships to venomous snakes. Rather than relate in violence, the Hopi incorporates the rattler into ceremonial and spiritual life. Many tribes have devised a social system by which people who are homosexual may be accepted, if not respected, in the larger society. Through the establishment of relationships one seeks unity with all earthly and spiritual creation. Relationships are sought between events as well as things, especially those affecting the individual, or which happen at a meaningful moment.

The family goes beyond the nuclear family unit to include grandparents, aunts, uncles, cousins, and adopted family members. The family rates very high in the value system of Indian societies. Thus, you will often see in your work what John RedHorse (1978) and others describe in their article, "Family Behavior of Urban American Indians" as the "extension of several households representing significant relatives along both vertical and horizontal lines" and family transactions within a community milieu. This is important (he says) for professionals to remember so that mislabeling may be avoided. Normal behavioral transactions within the network relational field, for example, may appear bizarre to an outside observer.

When you see an Indian client who suffers a number of stress-related symptoms, can't keep appointments because of no gas money or bus fare, yet you discover he or she is housing an assortment of what are to you, distant relatives, you will now understand why he or she may feel reluctant to ask them to leave. You will become more creative in your assistance to that person. Your intervention will consider the family unit, alternative support systems, and other ways in which you and the client can work together to alleviate the pressures in her life.

Personal self-determination is important in the Indian cultural value system, but in a way which is different from the Euro-American value system. In the tribal traditions of most American Indians, controls were exerted by a system of taboos. Rarely would you find written laws, or laws which were absolute in degree of infraction or the severity of consequence. Taboos were taught, or are taught, by oral tradition, often in the form of legends and by a complex semi-mystical system of conditioning. Part of the mystical system was the reliance on universal concepts of positive or negative forces which, it is believed, could be acquired by any and all through ceremonies, rituals, and their own personal relationship with their creator. If, in truth, there is a universal "good," and each one perceives similar ideas through the same source, then personal habits of correct behavior would naturally follow.

A system of taboos places a wide perimeter around an infinite assortment of behaviors, but cannot deal in specific individual behavior patterns, such as laws do. In other words, in a taboo system, the freedom to respond to individual, personal or spiritual directives in a variety of ways is not inhibited until the limits set by the taboo are violated. Even then, the action is sometimes tolerated because the nature of the violation is viewed as appropriate for that person at that time. The perimeter of a taboo system is flexible. When an unquestionably destructive act violated a taboo however, the consequences would be severe, and sometimes, irrevocable.

Implied in the taboo system is the idea of personal responsibility, personal power, personal aspiration and mobility. These are the positive aspects of a control system which are emphasized more frequently than the negative. The degree of self-determination within traditional structures could be limited only by the individual. Where the non-Indian service person often becomes confused is in trying to define "self-determination" or "self-reliance" or "me-ism." Instead, "self-determination" must be defined in the context of a tribal society of interdependent people who attempt to live cooperatively with others and their environment.

One can now begin to understand how an Indian client might respond to authority and directives. One can now see why the idea of submitting to innumerable sets of restrictions is abhorrent. Some Indian people have suggested that one of the problems in alcoholism treatment and recovery is that while a taboo may exist against some of the things an alcoholic does, there are no social sanctions against the choice to drink. Therefore, it's no one's business to say anything to limit choice, even if they see it to be potentially harmful.

There are other important values that Indian people might see as basic to the Indian views. There is, however, only one more basic value that I want to mention here. It appears to transcend all of the other values mentioned before and to determine their direction and function in Indian society. That value is harmony. Relationships are important, but it is harmonious relationships that are sought. Family is important, but it is harmony or lack of harmony, among family members which determines its role and rank in the larger society as well as its own sub-units. Self-determination is often assessed by the degree of harmony one sustains within his microcosm. Certainly one who moves harmoniously among creation is one who has himself in charge.

For a final comment on value systems, I would like to relate a legend. This story comes from the Pacific Coast of Washington. Once, many years ago, there was a fishing village where everyone depended upon the food from the beautiful river than ran along nearby banks. Every year, they would await the fish run and all the people would work together, setting their nets and preparing for the catch. Every year they would perform their "First Fish Ceremony" and give the first catch to one of the people of great wisdom and feed all the people in a great celebration of thankfulness. Then everyone worked together to clean and preserve the fish, and they all lived in peace and harmony together. One year a man named Tsah-bas came to live there. That year, before anyone else had a chance to prepare their fishing nets and other gear, he had stretched his tight net from one edge of the river to the other, upstream and downstream. When the fish came he caught them all, but a few little scrawny ones that slipped through his nets. Day after day, the people watched as he hauled in net after net full of fish and heaped them upon the bank. For days he feasted on his catch, never caring to offer any to the hungry people. But there were many more fish than he could ever use or preserve, so they began to rot. In just a few months, all the fish had rotted, and turned to an ugly slimy substance. One morning, when people looked at the river it was covered with the black rot from the spoiled fish, and no one could get rid of it. Months went by and the next fishing season was approaching, but still the river was covered and nothing would be able to live there. Finally, one young man was determined to find a way. He purified himself for many days before he dove into the river under the slime and swam all the way upstream to try to find a solution. Finally the water spirits felt pity for him because he was tired and beginning to need some air so they gave him a stick with fire on it. When he took it the fire made a hole in the slime where he could swim through and then he burned the whole surface so that the fish could run again and his people could live. Tsah-bas, they say, is the spirit of greed, and one must never, ever invite him to one's village because he will spread his slime all over everything and give a greedy spirit to all the people and no one will be able to survive. Although the desire to accumulate wealth is not unheard of, even Indian people who have never heard this legend find it difficult to be acquisitive and competitive.

3. Patterns of Belief

Rooted in these and other values, a set of basic beliefs emerge. Personally, I'm not sure that it is not the other way around, but to continue, I would first say that Indian, all Indian, culture is a spirit-oriented culture. Nearly every spiritual expression among Indian people, regardless of the faith they practice today, is performed against a backdrop picturing the spirit world as the real world. One daily encounters a shadow world. This is the world which only mirrors that which is real, that is, that which is spiritual.

Consequently, not only does everything we perceive through our senses have a spirit, including animals, trees, etc., but every thought, feeling and act also has a corresponding spirit. In a culture which lives this close to the spirit world, it is not considered pathological to "see" or "hear" spirits in our everyday life. Not every Indian believes this nor practices communicating with spirits. Nevertheless, the backdrop still exists and many people still play their spiritual roles close to the original scripts as they were written eons ago. Because of this spiritualism, nearly every Indian being assessed by the MMPI might be diagnosed "paranoid schizophrenic" through the way he/she responds to at least six questions.

In the DSM III manual which presents the diagnostic criteria prescribed by mental health systems nationally, there is a category of personality disorder entitled Schizotypal Personality Disorder. Under that, there is a list of eight characteristics which describe this disorder. At least five, and possibly seven, of those characteristics would be attributed to most Indians, immediately labeling them schizotypal, if not schizophrenic.

Specifically, it is a normal, expected and even admired event when an Indian person feels, sees or hears spirits. Sometimes these spirits have identity, such as an animal or an ancestor, and sometimes they are only spirits. Dreams are very important and may direct the lives of individuals and families and a great deal of effort is put into their correct interpretation. Visions are a frequent occurence and are sought, actively sought, as a means to determine the direction and purpose of one's life and its significant trends and events.

As in other spirit oriented cultures, the boundaries between entities are not as clearly defined as they are in the Euro-American culture. Consequently, it is believed possible, at some level, to "become" or seem to become, someone or something other than one's usual identity.

All things share in a spiritual existence. It follows that respect and reverence will become part of a belief system, enacted in a variety of tribally prescribed manners as well as one's own personal inclination. In these behaviors, there is a constant awareness of others, of other created things, such as the earth, and how, at any given moment, they are relating with the individual. For example, in most tribes staring is considered rude, and in some, prolonged eye contact is extremely disrespectful. In nearly every Indian tribal tradition is some sort of emphasis that it is wrong to embarrass another person or to make another feel uncomfortable in any way. Whenever someone "forgets" they are apt to be reminded. Often, the direct, personal questions found in intake therapeutic interviews offend in this way, especially when questions refer to the family.

All tribes teach some way in which the people acknowledge events in nature and ways in which to participate. For example, there are special ceremonies for each new moon, and special times when one should not do certain things in routine.

Traditionally, Indian tribes operated in a consumer economy. In other words, you would gather and accumulate only that which could be used within a reasonable period of time. In fact, even when things are free and may be new, few are prone to take more than they need or to not leave something for the next one. An example was seen not long ago in the Spokane Indian Clinic when a case of baby formula was left out with a sign above it saying, "Free, help yourself." It was about five days before it was all gone in spite of the fact that most people or their families have infants. On the other hand, it is not unusual for some people to try to "work" the system and theft among the street Indians is common.

As a way of distributing wealth and as a way to spiritually "cleanse" oneself, most tribes developed a form of "give-away." The coast tribes have a very complex way of providing equitable distribution of goods in what is called a "Potlatch." In most tribes people have other ways and times of giving, such as birthdays or naming ceremonies. The giving, however, goes the other way. The birthday family or the people giving and receiving names are the ones who do the giving, who share their good fortune with all the people who have come to celebrate. This is not an archaic practice of the past. Today's modern Indians are finding social, spiritual and economic value in ceremonial giving-away. Thus you find a basically sharing society, one in which people truly believe "it is better to give than to receive" and put it into practice, not once a year, but on a daily, minute-to-minute basis. As my grandfather once put it, "What's the good of having something, if you can't give it away!"

What has been pictured here may appear as an idealized society, a utopian world in which everyone is happy, contented and well-integrated. "But," you may ask, "what about the family in which there is incest? What about the lone alcoholic sleeping in moldy doorways? What about the two year old child, malnourished and neglected?" Some are concerned with the numbers of Indians appearing in Public Assistance lines or assorted instances of violence and suicide. Those who are already living closer to Indian society may wonder about internal quarreling and tribal rivalry. Where do these factual circumstances fit into a culture whose spirituality directs everyday behaviors, in which children are precious, and family relationships come before self-interest?

It is tempting to fault history, to remind the world of recorded historical events in which Euro-Americans enacted the role of victors over the conquered, where innocent masses become the victims of conquest. But in doing so, I, we, perpetuate the image of helplessness, dependency and impotence of the American Indian living in a society where only hostile forces control his fate. This is a false and destructive picture, and, I suggest, one that holds more than a brush-stroke of responsibility for the social anomalies human service providers see every day.

A better explanation comes from a great American historian, Dr. Albert Burke. Dr. Burke forms two circles, one representing Indian, the other Euro-American cultures.

On the perimeter of the Indian circle, he draws representations of animals, trees, rocks, mankind, rivers, etc., and in the center of the circle, something representing Primary Life Force, God, whatever your preference. On the Euro-American circle, he places Man in the center, all other created things along the perimeter and God coming from somewhere outside the circle altogether.

Can you image even the minimum implications from this conceptual image of our two systems? What follows if you pit one society, whose structure places man in brotherhood with all other created things against a society which sees mankind as the center of the universe with other creation as subservient, as usable and abuseable resources? It is natural, for the one to view with horror the indiscriminate slaughter of his brother, his Sustenance, his Spirit of Life — the buffalo. It is equally natural for the other to see only that the strip down the center of the buffalo's tongue is useful to run certain machines in his new industries. After all, animals were put here for our use. Neither side could even begin to negotiate with the other, bringing about bloodshed and loss for both.

Today there is still conflict over the acquisition of natural resources and the degree to which we can ignore our stewardship over our Mother, the earth. Although this has become not just an Indian/non-Indian issue, but one in which both groups are represented on either side, historically it was racially divided.

As these two opposing systems clashed, it was like a collision of meteors, the universe of both exploding in flame, molten masses being hurtled into space and others being ground into foreign soil by the pressures of the impact.

The people roaming our nation in pitiable circumstances or performing malevolent acts against each other, we are those pieces who survive the collision but have lost our rootedness. We are part of one mass being ground into the soil of the other. Part of us here, in this circle and part there, in the other. The remainder of either identity is lost, still groping in space. The same meteoric violence is continuing within each one of us, white and Indian alike. And this is the great pity of it all . . .it did not have to happen that way. We could have interfaced without polarizing.

We could have taken the time to define ourselves, our fears, our needs and our goals. We could have listened, communicated, and shared information upon which to establish a relationship in which there is harmony and balance. Perhaps we can begin today.

4. Service Delivery System

The implications in treatment need not be thought revolutionary. A non-Indian psychiatrist in Tacoma is respected and often in demand by Indian people there. His response to being questioned about his popularity centered around his own proclivity toward some of the Eastern systems, especially those which include meditation and the idea of giving up one's self-defenses and ego attachments. He spoke of his willingness to perceive a client's concept from the client's view and to explore those phases which he did not understand.

Another Caucasian psychologist told his client, "I know quite a bit about psychology, and I think I'm a good therapist, but I'm having a hard time understanding what it's like to be an Indian from an isolated reservation, just out of six months in prison and now in a strange city. If you would try to educate me on these things, I think I could be helpful to you."

Some therapists see themselves as expected to know everything, and therefore, must pretend to understand that which cannot be immediately understood. Do they think this pretense is not perceived by even the most dysfunctional client or patient? Edwin H. Richardson, in his very fine contribution to Derald Sue's (1981) book **Counseling the Culturally Different,** lists thirty-seven differences in Indian and Anglo values. Among the first of Indian values he lists "humility." It is important for a therapist to have the self-confidence to be humble.

On the other hand, a therapist interpreted as avoidance a client's efforts to let him know that he had other, even admirable, qualities besides his emotional dysfunction. The therapist needed to understand how difficult it might be for an Indian to be mechanical about his existence. How difficult to see himself as a car engine in which the carborator needs adjustment so you take it out, away from the rest of the car, fix it and put it back. The clients tend to see themselves and their dysfunction **only** in relation to their other parts and the environment in which they live.

Another therapist was concerned that an Indian client did not participate in group discussions or activities. All the therapist needed to understand was that his own expectations were not in alignment with the client's cultural expectations about group discussion and group paticipation. He needed to understand that his client **could** have been respectfully listening, or simply comfortable with silence. The client might not be comfortable with open discussion. The therapist could then begin to move into a space with his client where treatment efforts and their effects could be negotiated.

On the other hand, I was once involved in a case where an Indian mother and her son were being sheltered and helped by the generosity of a Caucasian woman. The latter identified the teenage boy as the client and did most of the talking in our first interview. At the same time she was describing the young man as "slow," "unsophisticated," "not capable of high grades" and never "college material," she was telling me that he was a chess-master in a local chess club, that he figured out the rubic-cube in a matter of minutes and other feats requiring developed intelligence. From former teachers, he was reported to have "superior intelligence" and a "brilliant mind." The same thing was happening that often occurs in schools, in job interviews and, unfortunately in counseling situations. The non-Indian has no difficulty accepting the "Indian-ness" of the other person, but finds it impossible to acknowledge intelligence, skills and competencies as qualities an Indian might possess.

As I see it, the primary function of a therapist or service provider is to empower his or her Indian clients and patients. Whatever treatment models are engaged in, they should be those which are designed to empower the clients to see themselves within the context of their own birth-rights, their history, and their perceptions of reality.

Except in crisis intervention, treatment models should be those which create an environment in which self-discovery and self-direction is encouraged and supported. They should be adapted to fit into the values and belief systems of the particular Indian being treated. More often than not, a holistic approach is best.

Depending upon the orientation of the client, it would be to the therapist's advantage to have a contact from the local Indian community. This contact could be helpful in many ways, but most of all if traditional healing methods are preferred by the client. The Indian view of wellness and illness is probably best described by the Navajo; "Healthfulness is being in harmony with the universe." In other words, when persons are "out of harmony" they get sick. Sickness can be physical, emotional, social or eventful, such as a series of "bad luck." The role of traditional healers is not only to administer healing to the immediate malady, but to restore harmony within the individual. They will usually place consider-able responsibility on their patient for his own condition. The healer may tell the patients, for example, that their illness is due to the anger they feel toward their relatives, and if they do not give that up, they will get sick again. Whatever is out of balance or harmony is usually something caused and sustained by the patients themselves.

Non-Indian practitioners need to grant credibility to these traditional methods of healing. The greatest example is Dr. Robert Bergman, who was the director of an NIMH project on the Navajo Reservation. The project was a training program for medicine men and women and he has written several accounts of healing he has witnessed. But the best example given to me, personally, was from a Caucasian psychiatrist in western Washington. We were on our way to lunch when he asked if I knew any medicine man who understood "Dog Power." I couldn't believe what I was hearing, yet, even as I saw this blond, teutonic, western-educated doctor, his question rang in the air. I conceded tenuously that I might be able to find someone, but why? Then he told me of a patient, a woman in her fifties:

> Angeline (not her real name) had been raised by her grandparents, both "medicine way" people and was being taught by her grandmother, since she had seen in Angeline some of the qualities that demonstrate spiritual strength. When Angeline was about twelve, some people from a church school came and took Angeline away to live at the school. There she was taught that the ways of her grandmother were evil and the work of the devil. They repeated to her that anyone who "saw" or "heard" spirits was insane. She was taught that only crazy people did the things she and her grandmother did — crazy or possessed. Angeline was admitted to a mental institution when she was about eighteen years old and spent more than half her adult life in institutions. During the times she was free, she married and had five or six children. Over two or three years she recently experienced divorce, the suicide of one daughter, the death of a son from drug over-dose, the institutionalization of another son, and most recently, the death of her youngest and dearest daughter who had been hacked to pieces. Through it all, she had held up admirably, but finally confided in the psychiatrist that before her grandmother died, another medicine person had put a curse on her and her family utilizing "Dog Power." Angeline believed that this curse was the cause of her own misfortune and that only another medicine person who also knew "Dog Power" could reverse its influence.
>
> The doctor did, in fact, locate a medicine man to reverse the "bad medicine" and now, whenever I hear from someone who has seen Angeline they have only good things to say about her activities and her general health.

There is one underlying theme which I ask you to keep in mind. Indian people, as a whole, do value their own heritage. Even after 400 years of contact, most of us do not see the superiority of the Euro-American systems. Many of us do not see the real benefit in replacing some of our old traditions with contemporary, non-Indian traditions, although many times we have made that sacrifice in order for our children to survive.

However, few if any, of the traditional Indian practices and philosophies remain pure. We have all been influenced by the Euro-American culture and sometimes in ways for which we might feel grateful.

It is only with the patience and understanding of people who willingly try to bridge the span between us that we sustain our faith in our eventual existence together in harmony.

REFERENCES

Bateson, G. (1969). *Steps to an ecology of mind.* New York: Ballentine.

Red Horse, J. C., Lewis, R., Feit, M., & Decker, J. (1978). Family behavior of urban American Indians. *Social Casework, 59,* 67-72.

Richardson, E. (1981). Cultural and historical perspectives in counseling American Indians. In D. W. Sue (Ed.), *Counseling the culturally different* (pp. 216-255). New York: Wiley.

Sue, D. W. (Ed.) *Counseling the culturally different.* New York: Wiley.

Waddell, J. O. (1981). Cultural relativity and alcohol use: Implications for research and treatment. *Journal of Studies on Alcohol,* Supplement No. 9, 86-92.

CHAPTER 7

CONCEPTUALIZING AFROCENTRIC AND EUROCENTRIC MENTAL HEALTH TRAINING

GERALD G. JACKSON

A FRICAN AMERICAN mental health professionals have been in the forefront in launching criticisms against the preparation they received to be psychiatrists, social workers, psychologists, and counselors (e.g., Bell, 1971; Funneye, 1970; Jones, Lightfoot, Palmer, Wilkerson, & Williams, 1970; R. Jones, 1980). Collectively, they have made recommendations to their respective professional groups and credentialing institutions to expand extant mental health theories, techniques and practices so that these elements of the mental health delivery system would be more congruent with the history, socio-economic and political experiences of African Americans. As advocates of African Americans, they have lobbied for the organization of a body of mental health professionals who would combat the systematic antecedents to mental disorders in the African American community (e.g., Butts, 1977; Green, 1974; Johnson, 1972; C. Pierce, 1970; W. Pierce, 1972; Williams, 1970).

If one closely examines the recriminations, models, proposals and recommendations of African American mental health professionals, as I have done and reported (G. Jackson, 1976a, 1976b, 1976c), one can find a strong reaction in their various forms of protestation to what I have termed culturalism (e.g., G. Jackson, 1979a, 1979b, 1979c, 1982). To reiterate and perhaps make more clear, culturalism is a social phenomenon that manifests itself in the rejection of another group's characteristic language, art, music, sex-role definition, family structure, style of dress, dance, religion, socio-economic and political institutions and

131

phenotype. More subtle forms of culturalism would be the denial of the target group's interpretation of history, mode of logic, measurement of progress, concept of human nature, communication style, concepts of time and space, and definition of group.

Carried a step further, the factors that propelled me to write this chapter were my observations of the limits of the psychological construct, "racism." The term did not, to my satisfaction, address two derivatives of culturalism, Eurocentrism and Afrocentrism. Briefly stated, Eurocentrism is the belief in the comparative superiority of Anglo American culture, in particular, and Euro-American culture, in general. Adherents affirm that what is normative for groups who either occupy or descend from European territories is a yardstick for evaluating other culturally distinct geographical groups. Specifically, proponents of Eurocentrism ascribe comparatively greater value to Indo-European languages, individualism, competition, classical European music, representational art, Judaeo-Christian religions, the cognitive domain, analytical mode of thought, Cartesian logic, a linear-progressive view of time, the separation of time and space, and Nordic physical characteristics. In contrast, Afrocentrism is the belief in the viability of people, customs, beliefs, and behaviors emanating from African lands. Proponents of this outlook advocate collectivism, cooperation, jazz, symbolic art, traditional African religions, African physical characteristics, the affective domain, relational mode of thought, spiral view of time, the integration of time and space, and diunital logic, a categorical mode explained more fully in the following section.

Conceptual Maps for Contextualizing Mental Health Training

A scientific community is composed of practitioners of a scientific specialty. To become members of such a community, one undergoes a similar education and professional initiation. The technical literature of this type of community sets its membership boundaries and the limits of its subject matter. Participants are viewed, as a consequence, as individuals "uniquely responsible for the pursuit of a set of shared goals, including the training of their successors" (Kuhn, 1969, p. 177).

Generally speaking, there are three levels in which such communities exist. The most global level is the community of all disciplinary scientists. The second level is the main scientific professional groups in which membership is demarcated by highest academic degree, membership in professional societies, journals read and the use of similar techniques. The last level is that of "schools" within the community, such as the behaviorist and psychoanalytic persuasions among mental health professionals.

In the same vein, African American mental health professionals have organizations, journals, conventions and the schools of thought which are counterparts of predominantly European Amerian mental health institutions. For example, among African American psychologists there are the "empirical" and "africanist" schools of Black psychology.

Viewed as a dialectical process, African American mental health professionals and organizations have made fervent attempts in the past and in the present to make their parent organizations more socially responsible and accountable to African American needs. They have advanced models of leadership and comradeship (Banks, 1971; Williams, 1970). Carried a step further, as guidelines for specific actions, some have identified shortcomings in assessment instruments (Buck, 1975; A. Hilliard, 1981; Hixon & Epps, 1975; Samuda, 1975; Taylor, 1975; Williams, 1974, 1975b), the attitudes and training of professionals, and the models governing the practice of social work, counseling and therapy (Better, 1972; Gilbert, 1974; Gordon, 1970; Gunnings & Simpkins, 1972). Lastly, some emphasized the need to get more African Americans trained to conduct therapy (C. Pierce, 1968; Williams, 1974; Wispe, Ashe, Hicks, Hoffman, & Porter, 1979).

In recognition of the societal dimension of the problem, a number sought to redress the global problems of African Americans by proposing models for dealing with institutional racism (Sedlacek & Brooks, 1973a, 1973b) and the legal or criminal justice system (Hilliar, Dent, Hayes, Pierce, & Poussaint, 1974; M. Jones & Jones, 1972). Some even went so far as to try to allay fears that trained African American professionals would abuse their power relationship with European American clients by publishing accounts of their successes with such individuals (Schachter & Butts, 1968; Curry, 1963; Grier, 1967).

In response to this "Black" assertiveness by African American mental health professionals, Comer (1970), an African American psychiatrist, recounted the "White" backlash. Researchers, he noted, viewed the charges against White researchers in the Black community as unjust and as part of a ploy on the part of certain Blacks to gain control of research and intervention program money. Some interpreted the negative attitude toward testing and research in the African American community as understandable but an excessive and self-defeating reaction to the historical Black-White relationship. Still others agreed that the reaction was healthy, and in some cases just, but would pass in time as African American people gained more success in all phases of American life.

Cobbs (1970), another African American psychiatrist, however, affirmed that psychiatrists and other professionals deny their culpability in the existence of White racism by assuming that they are exempt. He noted that it is precisely because so many people assume that they are excused that the climate of retaliation is present in the United States today.

One alternative to the schism depicted above is the concept of diunitality. Dixon and Foster (1971) proposed it as a means of lessening racial polarization and conflicts in America. Their review of race relations research revealed an implicit assumption in such research that everything falls into one category at the same time and they concluded that this philosophical orientation resulted in the placement of African Americans and European Americans into exclusive racial/cultural categories. Moreover, once placed into distinct categories the inference is made that they are "mutually exclusive, contradictory and antagonistic" (Nelson, 1975, p. 25). To resolve the problem stemming from a dichotomous mode of reasoning, the authors recommended the use of diunital logic and defined it as: "Di means 'akin to two' or 'apart.' Unital, the adjectival form of the world unit, means a 'single thing that constitutes an undivided whole.' Diunital, therefore, is literally something apart and united at the same time. According to this logic, something is both in one category and not in that category at the same time and in the same respect.' (Dixon, 1976, p. 76). The authors speculated that the state of diunitality would be achieved when "Black and White Americans accept the contradictions endemic in their cultural environments as mutually rewarding and mutually relevant" (Nelson, 1975, p. 26).

Consistent with the concept of diunitality, in the next section a conceptual map of training will be presented which is designed to be comprehensible to African American and European American professionals.

Clinical Training and Culturalism

Several authors have documented the culturalistic thrust and even the practice of White racism within the profession of psychiatry (e.g, Thomas & Sillen, 1972; Willie, Kramer, & Brown, 1973). What has been perhaps even more harmful has been the extension of culturalism into the theoretical and practical orientation of other mental health professions (Alvarez et al., 1976). For instance, Goldstein (1973) observed that social workers, based upon Freudian theory and techniques, departed from their earlier stance of doers and providers of concrete services to that of passive observers. In his assessment: "Prior manipulative approaches were disclaimed. The concept of a detached professional attitude emerged along with the admonition that practitioners should keep their feelings and activities in abeyance. Thus, practice of this type would have to limit services to those clients who could respond to and use a less active approach, to those whose problems did not require immediate action" (p. 31). In addition to structural and ideological barriers, the following discussion indicates some of the ways in which culturalism presents itself in clinical training.

Language

Since the charge of mental health professionals is not to teach standard English but to try to comprehend the manner in which clients communicate, I was initially astonished to discover language usage and acceptances in other areas of life as the explanation given by professionals for not supporting the use of Ebonics, the spoken language of African Americans (Williams, 1975a), in counseling and psychotherapy situations.

I now realize that the modal way in which African Americans use the English language is a controversial subject that pivots around the deficit hypothesis. On the surface, one could speculate that the resistance of mental health professionals to accepting the legitimacy of the Black Oral Tradition of using the English language (Smitherman, 1973), is based upon their socialization in a mono-lingual society; however, it is my hypothesis that the origin of this resistance is in culturalism. Acceptance of the Black Oral Tradition includes the recognition of traditional African culture as a viable source and recognition of racism as a force in the maintenance of a distinct way of communicating. Moreover, since most mental health professionals are ill equipped to deal with either racism or internalized oppression, attempts are made by trainees to avoid a full discussion of language practices. In particular, for African American professionals who have forcibly and painfully altered their communication pattern to conform to the demands of the majority group in American, and have had difficulty in communicating with ordinary "Black Folk" (Gwaltney, 1980), the language issue invokes in them a sense of their marginality in American society.

Art, Music and Dance

The African American aesthetic (Gayle, 1972) usually becomes an issue during the social hours of training situations. African Americans lambast having to endure Eurocentric music, scenery and dancing. The area is also a training issue because the "Black Aesthetic" is an integral part of the process of counseling and doing psychotherapy with African American clients (e.g., Pasteur & Toldson, 1979).

Relatedly, in a workshop I was conducting for an inter-racial group of counselors, I noted the importance of listening to words in "rappin" music. The African American participants agreed that it was important to comprehend the words in order to provide counseling to adolescents. In the midst of our exchange over the connection between the words in such music and the tempo of social conditions, I interrupted the flow of the conversation to ask one of the European American participants, who had a puzzled look on his face, if he understood the point being made. He responded that he could not hear the message in such music because he found the rhythm offensive. Thus, he missed the cross-cultural point and alienated himself from the other participants, who commented to me privately that he personified why African Americans needed African American counselors.

Sex Role Definition

The role and behavior of males and females is a crucial aspect of training programs for mental health professionals. In one training situation, in order to concretize the dynamics involved in inter-racial relationships, I had videotapes made of the interactions of a three-day training program. During one of our process meetings I showed the filming of the interaction between an African American male and a blond-haired European American female. Participants were asked to make comments on what they thought they had observed. The European Americans described the exchange as an argument while the African Americans thought the female was flirting with the male.

Sex role definitions can also be a problem in uniracial training situations involving visible minorities (G. Jackson, 1972). In one such training program for counselors of college students in compensatory programs, I suggested that the first step in the process might be the sharing of anxieties associated with one's sex role. The group agreed and the males started first by disclosing the anxieties behind their facade of "coolness." The female participants posed a multitude of questions to the men; however, when it was the latter's turn to self-disclose the females reneged on their commitment. Many claimed that they had been told by their mothers to "never tell a man everything that is on your mind." One female did go against the position of her gender group and shared with the men some of the games women play. Weeks later this individual met me in the street and bemoaned how she had been criticized, in the after group meeting of the women, for self-disclosing.

Religion and Church

At the close of a training session for psychiatric trainees at a South Bronx hospital an official of the group asked me if his interpretation of the meaning of a part of my presentation was correct. I had indicated that the religiosity of African Americans had to be taken into account when delivering mental health services and he had deduced from my statement that "God is alive in the Black community." After I agreed with his inference, he retorted, "God is dead in the White community." None of the European American trainees and officials protested his appraisal of their religious orientation. My rejoinder to his declaration and the silence of the group was that I was not addressing the religiosity of psychiatrists, I was noting a dimension that should be taken into account when administering mental health services to African American communities and individuals.

In another training situation in which a spiritualist was brought in to introduce to mental health trainees a culturally specific form of mental health practice in African American and Latino communities, an African American male participant was so impressed by the skill of the spiritualist that he sought the person out months later for "a reading." His behavior was consistent with the syncretic approach I have observed in many African American mental health professionals. They practice psychotherapy and counseling, however, when they experience depression or indecisiveness they seek out traditionally African American churches, sagacious family members, friends or spiritualists.

In European American culture the sacred and secular dimensions of life are separated, based upon Western philosophical and cultural traditions. Educational institutions, steeped in this cultural and philosophical tradition, produce mental health professionals who accept the division and who practice their profession according to secular parameters. The traditional African American church, as a sacred and secular institution, is incomprehensible to many trainees. It is difficult for them to fathom that this church is predicated in part on an African philosophical outlook that fused the sacred and secular and is based in part on the socio-political demands to be holistic in order to meet the needs of African Americans. The communication style of the traditional African American preacher (e.g., Pipes, 1981), and the media portrayal of him combine to denigrate an appreciation of his worth and the perception of his church as an adjunctive force in the delivey of mental health services.

Communication Style

Kochman (1981) observed the African American communication style represented involvement and was designed to "generate affect." It is, in his assessment, high-keyed, animated, interpersonal, confrontational, heated, and low. In contrast, the European American style is one of "detachment" and is "without affect." It is, as a result, low-keyed, dispassionate, impersonal, non-challenging, cool, and quiet.

Specifically my style has been categorized as "secular," that is, it is urban and Northern, and "tends to be more cool, more emotionally restrained than the sacred style" (Smitherman, 1973, p. 37). However, it shares, according to Smitherman's (1973) description, the following characteristics with the "sacred" or rural and Southern style, characterized by "Black" preachers:

Call and response. The speaker's solo voice alternates or is intermingled with the audience's response. The respose can take the form of a back-and-forth banter between the speaker and various members of the audience. Or the audience might manifest its response in giving skin (fives) when a really down verbal point is scored. Other approval responses include laughter and phrases.

Rhythmic Pattern. Refers to cadence, tone and musical quality. This is a pattern that is lyrical, sonorous, and generally emphasizing sound apart from sense.

Spontaneity. Speaker's performance is improvisational, with the rich interaction between speaker and audience dictating and/or directing the course and outcomes of the speech event. Since the speaker does not prepare a formal document, his delivery is casual, non-deliberate, and uncontrived. He speaks in a lively, conversational tone, and with an ever-present quality of immediacy. All emphasis is on process, movement, and creativity of the moment.

Concreteness. Speaker's imagery and ideas center around the empirical world, the world of reality, and the contemporary Here and Now. Rarely does he drift off into esoteric abstractions; his metaphors and illustrations are commonplace and grounded in everyday experience. Perhaps because of his concreteness, there is a sense of identification with the event being described or narrated.

Signifying. Technique of talking about the audience or some member of the audience in order to initiate verbal "war" or to make a point hit home.

With respect to using my style, some participants have expressed dismay over not being able to write down what I said and appeared only partially satisfied with my reply that I did not want them to write anything down but to simply hear what I was saying. Some have said that I should, as a side line, consider becoming a comedian because of my humorous anecdotes. Others have said that they found my ideas to be thought-provoking and enlightening and added that they got lost by my rhythm, physical movement around the room and convoluted line of reasoning.

There are several reasons why I am ambivalent about adopting a purely European American style of communication. First, trainees who receive information on the African American style would not get a true understanding. To illustrate, a group of module designers for a counselor training program met for drinks to get to know one another better. I did not pay attention to the silence of the European American until he interrupted the exchange between me and an African American female and said that he did not understand one thing we had been saying. He added that for years his students had been proclaiming a cultural difference in communication style but he did not know what they had meant until being with us. He added that he did not detect a misuse of the English language, we simply conveyed information in a manner that he could not comprehend.

Second, the use of a purely European American communication style by an African American speaker registers a different message to African American trainees. Take "signifin,' " for example: Smitherman (1973) noted: "The interesting thang bout this rhetorical device is that the audience is not offended and realizes—naw, expects—the speaker to launch this offensive to achieve his desired effect" (p. 38); and making one's point is a real expectation on the part of African American participants.

Third, a purely European American communicative style violates my cultural canons about being with people and not over them. What is clear to me is that I find it disconcerting to address a group for more than an hour and wait for my feedback until the end of my presentation. I need direction from the group to feel we are one.

Relatedly, in lecture situations in which European Americans are the majority, African Americans inhibit their call-response pattern; however, when they are sizable in number they give feedback and direction. In addition they tend to rate those lectures higher in enjoyment and learning that permit them to be an active part of the communication process of discussion.

Concept of Time

Recently, the magazine **Psychology Today** published two articles on how cultures and sub-cultures determine the time perspective of human beings (Levine & Wolff, 1985; Gonzalez & Zimbardo, 1985). However, I have been dealing with the implication of this fact for mental health treatment of African American for more than a decade, and I have published on how differences in temporal perspective influence the design and interpretation of mental health research results (G. Jackson, 1979c).

Most mental health practitioners are unaware of the cultural bias of their notions of time and have received little training in how to conceptualize and work with people who operate from a different peception of time. For example, a European American researcher linked my remarks on time to some erroneous assumptions he had made about the competency of visible minorities. We had both been in attendance at a training program to cultivate a culturally sensitive approach in researchers and program designers for substance abuse. The training was designed by a visible minority consulting firm and many of the presentors and workshop leaders were people of color. My colleague shared his dissatisfaction with the characterization of traditional research designs by the presentors but what disturbed him the most was the lateness of the events. He confessed that he had actively resisted the notion that visible minorities in power could not do things correctly but was beginning to change his mind, based upon his observation at this training program of how the workshops ran over time. When asked if the other participants appeared to be disturbed by the way time was allocated, he admitted that he had not really taken that into account. He used as his reference the stipulated time on the program and his culturally ingrained notion about punctuality.

African American trainees do not deliberately abuse time schedules and most would, if asked, verbalize a commitment of punctuality. What happens, however, in practice is a matter of culture. To illustrate, at the outset of a five-day residential training program for primarily visible minority counselors, the head trainer informed the group that the program would operate "on-time." He remarked that he would make certain that the stereotype of tardiness would not be a reality and the group agreed to assist him by following the schedule to the minute. What was ignored was the cultural need to be **"in**-time" rather than **"on**-time."

For the first couple of days the program moved according to the time schedule originally made, and concomitant with the group's adherence to the schedule was a growing tension that few wanted to consider because everything was going according to plan. What was not occurring, I observed, was emotional involvement in the learning and a genuine openness to exploring sensitive areas. I was not shocked, therefore, when the group of trainees rebelled and professed as one of their major gripes the "rigid" time schedule. Many claimed that the pressure to stay on schedule prevented them from fully engaging in the feelings and concerns generated by the program's structured activities. Rather than focus on temporality as a philosophical matter, time was bantered around as a symbol of much deeper psychological ills.

Concept of Space

There are several ways that the subject of spatiality can influence training, such as size of the room, furniture, and seating pattern. Visible minorities are particularly sensitive to messages conveyed by the use of space. For example, in a training situation in which groups were divided into "Black" and "White" categories, a European American female was accosted by the African American group for not coming to their group. She responded that she was "White" and remarked that she had been mistaken for a "Black" before, even though none of her physical characteristics were African. The group informed her that she did not act "White." She could not comprehend what they meant so some of the members indicated that what was meant was that she did not appear to be uncomfortable in the physical space of them. She still did not understand so I had her view the videotape of the first meeting of the participants. She saw that she had sat in the middle of the African American section. There were no visible boundaries drawn but she was in their midst and did not exhibit any signs of discomfort. In fact, she interacted with them as if she was a member of their group. In defense of her seating selection, she exclaimed that the seat she took was the only one available when she arrived and added that she was Jewish and originally from Bronx, New York, so coming into physical contact with "Blacks" was a natural thing for her to do.

Cognitive Mode

There is an African mode of thinking and logic and it can be shown to be operative in the manner in which people approach religion, family, group oppression, speaking, dance, art and learning (G. Jackson, 1982). It can also be seen in the way African American professionals in the field of mental health have organized themselves, and provided mental health services (G. Jackson, 1977, 1979c, 1985).

Several factors work against the success of this mode in the field of mental health. One inhibitor is the training process they undergo in order to get to positions of authority. They are taught to distrust their feelings and are reinforced to rely on thinking, to the exclusion of their feelings. By the time then, they reach a position of authority they have learned to dichotomize and have lost their capacity to develop programs and approaches that are based upon a complementary relationship between thinking and feeling. Second, "playing the game" results in an association of the thinking mode with work and the feeling mode with play or leisure time activities; therefore, their professional designs omit considerations that would emanate from a holistic appraisal system. Third, the gamesmanship they follow results in a private depreciation of approaches associated with European American professionals, such as research, conference presentations, evaluation and peer collaboration. Last, they have been trained to believe that the affective domain is fraught with punishments for African Americans and only a limited group of individuals such as athletes and entertainers are allowed to eke out a living in this area.

In conceptualizing culturally determined modes of thinking, I gained inspiration from the works of Robert Ornstein, especially his theorizing on cerebral dominance and time (G. Jackson, 1979c). I incorporated his thinking and research findings into my lectures and workshop. Of particular note, my extrapolations aided me in understanding the rivalry between different mental health professions and their preferred learning styles. Groups such as counselors and social workers are inclined to learn best from activities and presentations that engage their "affective" component whereas psychiatrists and clinical psychologists learn best from presentations that engage their cognitive domain. African American mental health professionals respond optimally when both domains are engaged and can maintain a connection between the two domains because they are divergent thinkers (A. Jackson, 1979).

Concentric Circles of Changes

In closing, the problem areas identified in this section will not be resolved by responding to each category as a distinct entity. Nor will the issues undergirding them be resolved by investigating the ontology, epistemology and axiology of mental health professions. Change may result from a realization that our efforts are designed to "convert" individuals and groups, and that this process entails more than the presentation of scientific data. It involves moving trainees through three concentric circles composed of culturalism, Eurocentrism and racism. For example, Torrey (1972a) suggested that Western therapists could actually learn from the "witchdoctor" to see the components of therapy systems in relief, could discover why they are effective or not effective, and could learn to be less arrogant about their own system of therapy. In support of his contention, he revealed how drug therapy, shock therapy, dream analysis and conditioning were used in non-Western cultures prior to their rediscovery and application by Western therapists (e.g., Torrey, 1972b, 1974). Similarly, Leff (1975) added elsewhere: "Principles of treatment that would be applauded by most Western psychiatrists have been utilized by native healers for centuries before psychiatry was recognized as a specialty in the west" (p. 128).

Dualistic thinking about cultures, bio-social groups, cognitive processes, verification of information and personal orientation would stifle acceptance of the information provided by Torrey and others. In general, Americans have been socialized and trained to believe in the comparative superiority of Western over Non-Western cultures, White over Black people, cognitive over affective domains, quantifiable over qualifiable data, individualism over collectivism and literate over oral cultures.

To illustrate, Anderson, Robinson and Ruben (1978) suggested that a fusion of Westernized medico-psychological approaches and Christian concepts of healing would avoid a dichotomous approach to health care and fulfill the comprehensive health needs of the population. Griffith (1983) added that such a collaborative approach would have positive implications for the type of mental health system that could be adopted in developing countries (see G. Jackson, 1976a). He also reported on a program that combined the two, as well as wrote about the therapeutic aspects of the African American church (Griffith, 1982; Griffith, English, & Mayfield, 1980; Griffith & Mathewson, 1981).

However, the issue is not one that is resolved by the presentation of evidence that falsifies dualistic thinking. Moreover, the division rests upon a Eurocentric ontology of material essence, individualism, independence, control over nature and survival of the fittest. It is based on an epistemology of object/measure, observation of experiences, rigidity and dualism. Last, it is grounded in an axiology of conflict/competition, control of life, ownership, and the acquisition of information. This philosophical base maintains the divisions and may be the reason why peoples of the world, such as Africans and their decendants, who are not fundamentally governed by it, propose and implement models that unite the two spheres. Most training programs do not address these bedrock issues because they entail a global perspective of the process of training individuals and groups, and such an outlook is beyond the pale of an analytical mode of thought.

Giorgis and Helms (1978), in an attempt to enhance the training of foreign students in applied (clinical) and academic psychology, expressed concern over the: (1) social science orientation toward the "White" Western world; (2) unilateral exchange of scholars; (3) Western perceptions and descriptions of other cultures in ethnocentric terms; and (4) limited number of psychologists in developing countries to provide adequate training. Based upon their experiences in such programs and an overview of the literature, they noted several barriers to the acquisition of culturally specific graduate training, and cultural differences that they believed were dimly appreciated by a majority of Western educators.

They cited language differences, practicum experiences among the middle class and the definition of graduate students as ignorant and dependent, as surmountable barriers. However, they indicated that not only were there many African languages that did not have a word for psychology, in many developing countries policymakers and administrators held the attitude that psychology had not demonstrated its usefulness. To rectify these problems, the authors advocated the use of para-professionals and technicians and a multi-disciplinary training model that included courses in economics, cross-cultural psychology, anthropology, etc. They felt that these additions would compensate for a limited number of professionals.

To minimize cultural alienation from the student's reference group, the authors recommended that contact should be maintained with their primary cultural groups; specifically, through an internship site in an area that contains a group similar to their group of cultural origin.

Along the same lines, they felt that students could be encouraged to use seminars and lectures to speculate about how traditional psychology is or is not pertinent to their indigenous culture. Relatedly, they suggested that training for foreign students in psychological testing should be extended to the area of test construction and theory, in the event that returnees should discover that the "standard" instruments do not work at home. One's dissertation or thesis, the authors affirmed, could be based on the suggestion by those in authority to collect data from the students' base country. Lastly, they suggested that trainees should be given a subspeciality in an area of immediate worth to the students' society. In this regard, they espoused that additional training as a medical assistant or paralegal aide could be used as an avenue to sensitizing their community to the new discipline and skill. Most central, the authors reported that for their contemporary needs the dyadic psychotherapy model regnant in the United States was the least efficient type of mental health care.

Returning to the United States scene, however, another group that has received inadequate attention is, perhaps paradoxically, the African American middle-income group. When most of the contemporary psychotherapists were trained, African American culture was portrayed as synonymous with lower-class culture. The percentage of affluent African Americans was small enough for most researchers to feel comfortable in leaving this group out of their research designs, despite the evidence by Frazier (1962) and Hare (1965) of the mental health problems of this group. Today, while the number of affluent African Americans has increased, training still uses a lower-class African American model. Similarly, few trainees are being prepared to assist either affluent or poor African Americans in handling the behavioral consequence of "modern racism," despite the literature on the problems of African Americans in corporate America (e.g., Davis & Watson, 1982; Dickens & Dickens, 1982; Fernandez, 1975) and the empirical and theoretical work on modern racism (e.g., McConahan, Hardee, & Batts, 1981).

These signs of the failure of affluence to eliminate the impact of group oppression on African Americans would not be seen as an anomaly in a paradigm that was experientially grounded, an outlook illustrated by the African American church (Pipes, 1981). It is eclipsed, however, by a paradigm that is based upon a social class model (Jackson, 1979c). In the words of Dr. James Turner (1985), ". . .the field of Africana Studies is a teaching and research enterprise that is committed to the interpretation and explication of the total phenomenon called the

Black Experience" (p. vi). A part of this experience is trying to be pro-Black and not anti-White and a part is attempting to eke out a living by being resourceful and ethical. Training individuals to assist individuals in this struggle can not be rooted in abstract notions; it has to be based upon a similar dialectical process.

REFERENCES

Alvarez, R., Batson, R., Carr, A., Parks, P., Peck, H., Shervington, W., Tyler, F., & Zwerling, I. (1976). *Racism, elitism, professionalism: Barriers to community mental health.* New York: Jason Aronson.

Anderson, R., Robinson, C., & Ruben, H. (1978). Mental health training and consultation: A model for liaison with clergy. *Hospital & Community Psychiatry, 29,* 800-802.

Banks, G. (1971). The effects of race on one-to-one helping interviews. *Social Service Review, 45,* 137-146.

Bell, R. (1971). The culturally deprived psychologist. *Counseling Psychologist, 2,* 104-107.

Better, S. (1972, Fall). The Black social worker in the Black community. *Public Welfare,* 2-7.

Buck, M. (1975). The multi dimensional model for the assessment of children referred for classes for mental retardation. *The Journal of Afro-American Issues, 3*(1), 91-102.

Butts, H. (1977). The psychoanalyst, the Black community and mental health. *Contemporary Psychoanalysis, 7,* 147-152.

Cobbs, P. (1970). White mis-education of the Black experience. *Counseling Psychologist, 2,* 23-27.

Comer, J. (1970). Research and the Black backlash. *American Journal of Orthopsychiatry, 40,* 8-11.

Curry, A. (1963). Some comments on transference when the group therapist is Negro. *International Journal of Group Psychotherapy, 23,* 363-365.

Davis, G., & Watson, G. (1982). *Black life in corporate America.* New York: Anchor/Doubleday.

Dickens, F., & Dickens, J. (1982). *The Black manager making it in the corporate world.* New York: AMACOM.

Dixon, V. (1976). World views and research methodology. In L. King, V. Dixon & W. Nobles (Eds.), *African philosophy: Assumptions and paradigms for research on Black persons.* California: Fanon Research & Development Center.

Dixon, V., & Foster, B. (Eds.). (1971). *Beyond Black or White.* Boston: Little, Brown.

Fernandez, J. (1975). *Black managers in White corporations.* New York: Wiley.

Frazier, E. (1962). *Black bourgeoisie.* New York: Free Press.

Funneye, C. (1970). The militant Black social worker and the urban hustle. *Social work, 15,* 5-13.

Gayle, A. (Ed.). (1972). *The Black aesthetic.* New York: Anchor.

Gilbert, G. (1974). The role of social worker in Black liberation. *Black Scholar, 6,* 16-23.

Giorgis, T., & Helms, J. (1978). Training international students from developing nations as psychologists: A challenge for American psychology. *American Psychologist, 33*(10), 945-951.

Goldstein, H. (1973). *Social work practice: A unitary approach.* South Carolina: University of South Carolina.

Gonzalez, A., & Zimbardo, P. (1985, March). Time in perspective. *Psychology Today,* 20-27.

Gordon, E. (1970). Perspectives on counseling and other approaches to guided behavior change. *Counseling Psychologist, 2,* 105-114.

Green, R. (1974). The social responsibility of psychology. *Journal of Black Psychology, 1,* 25-29.

Grier, W. (1967). When the therapist is Negro: Some effects on the treatment process. *American Journal of Psychiatry, 123,* 1587-1591.

Griffith, E. (1982). The significance of ritual in a church-based healing model. *American Journal of Psychiatry.*

Griffith, E. (1983). The impact of sociocultural factors on a church-based healing model. *American Journal of Orthopsychiatry, 53*(2), 291-302.

Griffith, E., English, T., & Mayfield, V. (1980). Possession, prayer, and testimony: Therapeutic aspects of the Wednesday night meeting in a Black church. *Psychiatry, 43,* 120-128.

Griffith, E., & Mathewson, M. (1981). Communitas and charisma in a Black church service. *Journal of the National Medical Association, 73,* 1023-1027.

Gunnings, T., & Simpkins, G. (1972). A systematic approach to counseling disadvantaged youth. *Journal of Non-White Concerns, 1,* 4-8.

Gwaltney, J. (1980). *Drylongso: A self portrait of Black America.* New York: Random House.

Hare, N. (1965). *The Black Anglo-Saxons.* New York: Macmillan.

Hilliard, A. (1981). I.Q. thinking as chatechism: Ethnic and cultural bias or invalid science? *Black Books Bulletin, 7*(2), 2-7, 30.

Hilliard, T., Dent, H., Hayes, W., Pierce, W., & Poussaint, A. (1974). The Angela Davis trial: Role of Black psychologist in jury selection and court consultations. *Journal of Black Psychology, 1,* 56-60.

Hixon, J., & Epps, E. (1975). The failure of selection and the problem of prediction: Racism vs. measurement in higher education. *Journal of Afro-American Issues, 3,* 117-128.

Jackson, A. (1979). Performance on convergent-divergent tasks by Black adolescents. In W. Smith, K. Burlew, M. Mosley, & W. Whitney (Eds.), *Reflections on Black psychology.* Washington, DC: University Press of America.

Jackson, G. (1972). The use of role playing job interviews with Job Corps females. *Journal of Employment Counseling, 9,* 130-139.

Jackson, G. (1976a). The African genesis of the Black perspective in helping. *Professional Psychology, 7,* 292-308.

Jackson, G. (1976b). Cultural seedbeds of the Black backlash in mental health. *Journal of Afro-American Issues, 4,* 70-91.

Jackson, G. (1976c). Is behavior therapy a threat to Black clients? *Journal of the National Medical Association, 68,* 362-367.

Jackson, G. (1977). The emergence of a Black perspective in counseling. *Journal of Negro Education, 46,* 230-253.

Jackson, G. (1979a). *Community mental health, behavior therapy, and the Afro-American community. Association of Advancement of Behavior Therapy Convention, Atlanta, GA, 1976. (ERIC Document Reproduction Service, No. Ed 159-501).*

Jackson, G. (1979b). The origin and development of Black psychology: Implications for Black studies and human behavior. *Studia Africana, 1,* 270-293.

Jackson, G. (1979c). The roots of the backlash theory in mental health. *Journal of Black Psychology, 6*(1), 17-45.

Jackson, G. (1982). Black psychology as an avenue to the study of Afro-American behavior. *Journal of Black Studies, 12,* 241-260.

Jackson, G. (1985). Cross-cultural counseling with Afro-Americans. In P. Pedersen (Ed.), *Handbook for cross-cultural counseling and therapy.* Westport, CT: Greenwood Press.

Johnson, S. (1972, December 18). Presidential memo. Association of non-White concerns. 1.

Jones, B., Lightfoot, O., Palmer, D., Wilkerson, R., & Williams, D. (1970). Black psychiatric residents in White training institutes. *American Journal of Psychiatry, 127,* 798-803.

Jones, M., & Jones, M. (1972). The neglected client. *Black Scholar, 1,* 35-42.

Jones, R. (Ed.). (1980). *Black Psychology* (2nd ed.). New York: Harper & Row.

Kochman, T. (1981). *Black and White styles in conflict.* Chicago: University of Chicago Press.

Kuhn, T. (1969). *The structure of scientific revolutions: Postscript* (2nd ed.). Chicago: University of Chicago Press.

Leff, J. (1975). "Exotic" treatments and Western psychiatry. *Psychological medicine, 5,* 125-128.

Levine, R., & Wolff, E. (1985, March). Social time: The heartbeat of culture. *Psychology Today,* 28-41.

McConahan, J., Hardee, B., & Batts, V. (1981). Has racism declined in America? *Journal of Conflict Resolution, 25*(4), 563-579.

Nelson, W. (1975). Review of *Beyond Black or White: An alternative America.* Contemporary Black Issues in Social Psychology. Washington, DC: E.C.C.A.

Pasteur, A., & Toldson, I. (1979). *Roots of soul: The psychology of black expressiveness.* New York: Doubleday.

Pierce, C. (1968). The need from Negro psychiatrists. *Journal of the National Medical Association, 60,* 30-33.

Pierce, C. (1970). Black psychiatry one year after Miami. *Journal of the National Medical Association, 62,* 471-473.

Pierce, W. (1972). The comprehensive community mental health programs and the Black community. In R. Jones (Ed.), *Black psychology.* New York: Harper & Row.

Pipes, W. (1981). Old-time religion: Benches can't say "amen." In H. McAdoo (Ed.), *Black families.* California: Sage.

Samuda, R. (1975). From ethnocentrism to a multi-cultural perspective in educational testing. *Journal of Afro-American Issues, 3*(1), 3-18.

Schachter, J., & Butts, H. (1968). Transference and countertransference in interracial analysis. *Journal of American Psychoanalytic Association, 16,* 792-808.

Sedlacek, W., & Brooks, G. (1973a). Racism and research: Using data to initiate change. *Personnel and Guidance Journal, 52,* 184-188.

Sedlacek, W., & Brooks, G. (1973b). Racism in the public schools: A model for change. *Journal of Non-White Concerns, 1,* 133-143.

Smitherman, G. (1973). White English in Blackface, or who do I be? *The Black Scholar, 4*(8-9), 32-39.

Taylor, H. (1975). Quantitative racism: A partial documentation. *Journal of Afro-American Issues, 3,* 19-42.

Thomas, A., & Sillen, S. (1972). *Racism and psychiatry.* New York: Brunner/Mazel.

Torrey, E. F. (1972a). What western psychotherapists can learn from witch-doctors. *American Journal of Orthopsychiatry, 42*(1), 69-76.

Torrey, E. F. (1972b). *The mind game.* New York: Emerson-Hall.

Torrey, E. F. (1974). *The death of psychiatry.* New York: Penguin.

Turner, J. (Ed.). (1985). *The next decade theoretical and research issues in Africana studies.* New York: Africana Studies and Research Center, Cornell University.

Williams, R. (1970). The Black professional's issues and tasks for the 70's. *Journal of Operational Psychiatry, 1,* 67-73.

Williams, R. (1974). The death of White research in the Black community. *Journal of Non-White Concerns, 2,* 116-132.

Williams, R. (1975a). *Ebonics: The true language of Black folks.* Missouri: Robert L. Williams and Associates.

Wiliams, R. (1975b). Moderator variables as bias in testing Black children. *Journal of Afro-American Issues, 2*(2), 53-60.

Willie, C., Kramer, B., & Brown, B. (Eds.). (1973). *Racism and mental health.* Pennsylvania: University of Pittsburgh.

Wispe, L., Ashe, P., Hickes, L., Hoffman, M., & Porter, J. (1969). The Negro psychologists in America. *American Psychologist, 24*(2), 142-150.

CHAPTER 8

A CULTURAL PERSPECTIVE FOR SERVING THE HISPANIC CLIENT

MERCEDES C. SANDOVAL and MARIA C. DE LA ROZA

Hispanic Presence in the U.S.A.

RECORDED HISTORY in the U.S.A. dawns in Spanish. The first Europeans to set foot and write about continental U.S.A. were Spanish-speakers. The Hispanic impact as explorers and settlers is widely reflected in the geographic names of vast areas, ranging from the Atlantic to the Pacific (Boca Raton, San Francisco); and from the Gulf of Mexico to Canada's frontiers (Pensacola, Mobile, Colorado, San Louis). Hispanics not only discovered, settled and founded the first cities in continental U.S.A. (St. Augustine and Sante Fe) but brought alongside the basic elements or foundations of western civilization. Thus, they greatly contributed to the economic (grain cultivation, livestock, metallurgy), social (acceptance of integrated relationships between Spaniards and Indians and greater assimilation of the latter), legal (Roman Law), and a multitude of other aspects of the so-called American experience. However, the contribution of Hispanics has been at best ignored. As voiced by Walt Whitman: "I have an idea that there is much of importance to the Latin contribution to the American nationality that will never be put in sympathetic understanding and tact on the record." Maybe this omission (official and unofficial) was at first caused by the legacy of centuries old rivalries between Spain and England; between Catholics and Protestants. This might have been exacerbated by Anglo racial supremacy ideation contrasted with Hispanic overt racial and cultural blending with American Indians and Blacks. The oversight undoubtedly was later fueled by American aggressive

151

geopolitical and commercial policies at the expense of their Hispanic neighbors. Whatever the reasons, historical reality has been denied and the many contributions of Hispanics to the American experience have not been properly recognized and much less reported. Unfortunately, today, in spite of current evidence of yet new contributions of Hispanics in all important areas of life, most Hispanics in the U.S.A. have not fully internalized the positive impact that their ancestors as well as their contemporary cultural peers have had in American society and thus, many still suffer from feelings of rejection and marginality.

Hispanics Today

The Hispanic population in the U.S.A. is presently increasing, in a disproportionate manner, if compared to other ethnic groups. This is caused by a high birth rate, as well as by increased immigration patterns of both legal and illegal Hispanics.[1] However, many estimates consider that Hispanics number approximately 23,000,000, if Puerto Ricans in the Island and illegal entrants are included. If the present trend were to continue, Hispanics will constitute the largest ethnic minority in this country by the twenty-first century.

In general, the living conditions and demographic profile of Hispanics are deplorable. Even though Hispanics constitute one of the youngest groups in the U.S.A. (42% of this population is below 20 years of age)[2] Hispanic children and youngsters attend substandard schools and exhibit the highest high school drop-out rate.[3] This situation is ever more serious if we consider the fact that Hispanics are significantly urban since 85% of this population are city residents. This is but symptomatic of the poverty-bounded situation of most Hispanics in this country.[4] Most Hispanics suffer from poor nutrition and inadequate housing caused and fostered by under and unemployment.[5] Furthermore, there is an alarming shortage of health care services accessible to Hispanics. Poor accessibility is related to underutilization of such services, which are only used in a fragmented fashion and crisis situations. Even though Hispanics' lives flow in endurance of high stress-producing situations, mental health care services are often either not available or at best inadequate.

Characteristics of Hispanics

Heterogeneity

A great diversity is exhibited among those various population segments which are labeled Hispanic. This heterogeneity is partly caused by differences in national origins. The largest nucleus, practically 60% of this population, is of either Mexican origin or descent. The U.S. Department of Commerce Bureau of the Census regards as persons of Hispanic origin or descent those who identify themselves as being Cuban, Chicano, Mexican, Mexican American, Puerto Rican or other Spanish/Hispanic.

Cubans number well over 1,000,000 and are primarily concentrated in Dade County, Florida, New Jersey and New York. Other Hispanics are either descendants or originally from Central and South America as well as Spain. The diversity manifested by Hispanics due to differences in national origin entails different cultural and historical experiences, stressors and resources, resulting in different adaptive strategies.

Hispanics also manifest great heterogeneity due to variation in racial background and mixture. The Hispanic color spectrum includes mixtures of Mediterranean Caucosoids with Amerindian and African genes which have produced a highly colorful palette. The great diversity to be found among Hispanics is also accentuated by the differences caused by socioeconomic background, and by the fact that many are from rural extraction while others came to the U.S.A. well equipped with urban skills.

Yet another variable which has affected the status, self-concept and success of Hispanics in the U.S.A. and which has contributed to heterogeneity, has been the conditions in which they found themselves when they encountered mainstream America. There are great differences in the types of acculturative shock experienced by those early displaced Mexicans, victims of the great expansionary policies of the U.S.A. during the last century; the shock of conquered Puerto Ricans; and the reactions of the officially welcomed Cubans who were fleeing communist tyranny. Again, there are also great differences in the chances for positive acculturation between an immigrant of professional background and an illegal migrant.

Common Characteristics

It is very difficult to identify the various cultural traits that make up the elusive and complex concept of being Hispanic. The most obvious and salient of those common denominators is the use of the Spanish language. Spanish is today by far the most commonly spoken language outside of English in the U.S.A. There are at least 13 T.V. and 18 radio stations as well as many newspaper networks catering to the Spanish audience. The tenacity with which Spanish clings in the American experience has resulted in the existence of many bilingual programs in different school systems in the U.S.A. These do not adequately meet the needs of youngsters born in this country who still retain their mother tongue as their primary means of communication. Linguistic differences among Spanish speakers are not profound, since all regional Spanish expressions only attest to the symbolic integration and assimilation of a rich variety of folkloric experiences, which never impairs communication. However, in spite of its importance, the Spanish language is not a universal one since many people who have a Spanish surname and are of clear Hispanic descent do not master the language.

On the other hand, Hispanics, regardless of their national, racial and social background, have in common a very strong family orientation. The important place that the family plays in the lives of Hispanics clearly overrides the importance of, loyalty to, and participation in other institutions most cherished by White Americans, such as the community schools, churches and clubs. The Hispanic family is an expanded network reaching out to relatives, in-laws and "friends of the family," involving its members in mutually supportive relationships of interdependence. This extended family offers its members economic and emotional support and enculturation assistance. It also provides great opportunities for social interaction and partially caters to the health care needs of the ill and the old.

Among Hispanics, personalism, which is probably derived from the strong family orientation, is also very prevalent. Personalism is a need to relate in personal terms in a warm-emotional fashion; a need to trust people. Conversely, it also entails ignoring and avoiding impersonal relations and situations, distrusting institutions, laws and expertise which might be too abstract. Due to personalism, individuals are assessed according to their behavior with family and friends and not just according to professional and public performances. Personalism is behind strong feelings of attachment and commitment to family and friends. Personalism is at the base of the perception that life is nothing but a flow of interactions with other people, and that those interactions are the ones which can make it full and meaningful or empty. Personalism might be manifested in a fashion that people from other cultures may consider overtly subjective emotional and sentimental behaviors. Personalism places great demands on Hispanics' use of their time as well as encroachments on their privacy. On the other hand, this philosophical stance facilitates caring relationships.

Closely related to the personalistic orientation is humanism. This is a condition, mode of thought or action in which human interests, value and dignity predominate as factors determining human behavior, at the expense of institutions, legalities, and the like.

Individualism, Spanish style, is the manifestation of the assertion and acceptance of one's Being, of one's self-worth, of one's uniqueness. Individualism entails the perception that one is special to either a mother, father, wife, children, household, friends, etc. Individualism means that, at least in certain grounds, one has no substitute, one is unique and important. This strong value orientation is very early enculturated in the young by the parents who repeatedly tell their offspring about the unique place they occupy in their lives. Individualism claims that others, if they love you, should accept you the way you are. Individualism, however, does not necessarily entail strong self-interest as directive of behavior. On the contrary, the acceptance and advocacy of one's Being is an unconditional manner surprisingly causes tolerance towards others' self-assertiveness.

Authoritarianism, the condition that favors compliance to that authority which is legitimized by the family and the personal context, is also found among Hispanics. Authoritarianism fosters the acceptance of advice and directives by parents, teachers, relatives and significant others. However, authoritarianism Hispanic style does not include the acceptance of or submission to directives of official authorities (police, government officials). On the contrary, impersonal authoritarian figures and directives can and are challenged by Hispanics. This is due to what can be described as Hispanic selective compliance with the law, which viewed as impersonal, is not deemed as essentially respectable or acceptable. This orientation is linked to Hispanics' perception of rules as general guidelines which can and should be changed, and to which exceptions are expected, when other more important priorities like family or an individual's self-worth are at stake.

Paternalism is also a very prominent cultural characteristic of Hispanics. It is a condition which entails the perception that people in authority should manage and deal with subordinates in a manner similar to that of a father dealing with his children. Paternalism can be manifested in authoritarian yet caring and committed directives, which are accepted in those terms.

Another cultural trait characteristic of Hispanics is machismo. Traditionally machismo could be translated as a superlative of masculinity.

Not all the traits generally associated with machismo are homogenously found in each of its manifestations. Yet, machismo clearly delineates the role of the male as the decision-maker and leader of the family. The female, as his complement, should be non-assertive, somehow passive, and even submissive. If these roles are compromised, it has to be in a way in which the authority of the macho, as head of the family and his status as breadwinner, is not challenged.

Machismo, in its positive manifestations, entails trustworthiness, moral courage, responsibility and honor. In its popular, lower class manifestations, the worth of the machista is dependent on his masculinity, which needs constant ratification by other males. These machos are tough, with an aggressive sense of pride and a tendency towards violence. They are daring towards other men and towards women, exercising control by emotional displays of aggressive behavior (shouting, yelling, throwing objects, quarreling). In some instances excessive gambling, wasteful spending, use of alcohol and even drugs are part of the macho behavior repertoire.

One of the more salient characteristics of machismo is the belief that a man, to be a whole male, has to have many sexual conquests, even if married. Nevertheless, and incongruently so, these males, who ascertain their masculinity at the expense of the honor of females of other families, are required to protect the virtue of the women of their family. Machos are acutely sensitive to shame, and have great concerns for the opinion of their male peers concerning their behavior and that of the females in their family.

Machos should not allow other men to intimidate them. Yet, in spite of the fact that machismo precludes the notion that there could be another man better than oneself, in reality it foster subjugation to a strong man. This contradiction is responsible for the following and admiration that caudillos (strong men) have elicited in Latin America.

In congruence with the strong family orientation, with paternalism and authoritarianism, there is, among many Hispanics, an exaggerated version and emphasis on Respect. It is manifested as unabashed deference to people in authority and to coequals who are not personally close.

Another philosophical orientation, which is commonly found among Hispanics, is Fatalism. The acceptance of fate, of things that cannot be changed, in some instances causes the perception that life is nothing but a challenge to be met by endurance. Fatalism does not necessarily entail a negative perception of life but rather the acceptance of human frailty and limitations. Concurrent with fatalism and complementing it is the prevalent belief in the manifestation of luck as an unpredictable force which actively interferes in human life. The fatalistic stance and unabashed belief in luck are but manifestations of a mystical personalistic worldview which is prevalent in the Hispanic culture. This mysticism presupposes the existence of supernatural forces which willingly interfere in human affairs. In many instances, mysticism among Hispanics has not been appropriately channeled through the Catholic religion — to which officially most Hispanics are affiliated — or through other Protestant denominations, which many of them are increasingly joining. On the contrary, and probably due to the fact that the Hispanic experience in the Americas has been one of merging, syncretizing and amalgamating with other cultural experiences, Hispanics generally do not hesitate to deal, worship and communicate with other unworldly entities and forces, even when such transactions are not sanctioned by the church of their preference. The mystical view of the universe fosters the attempts to engage these forces in an active fashion on behalf of the individual.

Finally, a thorough consideration of value orientation is needed before emphasis is placed on the unique characteristics of Hispanics in relation to mental health services. There are great differences in value orientation between mainstream America and the Hispanic population of the U.S.A. Values affect a society's worldview, existential philosophy and meanings as well as life expectations. Kluckhohn and Strodtbeck (1961) developed a theory on how value orientations influence normative behavior. They identified five universal problems which confront all societies and people and for which solutions need to be provided within a limited range of variations. A society's preference for a given solution — dominant value orientation — does not however, preclude the presence of variant solutions of values seen as essential to well-being. The problems identified by Kluckhohn and Strodtbeck are: (a) the temporal focus of life, (b) the relations of man to nature and supernature, (c) the form of man's relations to other men, (d) the modality of human activity, and (e) the character of innate human nature.[6]

In reference to the **Time orientation** or the temporal focus of life, societies appraise the importance of behavior in terms of either maintaining Past traditions, considering Future repercussions, or resolving Present problems.

Mainstream White America is generally Future oriented. This society is characterized by a youth, change, and long-range planning orientation. Experience and living for today is neglected at the expense of having control over the future. Part of the American experience is buying educational insurance for the newly born, and quite morbidly, buying a plot in the cemetary and paying for one's own funeral while still alive. In contrast, generally, Hispanic societies have shown a pronounced preference for the Present orientation. Concern for the here and now, with some regard for the past experience, override obsessive preoccupation with what is viewed as the uncertain future.

The **Man-Nature orientation** refers to a society's perception of its relationships with nature, super-nature, and with the social environment. In those societies where the subjugation orientation prevails people see themselves as helpless in the face of natural and super-natural forces. An acceptance of these overpowering forces causes a fatalistic posture and the prevalent belief in luck. In societies where nature is perceived as ordered by laws and principles which can be explained by science and harnessed by technology, humans perceive themselves as capable of mastering and controlling their relationships with it. Hispanics, in general, have manifested a preference toward the subjugation orientation. This subjugation orientation is manifested by a prevalent belief in curses, a mystical world view and a fatalistic acceptance of destiny. It also causes an exaggerated reliance on luck to explain unusual occurrences, the resorting to wishful thinking when in situations of lack of control. This orientation is verbalized in idiomatic expressions such as **"escupir para el cielo"** (to spit to heaven), which reflects the fear that a strong self-assertive stand might cause super-natural retaliation. A similar world-view is expressed in **"nunca digas de esta agua no bebere"** (never say I won't drink from this water). A too self-assertive stand might elicit super-natural retaliation which will force you to do exactly what you assertively thought you would never do.

A manifestation of the subjugation orientation can be seen in the social acceptance of man's lack of control over emotions. Phrases abound in Spanish expressing these situations. **"El no se pudo contener"** (he couldn't control himself), **"Le dio un ataque de rabia"** (he had a rabies attack, to mean, he had a fit of rage). Uncontrollable display of emotions, even rage, are captured in these idiomatic expressions.

White-American middle class preference is for mastery over nature. In this society, science and technology are emphasized at the expense of the arts and humanities. The behavioral sciences not too successfully attempt to use the rigorous scientific methods of the natural sciences, in mostly unfruitful attempts to predict human behavior, instead of just accepting and understanding its complexity.

The **Relational orientation** deals with the nature of a person's relations with other people. In societies which are Lineal oriented, authority is highly valued and it is conceptualized as flowing in a vertical hierarchical scheme. In those societies with a Collateral orientation people relate to others following a horizontal network and on a basis of inter-dependency. The Individualistic orientation leads people to relate to others according to the priorities of their own interests in an autonomous fashion disregarding vertical and lateral frames.

In most Hispanic societies, the lineal orientation is preferred; **"donde manda capitan, no manda marinero"** (where there is a captain the sailor has no voice). However, this orientation is tempered by strong collateral support systems and network. In White-American middle class society the individualistic orientation prevails. This entails the individual's reponsibility for its own life which should be realized in an independent fashion.

The **Activity orientation** deals with the way a society evaluates and perceives behavior according to the manner in which it is manifested. Those societies which are Doing oriented value the use of time engaged in activities with measurable outcomes. On the other hand, societies which are Being oriented highly value behavior which is expressive of an individual's existential yearnings. Hispanic societies generally have shown a preference towards the Being orientation. This is a reflection of Hispanic-style individualism and inner self-assertiveness: **"Yo soy el rey di mi casa"** (I am the king in my house), **"Yo soy como soy"** (I am the way I am — also meaning I'm not going to change). This orientation impacts Hispanic perception of personality as fixed, practically immutable, and deserving of acceptance and respect, unless manifesting blatant anti-social behavior.

The White American middle class generally has shown a preference for the Doing orientation. People are assessed according to what they accomplish rather than what they are in essence.

The **Human Nature orientation** expresses how society perceives human qualities in terms of essential goodness, evilness or a combination of both. Those societies which perceive human beings as innately Good have a positivistic, optimistic view of human nature, in spite of its being susceptible to corruption triggered by society's forces. Those societies which are Evil oriented see man as essentially Evil-but-perfectible. In societies which are Neutral oriented man is perceived as neither Good nor Evil but as highly susceptible to good and evil according to the circumstances. Hispanics and many of the Mediterranean societies have preferred the latter orientation. This is expressed in an ambivalent perception of human nature — full of conflict — but capable of equilibrium. This is also apparent in the acceptance of human vulnerability and mortality and the frailty of human nature. This causes more leniency and tolerance, at least in appearance, of other people's behavior. Expressions such as **"Ay! Que Dios no me castigue"** (Oh! I hope God doesn't punish me), following negative remarks about somebody else, express the need for the speakers to at least verbally place themselves in somebody else's shoes. (See Sandoval, 1985, for a description of differences in value orientation between Mariel arrivals and earlier Cuban immigrants.)

Barriers to the Utilization of Mental Health Services

It has been generally ascertained that certain geographic, economic and cultural barriers have curtailed the utilization of mental health services by Hispanics (Becerra, Karno, & Escobar, 1982; Ruiz & Alvarez, 1975). One of the reasons why Hispanics do not utilize these services is that, in most instances, they are offered far from the Hispanic ethnic enclave. Impoverished Hispanics lacking adequate means of transportation are discouraged from profiting from available but not too accessible services. On the other hand, economic constraints might negatively affect their ability to fully utilize these services when available and accessible. For instance, since many Hispanics only have temporary employment they do not enjoy fringe benefits such as insurance plans, sick leave, etc., which would allow them to be covered or absent from employment without penalty.

Furthermore, there are several culturally-related factors that interfere with Hispanics receiving adequate mental health care. The linguistic barrier in many instances is unsurmountable (Marcos, Urcuyo, Kesselman, & Alpert, 1973; Ruiz, 1982). Unfortunately, the number of trained mental health professionals who are competent in Spanish is very limited, and thus, the accessibility of services to monolingual Hispanics is greatly impaired. On the other hand, the use of interpreters is limited, and the inadequacy, in most instances, is appalling (Marcos, 1979). Even when trained interpreters are used, an inhibiting distance between client and therapist is established which causes misinterpretations and misdiagnosis and erodes the trust which is basic in a therapeutic relationship. Furthermore, research seems to indicate that intimate matters are better expressed in the mother tongue (Marcos, Urcuyo, Kesselman, & Alpert, 1973). When bilingual Hispanics are interviewed in English they are placed in situations of greater stress by cross-cultural, cross-language factors which can affect the therapist's perception of the client's mental status (Marcos & Alpert, 1976). Furthermore, as the patient is expected to communicate in the language in which he feels less competent, the therapist will be missing the full impact of the verbal communication and also the patient's non-verbal cues.

Cultural differences in perceptions of health and illness, etiology and treatment, are also reasons why Hispanics do not adequately use mental health services. Cultural interpretations of symptoms can lead a Hispanic to seek help from a medical doctor instead of a mental health professional. This might result in inadequate treatment or no treatment at all (psychosomatic illness). In many other instances, and within their cultural context, a Hispanic might attribute his symptoms to supernatural causation and will seek relief from indigenous healers (see Garrison, 1977; Ruiz & Langrod, 1976; Sandoval, 1977, 1979). Yet in other instances the potential client's unfamiliarity with mental health services will render him incapable of seeking appropriate help.

Cultural differences in personality perceptions might render therapeutic modalities as useless. Hispanic perception of personality in general is that of a fixed entity. This leaves little room for therapeutic modalities that solely deal in intrapsychic process and are aimed at promoting personality change, growth and awareness. Cultural differences which affect expectations concerning therapeutic outcome may render the services as irrelevant (Acosta, Yamamoto, & Evans, 1982). The therapist might be seeking to assist the client in effecting a great change in his life while the client is only seeking help to alleviate and adjust to the surrounding conditions affecting him.

The Ethnic Team Approach

There is a scarcity of mental health services available to Hispanics and great cultural barriers which impede the utilization of such services even when available and accessible to Hispanics and to other ethnic clients. For these reasons, there is a need to design models and strategies which would overcome barriers and facilitate the cultural appropriateness as well as accessibility of mental health services. One very successful model was designed by the Department of Psychiatry of the University of Miami (Lefley & Bestman, 1984; Weidman, 1983). This model was based on ethnic teams directed by a behavioral scientist or "culture broker" (Weidman, 1973), clinicians, psychiatrists and mental health workers of the same ethnicity as the population being served. The members of the team as cultural specialists engaged in different activities geared to promote mental health and to reduce stressors, as well as in treating the clients. The ethnic teams developed a useful data base through action oriented research and needs assessments. They were able to gather a pool of information and supportive documentation to be used by community agencies when planning and programming for these ethnic enclaves. This collective culture brokerage function is aimed at promoting programs and services that are consonant with the life styles and social reality of the ethnic group being served. This primary intervention is aimed at enhancing the social environment and promoting conditions which are conducive to good coping capabilities, and at changing those which impair them. This role of the ethnic team, effecting linkages between needy populations and appropriate resources, including the established power hierarchy, is that of an agent of social change and advocacy for those alienated from the mainstream of society. It includes consultation and training of professionals, public officials and community leaders on cultural variables of the population they represent. It also includes mediation and negotiation with potencial resources in the development of preventive programs which would enhance the coping capabilities of the community residents. It might also entail assisting in organizing community residents to promote their participation in community planning and decision making. This function also includes referral services on clients and information about the availability of community resources.

In addition, the ethnic team approach addresses the need for direct services. One of the ethnic teams developed by the University of Miami/ Jackson Memorial Hospital Community Mental Health Services was "La Norguesera" Mini-Clinic at the Cuban Unit in the Allapatah neighborhood in Miami (Sandoval & Tozo, 1975). At this mini-clinic, clients were offered diagnosis and treatment within their own ethnic enclave and in their native tongue. It was organized as a drop-in center where the emotionally upset and the mentally ill were offered recreation, psychotherapy, medical follow-up and ample opportunities for social interaction. The atmosphere was casual and like that of a social club. The professional and paraprofessional staff effected the therapeutic interventions aimed at client rehabilitation in the community without referral to outside agencies. In this model the clinician was responsible for the clients' initial evaluation, referring them for further diagnosis and/or treatment, including psychotherapy for those clients who would benefit from this treatment modality; for in-service training; and for clinical supervision of the paraprofessional staff. In turn these paraprofessional cultural specialists functioned as the front-line therapeutic team who offered clients support and assistance but did not become embroiled with clients' intrapsychic processes. This psychosocial model delivered cost effective services particularly to the chronically mentally ill, while also meeting the needs of less severe cases. The author feels that the ethnic team approach is an excellent model for the delivery of mental health services, not only to Hispanics, but to other ethnic minorities, since services are rendered within the ethnic enclave and are delivered in a culturally consonant fashion. The ethnic team services include mediation, interpretation, brokerage, and training, as well as treatment. On the other hand, the ethnic team is capable of designing specific clinical strategies which respond to the cultural characteristics and value orientation of the client.

The author observed that the Cuban ethnic team incorporated several clinical strategies which responded to Hispanic cultural characteristics and value orientation and which, in some instances, would not have been considered acceptable by White American mental health professionals. Some of these strategies were not purposely adopted but emerged as commonsensical and most effective, even when causing the trained mental health professional some discomfort and dissonance with their disciplinary training. In many cases what seemed the "natural" (culturally consonant) way of dealing with a client escaped conceptualization or open verbalization. Trained Hispanic therapists often were not aware of their deviation from standard clinical procedures. However, consciousness of this denial occurred when they were confronted with the cultural values which had elicited the change in clinical practices.

Hispanic Cultural Characteristics and Their Clinical Implications

The authors feel that a recollection of how the most salient characteristics of Hispanics affected treatment strategies at the Cuban team could give valuable cues to clinicians dealing with Hispanic clients. It is necessary to point out that these strategies responded to the needs of a specific Hispanic group: the Cubans in Dade County, who, in many ways, are unlike other Hispanics in the U.S.A. However, the examples given may be generalizable in terms of some of the modal characteristics previously discussed.

In our experience with Hispanics, we have found that, in general, they are skeptical about the validity of some of the findings and techniques of psychology, as well as the efficacy of psychotherapy. Even among those who accept the control of Nature by man's science, there is a prevalent disbelief in the ability of the behavioral sciences to come up with final answers concerning human behavior.

In the cultural context of the Hispanic client, life and man are perceived as very complex, mostly because they are affected by a multiplicity of factors beyond anyone's control. This perception warrants multiple strategies to manipulate as best as possible the factors involved in a situation. This is why, when confronted with a problem or task, Hispanics look for the way to **"darle la vuelta"** (turn around the factors involved). On the other hand, mainstream Americans generally, following their Control and Mastery orientation, tend to look at how to "handle" the problem or task. This latter approach perhaps may enhance the role or status of psychotherapy as a means of placing a problem under one's control. Among Hispanics, since life is perceived as very complex primarily because it is lived with others, therapy, when accepted, is perceived as one of the many things that can help. Psychotherapy, then, is viewed as a means to assist the individual adjust to his reality, to bring some balance to life and not as a means to bring about drastic changes in one's lifestyle. Thus, therapeutic modalities which entail changes in vital philosophy are generally suspect and not very well accepted. Furthermore, some of the techniques used by some therapeutic models such as sensitivity training and confrontation are perceived as non-effective and as somehow dangerous tricks and games which turn them off.

If we are to consider the complex social ambiance of the Hispanic client it would appear that the use of an eclectic approach to the therapeutic process is recommendable. Furthermore, it is safe to say that a psychosocial approach should always complement an intrapsychic intervention.

The Family

The strong family orientation would indicate that family therapy is the ideal treatment modality to deal with the Hispanic client. However, family therapy as understood in American clinical culture would face serious problems and be subject to great modifications, since family for the Hispanic could entail the extended version of family rather than the nuclear concept prevalent in mainstream America. Besides, very likely, the therapist might be faced with the refusal of some key members to participate, especially the males. On the other hand, since the client basically perceives and accepts himself as a person with an essential status and role within a family, the counselor needs to continuously assess and deal with the influence of family members on the client. The counselor has to assist the client in developing more appropriate ways to handle/ interact with them. Moreover, the therapist should help the client maintain the collateral network of support (Escobar & Randolph, 1982). In other words the therapist needs to accept the family as both the most important support system of the client and probably also his greatest sources of stress. The therapist should turn into a family broker even when not exposed to all the family members, and should use his expertise to enhance the positive aspects and ameliorate the negative ones. The following is an example of such brokerage (or single person family therapy) in a clinical case history:

> Carmen is a 27-year-old Cuban female, married with no children, who came to therapy complaining of feelings of sadness and lack of fulfillment. She felt that her marital relationship was deteriorating. Carmen explained that she was an only child who had come to the U.S.A. when she was eleven with her divorced mother. Carmen met a 21-year-old man who later became her husband when she was 18. Unfortunately her mother died one year after Carmen got married. At the death of her mother, Carmen's husband and his family because "everything she had." However, Carmen felt very ambivalent. She really enjoyed her husband's relatives. She loved them, but she felt that she and her husband never had time for themselves. It was difficult for her to understand why her husband had to get involved as mediator in a father/son conflict when the teenage son of one of his cousins threatened to drop out of school. Yet, Carmen's husband felt that the role he played was part of his responsibilities toward his family. Confronting her husband regarding his assuming responsibilities she considered excessive and irrelevant would certainly damage their relationship. Besides, she did not want to risk breaking with them either. She viewed her mother-in-law as a great source of support for her. The most viable alternative for Carmen to deal with the situation was to "darle la vuelta" (go around it). In other words, to find a compromise. It was suggested by the therapist that Carmen and her husband arrange for short weekend trips as well as longer vacations alone. Thus, the pressure resulting from interacting with other family members would be regularly, though temporarily, alleviated. The therapist became a family broker. While maintaining the extended family ties, Carmen and her husband would secure some private time of their own.

Therapeutic modalities which emphasize the achievement of self-fulfillment and realization, sometimes at the cost of separation from the family and the loss of interdependence, may run contrary to the Hispanic ideal of a familial network of support and interdependence. On many occasions the authors confronted the rejection of therapists by clients who felt that the therapist's insistence on them "doing their own thing" was a reflection of selfishness and an unacceptable egocentric stance. Furthermore, they were fearful of the repercussions of what they perceived as excessive self-assertiveness: being left alone in the world and even incurring retaliation by supernatural forces. For instance, it might be appropriate for a White American client to contemplate leaving his parent's home to assert his independence. It might also be appropriate to remove an aging parent whose demands are in conflict with one's lifestyle. When a therapist explores these alternatives with a Hispanic client, other variables come into play. Generally, the guilt ridden client wants the therapist to assist him in dealing in a more satisfying fashion with the domineering or overburdening parent. Normally, the Hispanic client is willing to try and engage in small changes (compromises) which might make stressful situations more bearable (adding a studio apartment to a single family unit might take care of a young adult's need for independence as well as an aging parent's need for support) (Szapocznik, 1978). In other words, generally, Hispanics view life in the context of interpersonal relationships and they accept conflict as part of the latter. The studio apartment alternative ameliorates conflict while preserving interdependence. Thus, the Hispanic client normally accepts his own need to depend on others and conversely others' dependence on him.

Generally, Hispanic parents lengthen the dependency period of their children way after the legal age. It is acknowledged that emotional and physical maturity doesn't occur at the same time or at the same age for every individual. The Mastery and Control orientation influences mainstream Americans into standardizing versus individualizing situations, qualities, and even development. This is a culture where tests have long been used to measure an entity as complex as intelligence and/or achievement. Even beauty in the U.S.A. has standard measures.

Thus, it is accepted by many that is is very useful and even necessary for teenagers to leave home at eighteen. It is felt that "doing their thing on their own" enhances their chances of maturing and becoming responsible (for their own lives). Little regard is given to whether the individual is ready to do so, and whether that will make the person happier or whether leaving home might precipitate overdependency on alcohol, drugs, unworthy peers, mates, or counselors. On the contrary, Hispanics feel that the process of maturity is a lifelong process which cannot be fully arrived at in the early years of adulthood. Furthermore, they feel that the need for even more emotional support from parents is not necessarily a sign of immaturity. It is only natural for one to depend on those who care for you and it will only be natural for you to care for them when they need you. On the other hand, and maybe due to their neutral orientation, viewing the essence of Human Nature as neither Good or Evil but susceptible to circumstances, Hispanic parents always try to "avoid" situations which could be potentially dangerous (a young adult being by himself without the care of his parents). They feel that total independence is a folly since people who care for each other are always dependent on each other regardless of age. The Hispanic client, aware of the complexity of his social context, is willing to accept a multiplicity of roles as father, son, nephew, friend, with the multiple responsibilities it might entail.

Extended family and interdependent network orientation is behind the Hispanic father's often loud and obvious supervision of young children. In grocery stores and other public places the mother is not inhibited from shouting directives to the young children to constantly remind them — even when engaged in no mischief — that her inquiring but protective eyes are on them. These displays are meant to say **"Estoy arriba de ti"** (I am on top of you watching and protecting you constantly). By loudly verbalizing their directives they also mean to engage others in the social control of their children, seeking a sort of consensus protection. [If I (the mother) were to see other children getting into trouble I would tend to them as if they were my own.]

Personalism

Hispanic culture's pronounced personalistic orientation permeates the whole realm of interpersonal relations and, of necessity, greatly impacts mental health service delivery. From the very start, when choosing a therapist, Hispanics will generally select an individual with very good personal references, rather than one with impressive professional credentials and/or a display of expensive office furnishings. In other words, the human quality of the therapist normally will outweigh academic credentials because Hispanics do not fully trust the efficacy of psychological training or of psychotherapy.

The Hispanic, not unlike other non-Hispanic clients, expects to build a relationship of trust and affection with the therapist. However, unlike other clients, for the Hispanic it is absolutely essential. Furthermore, the emphasis that Hispanic life style places on the importance and the intensity of human interaction, causes Hispanics to be quite sensitive in detecting the differences between professional warmth and support acquired through mastery of skills and techniques vs. the legitimate empathy and compassion expressed as the result of extensive experience with many close relationships.

When a Hispanic starts a therapeutic relationship, it will generally be quite evident that he has a need for the therapist to relate to him in personal terms, since it is the only way he — the client — knows how to relate. Thus, the personalistic orientation implies a high level of familiarity which normally develops as a result of the client expressing concern about the therapist's well being and that of his family. Personalism also implies that the therapist may be expected to do a certain amount of self-disclosure concerning non-conflicting or non-intimate aspects of his life. Self-disclosure allows the client to better assess the therapist as a person and enables the development of a necessary level of trust and confidence. It is also common for the therapist and client to identify commonalities shared, such as favorite foods, music, hobbies. This process of disclosure and discovery intensifies the closeness, identification and personal relationship necessary for a positive therapeutic interaction. An example of this is found in the following case:

> Gerardo, a 36-year-old male, Mariel Cuban, charged with loitering, was found to be in need of mental health services and was referred to the Community Mental Health Center. At intake, the client claimed that he did not need the services. He was not cooperative and the task of eliciting any answers was practically impossible. The client was getting increasingly restless and the therapist was about to give up, when it became apparent that both were originally from the same hometown. The therapist began to share information about her childhood and adolescence, such as street address and the name of the school she had attended while growing up. Slowly the client began to get involved in a conversation about the hometown which evolved into the questions required for a psychosocial intake interview. The client no longer perceived the therapist as an intruder because they had shared similar experiences while growing up. The relationship became more personal. He was helped to break his own resistance by the therapist's self-disclosure.

When dealing with the Hispanic client it is not uncommon that, in some instances, compliance with treatment is conditioned upon the established personal relationship between client and therapist. The client expects the therapist to have a personal commitment to him and, conversely, he feels that he should also reciprocate and be committed to the therapist. This is based on the acceptance, by both, of their human condition and that the therapeutic relationship is a contractual relationship in which both have an investment: a human commitment. It is understood that the therapist's regard for the client has limitations. Since the client values the therapist he cannot afford to let him down and risk losing his regard. Many times the authors have heard this situation voiced in the words of a therapist to a client: **"Tomate las medicinas; hazlo por mi"** (Take your medicine, do it on my account) and the response of the client: **"Yo no le voy a fallar"** (I won't fail you).

In the American clinical culture, generally, the motivation behind a client's offering a present to the therapist is highly questioned. The therapist is expected to assess whether the client's motivation is manipulation, which could negatively impact the therapeutic relationship. In the Hispanic cultural context, sharing is a manifestation of generosity which enhances networking and inter-dependence. In a normal, non-clinical situation, Hispanics are expected to offer other individuals, even when known only casually or not acquainted at all, cigarettes, coffee, etc. Consequently, they also learn to graciously accept other people's offerings even when not desired. A Hispanic client's present to a therapist doesn't necessarily have to be a manipulation, but more than likely, an expression of gratitude and generosity. If not accepted, the client's feelings of self worth may be hurt and distance would replace closeness. Thus, the refusal to accept the present, even though appropriate in mainstream America clinical practices, is outside the Hispanic cultural context. However, sensitivity to his manifestation of the personalistic orientation should not preclude a therapist from exploring possible manipulative motivation on the part of a particular client.

The personalistic orientation also enhances the value of emotional interaction and display vs. control and mastery of feelings. In the Hispanic cultural context, the expression of emotions is accepted, more so, therefore, in a therapeutic relationship. Moreover, expressions of empathy and compassion toward the client are expected, since the client perceives himself in a subordinated, needy position vis a vis the protective, authoritarian position of the therapist.

Individualism

As already discussed, individualism Hispanic style is very different from American individualism. American individualism is highly competitive as if one's self is measured in comparison to others. In many instances, individualism is understood as one's ability to obtain economic and professional success, if possible, without other people's assistance. Among Hispanics, individualism entails the acceptance that each person **"tiene sus cosas"** (has his own individual peculiarities). Hispanic individualism might cause conflict but not necessarily competition. The reason is that an individual's peculiarities can be manifested in many different ways, rather than in measurable economic or professional success. Since every person has his own peculiarities there is a need to be tolerant, acknowledging the possibility that almost every one has something to offer; that each personality has some worthy characteristic. This individualistic orientation leans towards compensation. A popular idiomatic expression, **"Soy feo pero simpatico"** (I am ugly, but engaging), says it all. In other words, there is always something nice about a person which might be of help, assistance or complement to somebody else, as expressed by: **"Siempre hay un roto para un descosido"** (There is always one more tear in an already ripped cloth). In many ways interdependent networking makes good use of the compensation aspect of individualism: "My Aunt Maria has no professional/job skills, but she is an excellent mother; thus, I will use her to babysit my children." In that fashion everybody profits; the children get her loving care, she gets extra money, and I am at ease because my children are well taken care of.

Individualism in a therapeutic relationship can negatively impact the process. There might be obstinance and resistance on the part of the client to disclose and/or change. This is because individualism biases the perception of personality as a self-contained, complex entity, which has many different traits, but which is not likely to change. This is manifested in a stance such as, "The therapist is not going to tell me what to do, because I know best who I am and what is best for me." The therapist, when encountering this situation, has to overtly accept a client's peculiarities, specially those which the client is more aware of and openly brags about. The therapist needs, in many instances, to avoid direct confrontation with the client and assist him in realizing small changes, even though it means "giving in" on occasions. An accepting psychoeducational approach can have salutary long-term consequences.

Julio, a 23-year-old male, was referred by the court to the community mental health center for residential treatment service. He had been picked up by the police because he was wandering on the streets. He had resisted arrest and was charged with assault and battery on a police officer. During the first therapy session, Julio volunteered that he had experienced a similar incident in Cuba which had also prompted referral for psychiatric treatment. Julio complained and claimed that he could not understand how he would be involved in an incident with the police in the U.S.A., a free country, just as he had been in Cuba. He said he felt despondent because he could not help being the way he was. He simply thought of himself as a person who could not stand "being bossed around or being taken advantage of" by anybody. These characteristics of his personality, he thought, were the reasons why he would get into trouble. Julio felt that neither the psychiatric treatment nor the medication would help him since basic personality traits are unchangeable. He expressed his feelings concerning the belief that the effects of "a few beers" didn't have much to do with his rebellious behavior.

Julio's situation, however, was desperate. He was unemployed; his wife had deserted him; his aunt didn't want him to stay at her home; he had no friends. He was very depressed and was bitterly complaining that nobody loved or cared for him; instead, people rejected him. He felt that if people really loved him they would accept him "the way he was."

The therapist's strategy was to sensitize the client to the fact that some of his antisocial behavior was not necessarily an intrinsic part of his personality. The therapist also assisted the client in realizing the consequences that erratic behavior could bring and had actually brought him, plus stressing that there were many aspects of his behavior that he could control. He was made aware of the ways in which, under the influence of alcohol, he would become verbally and physically abusive and the terrible consequences this brought to his family life. He was enabled to accept that, in many instances, his disruptive behavior was symptomatic of mental distress which could be ameliorated by medication. The client was able to internalize that the medication could assist him in controlling behavior that he had considered intrinsically idiosyncratic and unchangeable.

He realized that when he was anxious he became irritable and that without proper medication he could engage in behavior which brought him terrible consequences such as getting into a heated argument at work and quitting without giving a fair warning. The internalization by the client of the possibility of his gaining mastery of his behavior by controlling his use of alcohol and by taking his medication permitted Julio to realize that there were many aspects of his life that he could change. After several months Julio left the residential component and went to live on his own. He is still receiving therapy on an outpatient basis. Nowadays, he has a full time job and is involved in a satisfactory live-in relationship with a woman with whom he has a two-month-old daughter.

Authoritarianism and Paternalism

It has been discussed already that authoritarianism is an important trait of the Hispanic culture. However, in the personalistic context of this culture, authority, to be legitimized, has to be in compliance with personal qualities or relationships rather than with impersonal institutions or official legal directives. Thus, a therapist, in order to validate his role, has to demonstrate his sound personal qualities and his commitment.

Therapists have to learn to deal with the authoritarianism of their clients as well as that of significant others. Legitimized authority is best left without challenge. One of the ways to handle authoritarianism is to either persuade or cue the authoritarian persons to assume attitudes and behavior which do not really emanate from them, as if they had actually initiated them.

> Lourdes, a 13-year-old female, was brought to the center by her 70-year-old father. The father pleaded to the therapist to try to "bring some sense to this kid." The initial interview yielded the following situation. Lourdes was attending a local junior high school and one day the school called the parents to inform them that she had skipped school with her 17-year-old boyfriend. When Lourdes returned home her parents questioned her as to whether she had engaged in sex with her boyfriend. Lourdes denied having had intercourse but the parents decided to take her to a gynecologist for a physical exam.
>
> The medical report confirmed the parents' suspicion which prompted a family crisis between Lourdes and her parents. The physician suggested that Lourdes and her parents should seek counseling services and they were referred to the local hospital's mental health outpatient clinic.
>
> The father, distrustful of the school whose staff was unable to "control his daughter," refused to send her to school anymore. He also put a lock on her bedroom door, forbade her to use the telephone and only permitted her to leave the house when accompanied by an adult.
>
> The first therapy session was abruptly brought to an end by the father when confronted by the therapist's critical questioning of the harsh disciplinary measures he had used with his daughter. At this point, Lourdes had become very depressed, refused to eat and constantly cried. The family doctor recommended to the parents to again seek family therapy if they wanted to help Lourdes.
>
> The parents' concern about Lourdes's physical health prompted them to make an appointment with the clinician of a local community mental health center. The therapist at the center promptly realized that it was necessary to assure the father that his authority was not going to be challenged. It was the therapist's assessment that, to help Lourdes, it was necessary to win the father's trust. The therapist became a cultural

broker to bridge the gap between the Hispanic traditional culture of the father and the American cultural milieu in which Lourdes was participating.

The conflict was more accentuated by the great generational gap caused by the difference in age between Lourdes and her father. The therapist empathized with the father's concern but at the same time confronted him with the legal implications involved in forcing his daughter to drop out of school. The therapist and the father agreed on seeking another school for Lourdes as the best alternative. The therapist also prompted the mother to be more actively involved in the therapeutic process and to assist in facilitating the relationship between father and daughter. The therapist continuously acknowledged the father's concern, emphasizing to Lourdes her father's great love for her and his commitment to parental responsibility. During the second therapy session, a decision was made regarding registering Lourdes in another school. By the time the third therapy session took place, the lock had been removed from the door.

As therapy progressed, the parents and Lourdes began making small concessions to achieve a compromise that would benefit everyone involved. Lourdes began to gain more insight concerning her own feelings and behaviors, including awareness that her sexual encounter was prompted by curiosity and experimentation rather than by an actual need or wish to become involved in a meaningful relationship. Some therapy sessions focused on the need for a responsible stance when engaging in sexual relations. Lourdes began to understand her parents' attitudes better and to realize that their actions were primarily prompted by their love for her.

As therapy progressed, Lourdes became less rebellious and more understanding while the parents became more willing to make concessions to her. A healthier atmosphere of understanding and care became evident.

The therapist has to accept that some of the members of the extended family have a right to interfere in the lives of others, that it is very much their business to do so. Furthermore, even in those instances when the directives are seen as burdensome and inadequate and even unfair, the Hispanic client might express acknowledgement which does not necessarily entail compliance. The client might verbalize the conflict by saying: "I am not in agreement with what my grandmother wants me to do, but **ella puede** (she can); **tiene derecho** (has the right). What this actually means to the client is that he has to deal with how the grandmother feels about an issue since she can interfere because she cares. The therapist has to assist the client in dealing with the significant others in a fashion that will enable him to appropriately handle the conflict without breaking away from that person. Since paternalistic authoritarianism fosters disregard for directives emanating from an impersonal context, in many cases the therapist needs to assume a paternalistic posture towards the client.

In some instances, authoritarianism is manifested by conferring of degrees and status to those people whom the client respects. On many occasions clients will call "doctor" the mental health staff whom they identify as supportive, even when those individuals are only mental health technicians.

Machismo

Machismo is one of the Hispanic cultural traits which greatly affect therapeutic intervention, especially family therapy. Machismo might be the reason why the Hispanic male seeks help at a more advanced stage of deterioration than is typically the case with females. In the Cuban clinic normally the female patient load was twice as high as that of the males. Apparently the Hispanic male needs to be in greater pain in order to seek mental health assistance. Placing yourself in a needy situation is probably not perceived as the manly thing to do.

In other instances, machismo negatively influences the therapeutic process. There is a resistance by the male to get involved in couples or family therapy, since males generally perceive this involvement as having a deteriorating effect on their integrity and authority. Machismo causes males to have less flexible ego boundaries than the females, and, therefore, to feel and express compassion and empathy less fully than females.

Fatalism

Fatalism, the acceptance of things that one cannot control, also has important treatment implications. Fatalism, psychologically and culturally, prepares people for life's uncertainties and, thus, the acceptance of vulnerability and lack of control. It also, at least verbally, impresses people with the need to be more compassionate, understanding and tolerant of other people's failures, and less demanding of life and of human beings. Fatalism supports the perception that there is no protection against adversity and that anything that happens to anybody can happen to me.

Fatalism in many instances causes people's perception of life as, **"una prueba"** (a trial), **"una lucha"** (a struggle), and the expectation that the therapist has to assist them in adjusting as best as possible to whatever life has in store for them. Multiple idiomatic expressions reflect this philosophical stance: **"Hacer la vida llevadera"** (make life bearable) or, in a situation of crisis, **"capear el temporal"** (weather the storm). The same way that clients seek small concessions out of life to live it adequately, or to carry through situations of crisis, they expect the therapist to assist them in managing and manipulating these concessions to be able to get by as best as possible. This is what is called **"vadear la situacion"** (wade through the situation). The therapist has to constantly **"tantear la situacion"** (get a feel of the situation) and, as the patient's coach, move with and assist him in the present situation, rather than insist on achieving former goals that in present circumstances might seem meaningless.

Acceptance of fatalism, which is very much related to the Subjugation to Nature orientation, greatly affects the religious overview and behavior. A mystical stance might entail great commitment to institutionalized religion. In many instances, however, participation in institutionalized religion is just socially cosmetic. While officially Catholic, many feel that in order to deal with supernatural forces, rituals other than Catholic ones will be effective. A more magical, manipulative approach to the supernatural. **(Santeria, Curanderismo)** might be preferred and perceived as obtaining better results than the impersonal, orthodox approach. There is a need for mental health professionals to understand the belief systems of their clients and to reach out to indigenous healers to seek out their cooperation with the treatment. In many instances, indigenous healers have been used with success in mental health settings, and in other instances, when contacted by the mental health professionals, they have cooperated effectively on behalf of their clients (Sandoval, 1977, 1979).

Cultural differences in value orientation between the therapist and the client greatly affect their perception of their respective roles as well as the therapeutic outcomes and processes (Szapocznik, Scopetta, Aranalde, & Kurtines, 1978). We are now going to discuss the clinical implications caused by the differences in value orientation between Hispanics and mainstream Americans.

In reference to the Time orientation, Hispanic preference for the Present clashes with the Future orientation or mainstream America. The preference towards the Present is apparently responsible for the fact that a majority of Hispanics who actively seek mental health services, are responding to a situation of crisis. In some instances, once the crisis is over, treatment is neglected. This is caused by a concern with solving the here and now, with little regard for the therapeutic outcome as it pertains to the future. Furthermore, the Present orientation is also manifested in a lack of interest in long term therapy. Hispanics assess therapeutic outcomes in reference to symptom amelioration, and not as a long process affecting personal change and growth. On the contrary, mainstream America's Future orientation has influenced clinical culture by emphasizing long range plans and future goals. On the other hand, the Present orientation allows little room for planning, particularly one's own time. This might be one of the reasons why Hispanic clients so often fail to keep clinical appointments (no-shows, coming too early or too late).

In general, however, there is greater acceptance and less demands imposed upon mental health clients, as well as the old and the feeble in societies which are Present oriented. Societies with a strong Future orientation have little regard for people who cannot plan future achievements.

In reference to the orientation concerning the relations of Man to Nature and to Super Nature, again, there is a clash between Hispanic and mainstream American preferences. Again, the role of the mental health client among Hispanics, as well as among societies that are Subjugation oriented, might be more socially rewarding than in societies which are Control or Mastery oriented, as mainstream America is. This is so because in Subjugation oriented societies, lack of control and/or Mastery is perceived as part of human nature.

Mainstream America's preference for Mastery has greatly influenced mental health professionals, who, sometimes, plan unrealistic therapeutic goals which are aimed at giving the clients control and mastery over their lives. This Mastery orientation sometimes heavily burdens the role of patients, specially the chronically mentally ill, as well as the aged, whose possibility of achieving control over their lives is remote. In addition, members of Mastery oriented societies, mental health professionals included, have less tolerance for unrestrained and uncontrolled emotional display than those societies which are Subjugation oriented.

In reference to the form of men's relations to other men there is again a value conflict between mainstream Americans and Hispanics. Mainstream America's preference for the Individualistic orientation negatively impacts the role and self perception of the despondent patient. Moreover, the Individualistic orientation in many instances influences therapeutic goals which reflect unrealistic expectations of a client's capability for self reliance and self motivation. These expectations in many instances increase clients' stress and again negatively impacts their self-perception, since they are placed in frustrating, no-win therapeutic processes.

The Lineal orientation among Hispanics influences counseling since in most instances clients expect the therapist to give them clear cut directives. On many occasions at the Cuban unit, clients bitterly complained about therapists who, after a long session, would confront them with several choices or courses of action as responses to a specific situation. Clients used to voice their grievances complaining that if the therapist knew his job, instead of offering choices he would directly tell them which was the best. "If he has a Ph.D., why doesn't he tell me which is the best choice?" Followed by, "What is the matter with him? Is he afraid of making a mistake? Is he afraid of committing himself?"

As has been pointed out before, the Collateral orientation among Hispanics is a strong second place choice. The Collateral orientation impacts positively the role of the despondent client, as a person who is in great need of support and care.

In reference to the modality of human activity orientation, again there is conflict between the Doing preferred by mainstream America vs. the Being orientation preferred by Hispanics. Generally, the Doing orientation negatively impacts the role of those members of society who can no longer engage in materialistic pursuits, such as the aged, the feeble, and the mentally ill. In Hispanic society their role is more socially acceptable since people are assessed according to who they are, and not for what they can do. The Doing orientation has also impacted clinical culture as reflected in generalized treatment outcome expectations geared to making the client more self sufficient and autonomous, and measuring progress according to this capacity to do measurable chores independently. In Being oriented societies the self-worth of a person doesn't suffer as much if he is dependent on others to do things for him. On the other hand, there is much more acceptance.

The Doing $>$ $<$ Being orientation can cause different assessment of when a person is perceived as having mental health problems. Generally, in the U.S.A., when a person is not functioning well in his job or cannot keep a job, this non-functionality is perceived as possibly caused by a mental health problem. In Hispanic society the assessment in many instances is done in a social context where that person's behavior becomes **"inaguantable"** or **"insoportable"** (unbearable) or **"insufrible"** (unsufferable) to others, mainly the family and friends.

In reference to the Human Nature orientation, again there is some conflict between the Good and Evil orientation which is preferred by most Hispanics, and the Evil-but-perfectible orientation preferred by mainstream America. The Evil-but-perfectible orientation's impact on the clinical culture translates into higher expectations of the clients, less flexibility about treatment outcomes, and more rigid treatment plans. It demands more control. The Evil-but-perfectible orientation perceives maturity and responsibility as synonymous with man's ability to control emotions and to use reason as the means for man to become perfectible. The Good and Evil orientation preferred by Hispanics justifies the occasional lack of control and the ensuing display of emotions. It stimulates more compassion and understanding in the clinical setting. It allows less rigid treatment plans and more flexible treatment outcomes. It excuses failures and lowers the expectations of clients.

Concluding Remarks

Hispanic culture in the U.S.A. has demonstrated great survival qualities. Unlike other ethnic collectivities, Hispanics in this country have tended to cling to their culture and language. There are many reasons for this cultural persistence. One of them is the very early presence of Hispanic culture in the American experience, and the manner in which Hispanics became a conquered and partly disenfranchised people who were not allowed to participate or be fully involved in mainstream society. Thus, culture and language become the source of group identity and ego strength for this somewhat marginal group. Furthermore, many of the Hispanic groups which migrated to the U.S.A. and some of those who were displaced during the wake of White American expansionism, were not allowed to assimilate to the dominant culture because of racial considerations. However, as a group they were not subjected to the deculturating effects that slavery has had on American Blacks. Yet, as excluded, non-mainstream people, their culture became the core to which they rallied in search of group identity, ego strength and self-esteem.

Other important factors that have impacted the continuous strong presence of Hispanic culture in the U.S.A. is the geographic proximity of Hispanic America, the strong commercial ties between the latter and the U.S.A., as well as the steady flow of people to and from the Caribbean and the Southern half of the American continent. In any event, the strong Hispanic presence and the fact that the Hispanic population in this country continues to grow at an unprecedented rate, merits the attention of human services deliverers, especially those in geographic areas where there are large concentrations of Hispanics. Notwithstanding the acknowledgement of individual differences and diversity among Hispanics due to factors previously described, the mental health services providers, in order to be effective in a therapeutic relationship, need to know Hispanic culture and cultures, and to understand the role that culture plays in the lives of clients of Hispanic origin.

Understanding Hispanic culture will enable counselors and therapists to have a better grasp of those personality traits which are patterned and rewarded by Hispanic culture. It is important for providers to have an understanding of the resources which Hispanic culture makes available to its members as well as those stressors which are more commonly found in that culture. This knowledge will enable them to better utilize the resources of the culture and also to more effectively ameliorate its stressors on behalf of the client. This understanding will allow mental health service providers to delve deeper into the Hispanic psyche, to respect its peculiarities and strengths, and thus develop better empathy and communication with their clients.

NOTES

1. In 1980 the U.S. Bureau of the Census reported 14.6 million Hispanics in the U.S.A. mainland. This is an increase of 61% from the 1970 census and represents approximately 6.48% of the total population. See U.S. Department of Commerce, Bureau of the Census, 1980 Census of Population, Volume I Reports, *Characteristics of the Population,* "General Population Characteristics," Series PC 80-1-B1.
2. According to the U.S. Bureau of the Census, the median age in the U.S. in 1980 was 31 while 23 was the median age for the Hispanic population. See U.S. Department of Commerce, Bureau of the Census, 1980 Census of Population, Volume I Reports.
3. In 1981, 36.4% of 18 and 19 year old Hispanics were high school dropouts, more than double the national figure (16%) and significantly higher than Blacks (19.3%). They also experienced a high rate of grade-level advancement problems. While fewer than one out of ten White American students 14 to 20 years old were two years or more behind their age group, one out of four students of Puerto Rican or Mexican origin lagged behind. Only 17% of Hispanics 18 to 20 years old were enrolled in college as compared to 20% of Blacks and 26% of Whites. See U.S. Department of Commerce, Bureau of the Census, "School Enrollment--Social and Economic Characteristics of Students: October, 1981," *Current Population Reports,* Population Characteristics Series P-20, No. 373, February, 1983.
4. Hispanics' income falls between that of Whites and Blacks. In 1982, the median family income of Whites was $24,603; Hispanic family income was $16,227; Blacks was $13,598. However, Puerto Rican median family income was lower than Blacks. See U.S. Department of Commerce, Bureau of the Census. *Money Income* and *Poverty Status of Families and Persons in the U.S.: 1982,* CPR Series P-60, No. 140, 1983.

5. According to the U.S. Bureau of Labor Statistics, 1983 annual averages regarding the employment status of those 16 years of age and older, the rate of unemployment for the total population was 9.6%. However, among Whites, only 8.4% were unemployed while among Hispanics the figure was 13.8% and among Blacks 19.5%. See U.S. Bureau of Labor Statistics, *Employment and Earnings,* Vol 31, No. 1, January, 1984, p. 201.

6. Comparative research on value orientations and health beliefs and practices among Black Americans, Bahamians, Cubans, Haitians, and Puerto Ricans residing in Dade County, Florida, was conducted by Dr. Hazel Weidman and collaborators. See Weidman (1978) and Egeland (1978), *The Miami Health Ecology Project Report,* Vols. I and II. Miami: University of Miami School of Medicine.

REFERENCES

Acosta, F. X., Yamamoto, J., & Evans, L. A. (Eds.). (1982). *Effective psychotherapy for low-income and minority patients.* New York: Plenum.

Becerra, R. M., Karno, M., & Escobar, J. I. (1982). *Mental health and Hispanic Americans.* New York: Grune & Stratton.

Egeland, J. A. (1978). *Ethnic value orientation analysis: A research component of the Miami Health Ecology Project* (Vol. 2). Miami: University of Miami School of Medicine.

Escobar, J. E., & Randolph, E. T. (1982). The Hispanic and social networks. In R. M. Becerra, M. Karno, & J. I. Escobar (Eds.). *Mental health and Hispanic Americans: Clinical perspective* (pp. 41-57). New York: Grune & Stratton.

Garrison, V. (1977). Doctor, *espiritista,* or psychiatrist? Health seeking behavior in a Puerto Rican neighborhood of New York City. *Medical Anthropology, 1*(2), 65-191.

Kluckhohn, F., & Strodtbeck, F. (1961). *Variations in value orientations.* Evanston, IL: Row Peterson.

Lefley, H. P., & Bestman, E. W. (1984). Community mental health and minorities: A multiethnic approach. In S. Sue & T. Moore (Eds.), *The pluralistic society: A community mental health perspective* (pp. 116-148). New York: Human Sciences Press.

Marcos, L. R. (1979). Effects of interpreters on the evaluation of psychopathology in non-English-speaking patients. *American Journal of Psychiatry, 136*(2), 171-174.

Marcos, L. R., & Alpert, M. (1976). Strategies and risks in psychotherapy with bilingual patients. *American Journal of Psychiatry, 133*(11), 1275-1278.

Marcos, L. R., Urcuyo, L., Kesselman, M., & Alpert, M. (1973). The language barrier in evaluating Spanish-American patients. *Archives of General Psychiatry, 29,* 655-659.

Padilla, A. M., Ruiz, R. A., & Alvarez, R. A. (1975). Community mental health services for the Spanish-speaking/surnamed population. *American Psychologist, 30,* 892-905.

Ruiz, P. (1982). The Hispanic patient: Sociocultural perspectives. In R. M. Becerra, M. Karno, & J. I. Escobar (Eds.), *Mental health and Hispanic Americans* (pp. 17-27). New York: Grune & Stratton.

Ruiz, P., & Langrod, J. (1976). The role of folk healers in community mental health services. *Community Mental Health Journal, 12*(4), 392-398.

Sandoval, M. C. (1977). Santeria: Afrocuban concepts of disease and its treatment in Miami. *Journal of Operational Psychiatry, 8*(2), 52-63.

Sandoval, M. C. (1979). Santeria as a mental health care system: An historical overview. *Social Science & Medicine, 13B*(2), 137-151.

Sandoval, M. C. (1985). *Mariel and Cuban national identity.* Miami: Sibi Editorial.

Sandoval, M. C., & Tozo, L. (1975). An emergent Cuban community. *Psychiatric Annals, 5*(8), 48-63.

Szapocznik, J. (1978, October). *A programmatic mental health approach to enhancing meaning of life of Hispanic elders.* Paper presented at COSSMHO's National Hispanic Conference on Families, Houston, TX.

Szapocznik, J., Scopetta, M. A., Aranalde, M. A., & Kurtines, W. (1978). Cuban value structure: Treatment implication. *Journal of Consulting and Clinical Psychology, 46*(5), 960-970.

Weidman, H. H. (1973, March). *Implications of the culture broker concept for the delivery of health care.* Paper presented at the annual meeting of the Southern Anthropological Society, Wrightsville Beach, NC.

Weidman, H. H. (1978). *The Miami Health Ecology Project Report* (Vol. 1). Miami: University of Miami School of Medicine.

Weidman, H. H. (1983). Research, service and training aspects of clinical anthropology: An institutional overview. In D. Shimkin & P. Golde (Eds.), *Clinical anthropology: A new approach to American health problems?* (pp. 118-151). Lanham, MD: University Press of America.

CHAPTER 9

MENTAL HEALTH SERVICES FOR HAITIANS

CLAUDE CHARLES

T HE HAITIAN COMMUNITY in large U.S. cities such as Miami, New York, Boston, Chicago, Philadelphia and various cities in New Jersey, is relatively diverse. Older ports of entry such as Boston have large enclaves of Haitians who have been in the U.S. for 20 years or more. The community is thus divided among those characterized by job stability, higher socioeconomic status (SES) and permanent residence or citizenship, and newer entrants characterized by lower SES, joblessness, and ambiguous legal status. The early Haitian migration, like that of the Cubans, was based on a mentality of impermanence. Both economically and politically induced, this migration was based on the premise that the sojourn in the U.S. would be temporary; that wealth would be accumulated and used advantageously in a return to Haiti. Although many were not active in political movements, their expectation was that the political situation in Haiti would change and offer greater opportunity when they returned. Such Haitians were often unwilling to participate in American life. Psychological disorders in this group were often rooted in a situation in which they deliberately impeded their own adaptation to U.S. life, without compensatory tools for broadening their perspectives. Many in this group led a deliberately restricted life without attempts to assimilate. A substantial number were working in the U.S. cities but educating their children in Haiti. Not interested in acculturation, separated from their families, they were consciously sustaining an inadequate and unsatisfying way of life. With the death of Papa Doc and election of Jean Claude Duvalier as President for Life in 1971, many began to come to terms for the first time with the eventuality of non-return to Haiti. The realization that there was no hope for change in the immediate future evoked various types of response. Massive denial, passive aggressive behavior, depression, feelings of loss of mastery, and self-deprivation, together with fantasies of return to a former life are behaviors frequently seen in clients from this older group of Haitian exiles.

The newest group of exiles is composed of Haitians who have arrived during the presidency of Jean Claude Duvalier. There are some people who came for reasons of family reunification, rejoining their relatives in the older exile group. Many, however, come on a legal basis with student, tourist or commercial visas and remain illegally after expiration of the visas, resorting to the usual means of survival of illegal aliens getting lost in the crowd. When they reemerge, with a sponsor, marital partner, or work permit, they can establish grounds for permanent residence. These people have a certain level of skill and are able, despite their illegality, to be employable and survive. The anxieties that evolve during the period of limbo, however, are often retained even after legal status becomes a possibility. Many feel frustrated and rejected by perceived non-support of the older Haitian community. Jealousy and ever-present paranoia, based on fear of persecution by the U.S. criminal justice system; denial of real causes of failure; and massive projection, are common defenses.

In cities such as Miami which serve as entry points from the Caribbean and Latin America, the new wave of arrivals after 1971 included those characterized as boat people. These people come without visas or any proper documentation and try to enter the country illegally. Tides of Haitians come either directly from Haiti in small boats or indirectly from other Caribbean islands. After the Mariel boatlift, Haitians as well as Cubans were given the status of entrants. An entrant is someone who enters the country illegally but is given a temporary status pending court determination of status. All Haitians entrants are considered excludable or deportable. If they have been caught by INS or other offical agencies after arrival in the U.S. they are deportable. But if they have been rescued at sea and escorted to a U.S. port they are excludable, i.e., they are less likely to obtain asylum because they are not considered to have entered the U.S.

Many Haitians in the U.S. manifest the refugee phenomenon of shattered expectations. With Haitians, however, the anxieties are even greater because most come into the country without proper legal documentation. Then they become either illegal aliens or entrants. There is a saying in Haitian Creole, "Kouri pou labli tonbe nan granrivye," "You al Health Services for Haitians 185

run to avoid the rain and you fall down in the river," a saying similar to "out of the frying pan and into the fire." This statement is used by many refugees to describe their entry experience in the U.S., when, instead of jobs, many find themselves incarcerated in a detention camp, with ambiguous legal status and the possibility of deportation.

Three Types of Haitian Clients

Haitian boat people who endure congested conditions in old leaky boats, with tremendous fear of their reception on both shores, travel and arrive under extremely traumatic conditions. Debilitated when they reach the U.S., exposed to sun, heat, lack of food and water, they will often exhibit symptoms such as nightmares, apnea, shock, or tremors. Nevertheless, they face harsh treatment in processing by INS and screening for communicable diseases, and are usually interred in jail or detention centers without receiving mental health treatment.

It is after their release into the community that their adjustment problems surface, and many become clients of the mental health system. These new arrivals must be divided into three groups: (1) those who come in the normal process of family reunification to rejoin relatives; they have a natural support system, (2) those without relatives who have been encouraged to come by close friends; they can still find a support system in the community, and (3) those on their own. They are the first immigrants from their families; they have no friends and a meager or nonexistent community support system.

The two former categories can afford a certain period of adjustment. The third category is required to become quickly self-supporting. The pressure is intense for personal survival and the demand to provide for and send for other family members left behind. The combination of a non-welcoming environment and intense need generates strong feelings of failure when work is unobtainable. If such entrants become incapacitated, they must depend 100% on the available human service agency — in this case the community mental health center (CMHC) — to provide them with shelter, rehabilatative treatment, and economic assistance.

In the two former categories, individuals dealing with adjustment or hardships will experience frustration, rejection, depression, and occasionally paranoia. There is still a pivotal base for survival and their reality problems can be resolved in group or family context. But with the category of lone individuals, the CMHC must assume complete responsibility for education, acculturation, and human support system. The

CMHC becomes the family. This means the provision of residential and social care as well as treatment. This treatment approach in the U.S. is a far remove from mental health treatment in Haiti. Before going into specific diagnostic and treatment issues, an overview of the mental health system in Haiti is in order.

Mental Health Care in Haiti: Problems of Haitian Identity

In a country 85% rural and 15% urban the majority of people live without any conceptualization of psychiatric care. The society, family and supernatural belief system provided resources for dealing with stressors that impinge on mental health. People with overt psychiatric disorders — **les fous** — were, like the medieval **bouffons,** a source of entertainment and of pity for the populace. **Fous** were accepted and fed by the people. When they became violent or dangerous they were taken into institutional settings. The primary asylums **(asyles)** were 18th century type institutions. Two institutions, one in Beudet and another in Signeau were custodial and the primary objectives were to isolate and penalize rather than to treat.

In Port-au-Prince the Centre Psychiatrique was developed in the 1960s. Psychologists and psychiatrists were few and located in the city. Haitian M.D.s were generally not interested in becoming psychiatrists. Mental health professionals tended to be psychoanalytic in orientation. Although these professionals had some influence on alerting teachers in the school system to psychological issues, mental health care was generally limited to the affluent and educated. Nevertheless, such care is considered stigmatizing and many affluent Haitians still come to Miami for psychiatric treatment rather than seeking it in Haiti.

The Haitian situation itself, however, is intrinsically traumatizing. The Duvalier regime has perpetuated a paranoia-inducing atmosphere of fear and ambiguity. The victimized are directly affected by the system; but those within the system are also victimized by their own uneasiness and instability. Many affluent Haitians, both within the government or protected within the private sector, must remove themselves from the oppressive environment in their search for psychiatric care and many are now found in the caseloads of Miami physicians and psychiatrists. Low self esteem is associated with awareness of low Haitian prestige in the world.

There is a loss of self in the growing rejection of Haitian identity. A novel published in 1981 by Marie Therese Colimon entitled, "Le Chant des Sirenes," tells of a little girl, Haitian born and bred, writing a letter to her mother in N.Y. She asks her mother to accelerate the process for her obtaining an American visa. "I want to rejoin you at home in N.Y. because I am languishing in my exile in Haiti." This territorial alienation exemplifies the erosion of national pride that underlies diminished sense of self and identity of many Haitians. Physical debilitation among the majority of poor Haitians also accelerates the depersonalization. The issue of self-perception is discussed further under treatment issues.

Rejection and/or denial of national identity, a profound sense of loss and internalized aggression have generated a rise in suicide among Haitians. Externalized aggression is manifested in intolerance, violence and physical abuse of spouses and children.

Among those with greater ego strength, individuals formerly deprived in Haiti become preoccupied with achieving and maintaining material possessions. These are viewed as extensions of the personality to such an extent that we see cases of personality collapse with the loss of such acquisitions. Criminality and violence are unusual developments in Haitian life directly linked to maintaining newly acquired wealth. Cases of battery, robbery, drug deals and other nontraditional behaviors now are seen as means of establishing identity through possession of material goods. This emphasis on materialism is paradoxically, a symbol of the Americanization process — of greater adaptation to life in the U.S. Today, **Vodou,** the Haitian supernatural belief system, is sometimes used for purposes related to acquisition or maintenance of material goods. This was not typically the case in Haiti, where **Vodou** was more often used for satisfaction of spiritual and emotional needs.

Vodou as a Therapeutic System

Vodou, a religion of African origin, shapes the general belief system of Haitians. According to Vodou, the universe is an interaction of forces. All the forces emanate from a single original source, a supreme almighty entity, called in Haitian Creole, Gran Met. Gran Met is all powerful, all knowledgeable, eternal. After creating the universe, He shared his powers with lesser deities or spirits called loas. Human beings in their everyday lives are in constant interaction with the loas and are forced to make deals with them to control the events occurring in their lives. The loas are perceived pragmatically as instrumental in conducting one's life. As power brokers, loas are basically amoral. It is up to humans to interact with and use a loa according to their needs and hopes.

Loas also are masters of parts of the human body. Certain aspects of human anatomy and/or physiology are specific territories or domains of appropriate loas. As all parts of the body are controlled, the brain too is controlled by a loa; mind, intelligence, and other brain functions are controlled by specific loas. Thus, problems of the mind are easily interpreted as having a supernatural cause.

In South Florida, we have seen an increase in the demand for spiritual healers or Vodou priests (houngans, male or mambos, female) to address the needs of people with mental or emotional problems which are assumed to be supernaturally caused. Observations of the interaction between mental patients and Vodou priests, indicate that there are three categories of intervention. As spiritual healers, Vodou priests use the following approaches:

Spiritual reshaping is the technique used for depressed clients with a high level of anxiety, who also report sensations of weakness and vulnerability. Spiritual reshaping is aimed toward obtaining three res0ults. First, fight the depressive mood by counteracting the **Bad Luck** (Guignon) that caused it. Second, after removing the Bad Luck, try to restore the client's self-confidence by convincing the client that there are no more obstacles to recovery. Third, reinforce the coping strength of the client by providing him with a greater sense of personal protection.

The instrumental techniques for achieving the objectives include: (a) cleansing the person, with ointments, oils, and magical lotions, and baths with plants, wines and perfumes; (b) cleansing the person's environment — typically the house — wtih incense, candles, and magical waters; and (c) construction of an amulet that the client will have to wear for personal protection. Sometimes there is the addition of a magical potion which the client drinks to give him greater strength.

Supernatural strengthening is the technique used for clients presenting with phobias, hysterias, and overtly paranoid delusions of persecution. The spiritual healers usually diagnose these conditions as caused by retaliation from the spirits (loas). Either the client failed to keep a specific commitment with a loa, or he/she has discontinued worship practices. The techniques focus first on renewing alliances with the loas and second, on appeasement of the angry or offended spirits. In this case, the spirits may be protector loas, but also dead ancestors or guardian spirits who have been neglected by the client. These offenses occur through violations of taboos or special traditions which involve commitments called angajman (engagements). Treatment will focus on complicated ceremonies with rituals that are aimed toward the following:

(a) bringing back the spirits to make their grievances known; (b) paying tribute or homage to the spirits in order to move them toward forgiveness and reconciliation; (c) consolidating the reconciliation through an exchange contract. The clients regain full mental equilibrium in exchange for fulfilling vows and promises to the spirits.

In the rituals we find ceremonies that involve use of foods, animal sacrifices, and cleansing baths. They end with an operation called the "paying back." For example, after the ceremony, everything that was used — food, animals, and also the underclothes the client typically wears during the bath — all must be destroyed. The ceremony always ends with the ritual of the client throwing seven pennies into the waste to be discarded. While throwing the pennies, he always must repeat the formula: "Now I am paying for all my past debts. Now I do not owe anybody anything. I want to be free again, to continue a decent life as a normal human being." The Vodou priest then takes all the waste and discards it, typically in the wilderness, but sometimes in a junkyard or a cemetery.

Exorcism is the third technique. This is the "heaviest" technique — considered the treatment of choice for clients presenting with hallucinations, hostile delusional systems, unremitting paranoid ideation, pronounced thought disorders, unprecipitated assaultive behavior or other florid symptoms typically associated with schizophrenia. These symptoms are believed to be caused by a curse or by the possession of the client by malevolent spirits. The curse can be externally caused by a malevolent spirit. However, it also can represent the loss of self protection because of the erosion of the individual's supernatural shield — which every human being is assumed to have.

The supernatural shield is believed to maintain a balance between positive and negative influences and to constitute a magnetic envelope that protects one from harm. "Envoutement" is the process used in penetrating the shield. The pin technique — sticking pins into a doll which is the representation of the person — is an example of envoutement. It is a means of breaking the protective shield around the ego.

Suicidal and homicidal ideation are considered a result of envoutement — the loss of protection of the self, the loss of control over one's own ego. Under envoutement, all psychological malaise can be somatized as physical debilitation and weakness, or sensations of being flaccid and lifeless. If the case is a curse caused by envoutement, the intervention will focus on making a deal with benevolent spirits that can become protectors of the client and therefore work to restore his supernatural shield. If the curse is caused by invasion of a malevolent spirit the intervention will consolidate the client's personal space or life field so that he cannot be invaded any more. Avoidance of relapse or decompensation is accomplished by creating an inviolate territory around the person.

Exorcism usually involves three stages of treatment. In stage one, there is the cleansing and ejection of the curse of the malevolent spirit. This typically involves a cleansing, banquets, animal sacrifice, and the "paying back" ritual. The second stage involves spiritual strengthening or recharging the body with positive influence using baths and ointments. The third stage involves a consecration to preclude relapse. In this stage there is use of amulets, magical potions and specific spiritual techniques. An example is the client's recitation of magical formulas or words whenever he or she experiences a feeling of relapse. At other times there are special mandates to be followed, such as burning a prescribed number of candles, paying a visit to the church or cemetery, or making a charitable gift.

These phenomena are reactive rituals of Vodou, involving the undoing of harm to the individual. The Vodou religion, however, has proactive elements. The descriptions to this point indicate therapeutic modalities used with mental and emotional illness. Trance and possession are proactive aspects which help to maintain mental health. These operate to maintain equilibrium by dealing with ordinary life stresses and frustrations.

Trance and Possession

Trance is like psychodrama. In a special ritual involving incantation of drums, singing and powerful environmental suggestibility, the individual enters into trance. Under the stress of psychological problems, the physical body tenses, By entering into trance the body expels these pressures through shaking and convulsions. It is a process that appears similar to reactions to electroshock. The tremendous vibrations of trance are accompanied by the individual's interpretation that the spirits have visited that person, who acts in the capacity of medium, and have created the vibrations that shake the body. The individual then perceives at an unconscious sensory level that the spirits have heard the problem, entered the body, and are ready to help. Thus the person can get rid of all inhibitions that were keeping him or her anxious and physiologically locked. Frustrations are now released. After trance the person feels relaxed. The meaning of what occurred during trance is then interpreted by the senior cult members. The latter indicate that the person should now feel better because the spirits have heard the grievances as evidenced by their manifestation. The person can now face life feeling relieved of these pressures. He also has regained the security of knowing that he will find a solution for the problems since he is now assured of divine assistance.

Possession. First, possession for the individual is a direct communication with the spirit. The spirit enters the body, speaks and acts, communicating what should be done. There is a direct intrapsychic intervention by the spirit. Also, in true possession, new deals can be established by the spirit. This is similar to a treatment plan with prescribed goals, because the spirit can prescribe the new pattern of behavior that is required to regain equilibrium and remove problems. Third, the spirit can act as a mediator. Like a counselor, the spirit can stipulate what should be done to reduce tension between the patient and significant others, indicating the steps for reconciliation of conflicts. The spirit can indicate how a person should get out of intolerable situations. Spirits can unblock behavior and can give approval for alliances or relationships. They can convince the family members present to accept relationships they presently oppose or to reject relationships they previously wanted to foster. Through possession, spirits can warn about possible harmful encounters in the future and foster preventive behavior. They can unveil mysteries and clarify events for members of the group. They can also resolve interpersonal conflicts that have become maladaptive. For example:

> A man died, and his family suspected the wife was responsible through curse or poisoning. Because the wife was perceived as a witch, she had problems relating to the family, even though for the sake of the children she wanted a good relationship. In trance, a hostile family member was possessed and the loa was able to remove suspicion from the wife and effect a reconciliation.

Treatment Issues

Although most Haitians use supernatural explanatory models, prior to the 1970s, when individuals from the older exile group experienced hardship or failures, they would resort to supernatural interventions as a booster to maintain hope and morale. The supernatural was used for luck. After the 1970s, however, paranoia developed creating a condition of constant fear (fear of deportation by INS, of being returned to Haiti).

Feelings of persecution were accompanied by individuals' perceptions that their problems were due to a curse or the malevolence of others, either in Haiti (because they were jealous of the person's U.S. residence) or Haitians here who feared competition from newcomers. Thus the supernatural was now invoked reactively to establish relief from the curse rather than the proactive use of bringing good luck.

Clients in this group will often accuse close relatives of malevolent jealousy. Paranoia is used as an escape strategy to avoid personal responsibility. For example, cases of family conflict often revolve around the provision of shelter to relatives. The ordinary expectation of the shared payment of household expenses may be seen as a punitive demand from a jealous brother or sister who doesn't want the new exile to advance. In the U.S., the former easy flexibility of the extended family system with regard to household expenses no longer obtains. People are expected to pay their way. If a person cannot pay and is evicted, the explanation is turned upon the perpetrator in the following twisted logic: "I couldn't find a job because my own family members put a curse on me so I would be subservient to them and not advance the way they did." The consequence of unemployment is thus explained in terms of an antecedent curse. Failure and economic adversity are thus projected onto the persons who originally offered and then withdrew sustenance.

While anger might occur with an American or other non-Haitian evicted under similar circumstance, projection of a curse would not be likely to occur.

Treatment in these cases consists, first, of ventilation of frustrations. The second stage is a direct attempt to recapture historically the events that happened and to order them in comprehensible sequence and meaning. Problem-solving techniques, budgeting skills, and other stabilizing measures preceed the ultimate move toward family reconciliation.

Many Haitians have learned to respond to severe adversity with denial and projection. Thus there are rarely symptoms of severe depression or guilt because in many instances clients attribute their own personal deficiencies to the system or to other uncontrollable forces. They are not responsible because they are not in control. There is the expectation of receiving support and assistance from a godfather, a "bon papa," who **is** in control and will intervene in their behalf. This dependency on an authority figure is derived from the historical oligarchical system in Haiti. However, it has profound implications for therapy because it means that (a) the therapist must begin with some kind of directive stance and also function as a resource agent, and (b) one of the major tasks of treatment is to slowly educate these clients to understand the need to assume responsibility for their own lives. This is a different type of dependency from that usually arising from transference, since it is culturally-based and must be addressed in culturally syntonic terms.

In the following section we will deal first with problem areas, and second, with cultural strengths that should be highlighted in any training program for counselors of Haitian clients.

Reality Problems

In addition to the problems typically endured by people with a low level of literacy and few marketable skills, Haitians confront problems of special legal status previously discussed; fear of deportation; exploitation by employers; and substandard living conditions which generate health hazards. These conditions are different from those experienced in Haiti, since in an urban technological setting, poverty and congested households tend to erode traditional cohesiveness and mutual support. Absence of the extended family system not only removes emotional support, but also intensifies the experience of financial hardship when there is no work available.

New Acculturation Problems

The new culture rather quickly effects changes in sex roles. Living in exile makes both males and females in all SES brackets reevaluate their role; most were not prepared to do this. For example, in Haiti, a middle class woman, whether working or not working, had household help. Now she has to fulfill the cultural role of being "queen of the household" and hold a job as well, so she becomes overwhelmed. Helping out in the household has never been part of the Haitian male role. Making decisions has not been typical of the female role. Many women will refuse to make decisions even about household policy because the cultural tradition was for men to take this responsibility. Alternatively, some women may use this refusal as a manipulative device to test the man's concern about them. When that fails, the woman may become severely depressed because she is not only overwhelmed by role strain but by the need to assume an executive function for which she is not prepared. The failure of the man to make household decisions may also be seen as rejection. Alternatively, men who appear to accept the sharing of household burdens may manifest anger and irritability at the imposition of this unfamiliar role.

Haitian men are street people; Haitian women prefer to stay at home. In Haiti the male takes care of all major decisions; women ran their households but with assistance of many relatives and servants which protected them from loneliness. In the U.S., the woman uses projected decision-making and involvement in household affairs to involve her husband in the social support function formerly fulfilled by household help and relatives.

The acculturation process itself often provides a basis for marital conflicts in the household. The Haitian male perceives the U.S. female as more independent and compares Haitian partners—seen as dependent and exigent—adversely. Thus when reasonable demands are made, the male may react angrily.

In family therapy, Haitian males will acknowledge they feel more satisfied with American girlfriends; fewer demands are made on them. They resent the perceived possessiveness and dependency of Haitian women. There are increasing cases of women feeling frustrated, neglected and unappreciated. Drinking problems and child abuse are on the rise.

Men are not prepared to live in a small nuclear family unit at home with their wives. In Haiti there was much more outdoors living and companionship with male friends. Women had the extended family with whom to interact. These relationships are often missing in the transplanted life in the U.S.

Haitian males have a macho attitude. Males want to be taken care of, to be the major focus of attention. They also were used to multiple lovers, whether married or not. This is no longer affordable. Many men want control over their wife's wages for extra money in their pockets. There are many conflicts about money. Control of money is a compensation for lost status and prerogatives for many males. It is also a means of keeping their wives at home and assuming liberty for themselves.

Child abuse and incest are sometimes problems because of the new opportunity for such abuse. Some males were not used to living in close quarters and privacy with young children without other adults present. With the situation of the mother working at night and the father staying with the children, opportunities for incest increase. Incest in Haiti was considered an abomination, but it is found more and more in Miami, particularly with stepfathers. It was rare in Haiti because men did not work shifts or were not likely to be in a caregiving role while the wife was away. The wife was always in the home as a deterrent. People were not prepared for these situational changes in the U.S. Overall, the dilemma is one of rapid transition from a preindustrial to a technologically advanced society.

In any role conflict, and particularly in child abuse and incest cases, the counselor is faced with the dual objective of protecting the client from harm and keeping the family intact. Many interactions of mental health professionals and Haitians involve state health and welfare services which may seek to separate parents and children. In cases which offer a threat to the continuity of the Haitian family, the following steps should be taken: (1) explain the full situation and legal implications, (2) discuss options and alternatives, (3) give comfort, assuring that this particular situation is not the end of the world, (4) convey to the client that he/she is not alone, (5) don't take sides; family therapy techniques of reforging alliances are inappropriate in these cases, (6) try to see the man separately before addressing the problems of the family unit as a whole, and (7) set up goals and objectives for the family.

Ethnic Self-Depreciation

Haiti is associated with hardship. Haitian identity may be equated with low value. When Haitians are well established in the U.S., some try to bury the past and will flagrantly reject their Haitian identity. If, in turn, they experience unexpected hardship, they will have lost their support system.

The issue of ethnic self-esteem is very difficult to treat. This type of client comes with anger and self-hatred, and may reject Haitian counselors. There is negative transference and paranoid projection onto the community. Such clients may accuse all Haitians as responsible for their problems. They see it in males and females, adolescents, young adults, and even some elderly. This condition is mostly seen in adults who have suffered some status reversals, but is also seen in some adolescents. A particular poignant example of ethnic self-depreciation occurred in 1984 with the death of a 17 year old Haitian, whose name was anglicized as "Fred." A high achiever, Fred appeared to be a popular, successful young man with good school grades, an American girlfriend, a job, and bright prospects for the future. He spoke unaccented English and everyone thought he was Black American. One day his sister visited him at the fast-food restaurant where he worked and, in front of his girlfriend, spoke to Fred in Haitian Creole. Fred responded with violent anger. Following this episode he was very withdrawn, and a few days later he went to a vacant parking lot and shot himself. The newspaper accounts indicated the suicide was a direct sequela of exposure of his Haitian ethnicity. Discussion with his counselor indicated that Fred's perception was that the only way for him to succeed was to identify as an American, and everything about his Haitian identity was an impediment to success. Although there were obviously other problems—depression, and perhaps incipient decompensation in an overstriving adolescent— mental health professionals who knew Fred as a Haitian volunteer youth worker felt that his suicide could well have been avoided if the issue of ethnic identity had been acknowledged and explored.

Coping with Mental Illness

In any case of mental illness, a Haitian family will try to be support- ive until the behavior becomes intolerable. There is however, a tendency to deny the seriousness of problems. Family members are able to deal with cases of temporary depression and anxiety, but cannot deal with more severe neurotic reactions nor with overt mental illness. They will try to extrude the afflicted person. Because of this, even in cases of mild depression, the CMHC may try to find accommodations for a client outside the family setting. Among Haitians, the pressure to minimize any kind of disability is very great. There is a powerful incentive not to return to any previous low socioeconomic status, not to slide back to a primitive level of survival. A handicap will limit a person's opportunity to make money and achieve. So Haitians often view the dependency im- posed by a handicap as a life-threatening situation.

For the afflicted client the loss of material things that connoted status may precipitate a reactive depression. This sets up a vicious circle; the client will lose not only material things but human support.

Strengths and Adaptive Strategies

There are multiple categories of strength that are important to know in training counselors to work with Haitians:

(a) **Identity and Moral Pride.** In contrast to ethnic self-hatred that is a pathological sign in some Haitian clients, more Haitians feel a sense of pride in a value system associated with Haitian tradition. "I am Haitian—I won't lie; I won't steal." A counselor can establish a base- line of moral behavior to negotiate treatment goals. A moral con- tract gives a basis for negotiation. For example, property destruction or stealing are perceived as degenerate by many Haitian clients. A counselor can establish rapport and open dialogue by using such values as motivators for enhancing self-esteem and even for developing marketing skills, since stealing for survival is an unacceptable alternative to working. The depressed patient, particularly one who has had difficulty finding work, can be stimulated to attend vocational rehabilitation training through a moral imperative to avoid becoming a thief. These values can also be used to insure compliance to community rules in a group setting.

(b) **Family.** When there is a strong concerned family system, the family provides this basic moral code in addition to social support. The Haitian community also provides surrogate families for individuals without kin. If there is a common friend, a family will accept a stranger into their household or supportive network simply because of the referral of a third party known to both. People from the same town or locality will also provide a kin-like support system.

(c) **Tradition.** For Haitians, the ability to attach themselves to a past history gives a sense of pride, stability and continuity. Haitians recognize they had a culture and a place, and there is a strong historical and political commitment to home. They can rationalize that this is a transitional phase and someday they may be able to go home. The long history of Haiti as an independent country under Black control is another factor of pride for many Haitians.

(d) **More Flexible Margin for Survival.** Haitian entrants are used to subsisting on very little. For example, some Haitians can survive on one meal a day because they have been accustomed to it. Some Haitians can survive with unemployment four or five months because they have a precedent for that in Haiti. Haitians can survive and deal with hardships with minimal supports far better than people used to more creature comforts. A case manager who can find one meal a day for a Haitian is in a strong position to negotiate other goals.

(e) **Achievement Orientation.** Haitians have aspirations for the future. They are people who know why they are here and will seize opportunities. Most Haitians are not passive, blase, or blocked by inertia. They are immigrants who are always looking for ways of upgrading their opportunities. They will take courses, try to acquire skills, move to wherever jobs can be found. There is high frustation tolerance because they expect to encounter hardships.

(f) **Group Commitment.** Criminality is not a way of life. Haitians come from an island society, with open doors. Most are committed to others, not narcissistic or self-oriented. They are interested in the advancement of their children and their community.

(g) Cooperation. Haitians clients generally will be willing to cooperate with the counselor when the counselor is perceived as culturally sensitive and with problem-solving potential. Explanations will generally be well accepted and resistance minimal.

In dealing with Haitian clients counselors should be aware that they can appeal to these strengths to optimize case management strategies. The family is not always there. When they are, families are typically very supportive and show a strong sense of obligation and duty. Counselors need to focus on these strengths rather than to see family interactions in a pathological light.

REFERENCES

Colimon, M-T. (1979). *Le chant des sirenes* (Chant.). Port-au-Prince, Haiti: Les Editions du Soleil.

CHAPTER 10

ISSUES IN THE TRAINING OF COUNSELORS FOR ASIAN AMERICANS

MARIA ROOT, CHRISTINE HO and STANLEY SUE

Introduction

ETHNIC MINORITIES have received little tailoring of the mental health care system to meet their specific needs. Asian Americans in particular represent a diversity of groups whose bicultural and bilingual needs pose a challenge for the mental health system. For example, Chinese, Japanese, Korean, Pilipino,[1] Pacific Islanders, Vietnamese, etc., often require services that are unavailable in the mainstream system. The deficit in appropriate services may stem in part from the stereotype of Asians as a well adjusted and model minority. Problems of delinquency, drug abuse, and marital strife have been reported at much lower rates than for other cultural or ethnic populations, resulting in minimal efforts to respond to their mental health needs. Obviously, to the extent that the services are inappropriate, Asian Americans tend to avoid mental health facilities, prematurely terminate therapy, or seek alternative help-systems (Sue & Morishima, 1982). The fact that Asian Americans are underrepresented as clients in the mental health system has traditionally served to perpetuate the stereotype that they are relatively free of mental disturbance. Only recently has there been recognition that Asian Americans experience significant mental health problems despite the low utilization of services offered in the mental health system (Sue & McKinney, 1975).

The President's Commission on Mental Health (1978) **Report to the President** succinctly summarized the magnitude of the unmet needs of

Asian and other minority populations. As a result, changes in policies to ameliorate these problems have been initiated. For example, the National Institute of Mental Health has specified that special populations which include minority groups become a priority. The American Psychological Association has required an assessment of clinical programs' sensitivity and responsiveness to addressing training needs for serving minority populations.

This chapter is dedicated to an overview of the Asian-American needs and the steps that can be taken in the training of counselors to work with Asian Americans. It is suggested that an awareness of the culturally specific needs must be integrated into current conceptions of mental health care. Only then can there be an increase in the utilization of services and the reduction of the dropout rate in treatment. Our emphasis is on the need to train mental health professionals and paraprofessionals to meet current and future needs in the assessment and delivery of services to one of our most rapidly growing ethnic minority populations.

Cultural Factors and Treatment

One problem in the delivery of mental health services to Asian American-Pacific Americans (AAPA) is the failure to recognize cultural factors and conceptual differences between Asians and Westerners. This problem is further compounded since training practices consistently neglect to provide training, education, and experiences in dealing with ethnic minorities. As noted by Sue and Morishima (1982), this insensitivity to cultural factors influences all phases of psychotherapy including the assessment of problems, therapeutic interventions, process, and outcome.

The assessment of problems is biased since mental health professionals do not recognize AAPA cultural values, behavioral patterns and traditions and do not distinguish these from behavioral patterns often considered deviant in Western cultures. For example, traditional Asians place great emphasis on the family and behave in accordance to their roles and statuses within the community. The emphasis on the family in AAPA groups may be misinterpreted as overly dependent from a western conceptualization which views independence from the family of origin as the appropriate behavioral pattern.

Communication styles of Asians are often subtle and reserved. Variables such as age, sex, status, role, familiarity, concept of obligation, respect, shame, and "loss of face" often govern the style of communication of AAPA individuals. The customs are so important that AAPA individuals frequently use indirect forms of communication. For example, a third person may be brought in as a go-between in situations of confrontation or conflict in order to avoid loss of face for both parties involved. Unfamiliar with these customs and values of AAPA's, mental health professionals assess AAPA clients based on western standards of interaction which rely primarily on direct verbal communciation. Because of this, AAPA's are often mislabelled as non-expressive, quiet, passive, resistant, and uncaring.

Many AAPA's, especially those who are recent immigrants, do not speak English or speak it poorly. Clients may answer affirmatively to be polite when they do not understand the interviewer's questions. The interviewer, on the other hand, may place more emphasis on the choice of words or word order than is intended by the client. The language barrier and communication styles can therefore directly interfere in the adequate assessment of problems.

Cultural factors also influence therapeutic processes. Traditional psychotherapy is typically insight and feeling oriented. Therapists help clients explore their feelings and understand their problems. Asians, on the other hand, frequently perceive therapists similarly to medical doctors. They seek concrete advice, structure, guidance, and directions to deal with problems. Indepth personal questions by therapists may cause intense discomfort and disillusionment. In turn, these actions and the lack of concrete solutions may contribute to high rates of premature termination in AAPA clients.

Not only do cultural factors affect the assessment of problems and therapeutic processes, they also have tremendous impact on goal setting. For example, traditional western therapy often strives for individualism as an implicit goal of therapy. This goal, however, is likely to be counterproductive with many AAPA clients because it is in direct opposition to the cultural priority that stresses family over individual rights.

D. Sue (1981) suggests that the differences between Asian and Western conceptualizations can be perceived as language-bound, class-bound and culture-bound processes. Most AAPA's have bilingual and/or bicultural backgrounds. Even if they are brought up speaking primarily English, they are influenced by their parents who are bilingual and/or speak poor English. The heavy reliance on verbal interaction in psychotherapy can hinder not only accurate assessment of the character and motive of clients, but also rapport and therapeutic outcome.

Many AAPA persons do not fit the ideal middle-class YAVIS (young, attractive, verbal, intelligent, and successful) type of clients who are preferred by therapists (D. Sue, 1981). Unlike middle-class clients, they expect concrete and tangible advice which deals with their immediate concerns. They are often uncomfortable dealing with ambiguity, prolonged verbal exchange, and long range goals involved in traditional therapeutic situations. The relationship is further strained since most therapists are of middle-class or upper-class background. Clients may be likely to mistrust an authority from a different class.

As mentioned earlier, traditional AAPA culture differs from western cultures in that Asians tend to place great emphasis on the family as the central unit rather than the individual. In contrast to western culture where independent thinking and emotional expressiveness are encouraged, AAPA's behaviors are structured according to their role and status in the family and society (Hsu, 1970). Their interaction is well defined. Communication tends to be one-way from authority figures to the person. Expression of feelings in public is discouraged. When problems arise in the individuals, they are encouraged to keep them within the family. Since individuals are viewed as representatives of the family, exposing problems to mental health professionals would bring shame into the family and cause it to lose face in the community.

Cultural differences concerning non-verbal communication are also significant. For example, D. Sue (1981) pointed out that traditional silence is a sign for respect for elders in Chinese and Japanese cultures. The use of silence by AAPA's may be used to highlight a significant point instead of to signal others to join in the conversation.

Eye contact in the western culture is considered as an indication of attentiveness, although in the Asian culture, it may be viewed as a sign of lack of respect or deference. Likewise, volume, speed and directness in conversation also communicate different meanings in the two cultures. The western emphasis on directness in speech may alienate many Asians. Indirectness in speech is preferred since it avoids direct confrontation which may cause loss of face.

The previous discussion of cultural differences provides a context within which to understand AAPA behavior. As a note of caution, the context must not be confounded with the individual. AAPA's are a diverse group of individuals representing a heritage from various Asian countries such as China, Japan, the Philippines, Korea, and Pacific Islands. Personalities are influenced by the individual's unique cultural heritage and experiences. Mental health professionals need to appreciate the uniqueness of the ethnic individual and to utilize cultural differences to strengthen their understanding of the person.

In order to understand AAPA's, training practices need to provide sufficient information and knowledge of Asian and Pacific American culture, and allow actual experience working with Asian American clients. Current training practices do not provide adequate knowledge and experience with ethnic minorities. Recently, Bernal and Padilla (1982) conducted a survey of all fully and provisionally accredited APA clinical psychology programs in the United States. Of 106 programs, 76 programs offered replies to a survey that assessed the presence of curriculum and practicum experiences relevant to ethnic minority groups. They investigated the presence of five types of courses containing content relevant to broadening knowledge and cultural sensitivity: (1) courses that dealt exclusively with minority content, (2) cross-cultural clinical courses, (3) sociocultural courses, (4) cross-cultural research courses, and (5) other courses with minority content.

The findings of Bernal and Padilla's survey emphasize the need for a commitment to advancing efforts to enhance the training of future minority and majority professionals to serve minority persons. Thirty-one of 76 programs responding revealed a total of 57 minority related courses of which most were taught by 16 programs. Only 12 programs specifically offered courses that dealt exclusively with minority content. No program required a minority course for the Ph.D., while five programs required minority content in courses required for the Ph.D. The majority of programs did not provide courses to address sociocultural variables in behavior. Offering minority courses was unrelated to the presence or absence of minority faculty members within the department.

The implications of this survey are obvious. As of 1979, little was being offered in graduate training to prepare therapists and counselors to effectively work with culturally-dissimilar clients. Along with developing knowledge of the Asian culture, actual experiences dealing with AAPA's are crucial. Sue and Morishima (1982) pointed out that we must depart from discussion of AAPA's and their cultures on an abstract level and begin to apply knowledge on a concrete level. They suggested that only through actual contacts and experiences with Asian Americans can counselors develop appropriate skills.

What Can Be Done?

The overview of the inadequacies of the present mental health care system suggests directions in which to train culturally sensitive therapists. The model of intervention described in this chapter targets training of mental health professionals at three levels (Kim, 1981). The first level develops a knowledge base appropriate for the professional in his or her speciality such as clinical, counseling, or social psychology. The second level provides experience with a diversity of ethnic populations in order for trainees to appreciate the impact of cultures. Lastly, the third level of training integrates cultural awareness with therapeutic skills and knowledge for particular populations. The most attention is reserved for the last two levels of training since they contribute the most novel ideas for developing culturally sensitive mental health professionals.

The first level of training is a basic requirement for producing competent mental health professionals. It is at this level that one develops the knowledge base and psychotherapeutic skills relevant to being a counselor. Exposure to appropriate courses in clinical/counseling research and theory, assessment, treatment, psychopathology, community dynamics, prevention, and so on lays the foundation for professional practice. The academic training is so integrated with supervised field experiences in which trainees work with clients and community agencies. This first level of training is characteristic of most of the mental health training programs in psychology, psychiatry, social work, and psychiatric nursing. Unfortunately, many training programs do not advance much farther than level one training. The assumption in level one is that the development of basic counseling skills is applicable across cultures. As mentioned previously, there is now growing recognition that what may be considered as "basic" skills are often culturally-bound. The skills acquired are more appropriate for mainstream Americans.

Level two training is intended to provide trainees with an appreciation of cultural influences and of the status of ethnic minority groups. By offering courses or by incorporating ethnic content in existing courses on race relations, sociocultural factors and mental health, racism, ethnicity and adjustment, cross-cultural methods, etc., trainees can begin to discern those skills that are culturally-bound from those that have broader cross-cultural utility. In addition to curricular considerations, means must be found for trainees to work with a multiethnic diversity of faculty, students, clients, and community settings. Only through a multiethnic training environment can knowledge acquired through courses or workshops be applied and tested.

Level three training is especially geared for persons who anticipate working with particular populations such as AAPA's. While level two makes trainees more receptive to the importance of cultural factors in treatment and the dynamics of social structures in race relations, ethnic minority groups are quite heterogeneous: Knowledge of Black Americans reveals very little about the status of AAPA's, American Indians, or Hispanics. Even among the AAPA populations, it can be argued that, for example, Chinese are quite dissimilar to Pilipinos. In level three training, trainees (as in the second level) receive academic and field experience; however, the emphasis is on issues that are critical to a particular group. In the case of Asian Americans, immigration, overseas culture, the extended family concept, guilt and shame, values involving obligations, and historical experiences in the United States would be a few of the important topics to examine.

Two points should be noted in our discussion of the levels of training. First, the division of the levels does not imply that training necessarily involves a sequence in which an emphasis on ethnicity and culture (levels two and three) is simply added to the traditional kinds of skills found in level one. Ideally, level one should have ethnic and cultural considerations well integrated in the curriculum and in field placements for trainees. In practice, however, this is simply not the case. As indicated by Bernal and Padilla (1982), the inclusion of ethnicity and mental health contents has not occurred in a systematic fashion in most of the training programs. Our discussion of the three levels of training is thus used for heuristic purpose only, as illustrated in our later discussion of a training program for Asian Americans. Second, the analysis of the three components of training should not be perceived as relevant only to trainees who want to work with a particular ethnic group. While level three training is designed for specific expertise with a particular group, levels one and two are essential for any counselor. They prepare one to avoid ethnocentric bias. Even among White Americans, sociocultural factors are important to consider because of differences in social class, geographic background, sex, age, and cultural heritage.

An Asian-American Training Program

In view of the doubling of the Asian-American populations from 1970 to 1980 and the unaddressed mental health needs of these populations, it would seem reasonable to suppose that the training of mental health workers to meet the needs of AAPA groups would be a high priority. Unfortunately, this has not been the case. Because of stereotypes of Asian well-being and the lack of strong political advocacy in the mental health arena, Asian Americans were unable to receive much attention or aid in the early 1970's (Wong, 1981). Two Asian American social work programs were funded by the National Institute of Mental Health, although the programs primarily operated to fund Asian American social work students and to place the students for training in agencies that served AAPA populations.

The most comprehensive training program, the only one of its kind for Asian Americans in psychology, was the National Asian American Training Center in San Francisco. Funded by the National Institute of Mental Health in 1979, the Center served as a predoctoral internship for clinical or community psychology students. An analysis of the Center is instructive since it attempted to grapple with many of the issues presented in this chapter. Although no empirical evaluation of the outcome of the training program is available, the Center has served as a suitable internship for many students, and the mental health center which sponsored the program received full accreditation from the American Psychological Association. Five critical considerations were addressed: The model of training, critical mass of personnel, type of trainee, clientele and the community, and structure of the program (Sue, 1981).

Training Model. In trying to increase the availability of mental health manpower for AAPA communities, it was necessary to develop a model of training. The Center adopted a **speciality** model in that interns would be encouraged to develop general skills in assessment, intervention, research, etc., with a wide range of clients but with particular and specialized focus on AAPA groups. There were at least three major reasons for the adoptions of a speciality model. First, it was not practical to limit interns' experiences solely to AAPA clients. The community mental health center served a multiethnic clientele and the internship experience should reflect this diversity. Second, and more importantly, the Center maintained the philosophy that professional competencies could be developed only in the context of a multiethnic environment. For example, awareness and appreciation of Asian American cultural values occur only when there are non-Asian American groups with which to compare and contrast. Finally, if interns were trained to work only with AAPA's, they would be limited in the kinds of career options which allowed them to work with a special population. In selecting the specialty model, the Center intended to train competent psychologists who would have special skills rather than psychologists who could work solely with AAPA's.

Critical Mass. Specialty training is effective only when a critical mass of knowledgeable and skilled supervisors is available in the area of specialty. For AAPA's finding a sufficient number of supervisors was difficult. Asian Americans represented only a small fraction of the population and mental health professionals with expertise on these ethnic groups were difficult to find. Furthermore, since AAPA's represented many diverse groups (e.g., Chinese, Japanese, Pilipinos, Koreans, Cambodians, and Samoans to name a few), it was a major problem to locate bilingual/bicultural mental health workers for each group. Under the circumstances, the Center, located at the Richmond Maxi-Center in San Francisco, formed close working relationships with other facilities such as Chinatown Child Development Center, Asian Community Mental Health services, and San Francisco General Hospital. Interns could rotate to these facilities and be supervised by staff or other consultants with expertise on different AAPA groups, if such expertise could not be found at the Center.

Type of Trainee

Since the Center was funded by NIMH, it was limited to the selection of predoctoral students from APA-approved or NIMH-funded university programs in clinical or community psychology. At the time, the training program was not APA approved and it was unclear how many graduate students could be recruited for specialty training with Asian American populations. The Center itself maintained that the effectiveness of the program was highly dependent on the quality of its interns who would be required to devote one-year, full time involvement. Ideally, the Center sought students who were clinically competent (strong on level one functioning) with substantial interests in ethnicity in general (level two) and Asian Americans in particular (level three). All of these requirements and considerations would naturally limit the pool of prospective interns.

While recruitment was initially difficult, by 1981 outstanding interns were found from the University of California, Berkeley; Baylor University; University of Colorado; University of Washington; University of Denver; and University of Manitoba. This was accomplished through informal contacts with university faculty and through announcements sent to universities seeking assistance in identifying students who might be interested in the training program.

Clientele and Community

The National Asian American Psychology Training Center was located at the Richmond Maxi-Center, a community mental health center in San Francisco. With a catchment area composed predominantly of Asian

Americans, interns would be assured of access to Asian-American clients. Moreover, the rotation allowed additional exposure to a wide range of clients. About half of the clients seen by interns were from AAPA groups.

Program

As an internship program, the Center helped students to develop clinical-therapeutic skills, an awareness of community dynamics and intervention strategies, and research skills. These were accomplished not only through supervised contact with clients but also through case conferences, seminars, and involvement with community agencies. Particular attention was paid to the cultural backgrounds of clients, the influence of their background in interpersonal behaviors, the importance of family and community, and therapeutic strategies that were consistent with the lifestyle of the clients. One innovative aspect of the program was the development of a videotape library. Individuals with expertise on Asian Americans are small in number and distributed throughout the nation. In order to more directly expose interns to the ideas of these individuals, the Training Center videotaped lectures, symposia, debates, workshops, etc., of these individuals. Some of the videotapes were made of guests who agreed to appear at the Training Center. Others were taken at conferences, conventions, and presentations from throughout the nation. Topics on the videotapes included Asian American mental health, family, personality, stress, social support systems, cultures, etc. Thus interns could view the videotapes and discuss the issues presented. These videotapes could be available for future interns and others (university programs, internships, etc.) could also borrow the tapes.

As mentioned previously, no formal empirical evaluations were made of interns' outcomes as a result of training. Comments from interns about the training experience have been highly favorable (Tanaka, 1981) and the mental health center, largely because of the Training Center, was accredited by the American Psychological Association.

Summary and Conclusions

In this chapter, we have tried to indicate the inadequacies of the mental health system in the provision of services for AAPA groups. Asian Americans have not only been relatively ignored in the mental health field but also have been unable to receive effective services. Problems in therapy and counseling occur whenever mental health providers are unaware of the bilingual/bicultural needs, family dynamics, values and beliefs, and the communication patterns of AAPA clients. In order to improve mental health services, a number of strategies can be used. For example, certain skills training programs can be initiated (Pedersen, 1977) or teams of mental health workers with collective expertise on ethnic minority groups can be developed (Lefley & Bestman, 1984). We focused on the structure of an internship training program for postdoctural students. Such a program, of course, has to deal with a wide range of issues and problems such as the nature of the training, staffing, availability of clients, etc. The lesson learned from the program is that solutions to conceptual and practical problems in a specialty training can be found, if available resources can be pulled together and if innovative ideas are generated.

NOTE

1. Pilipino is the preferred ethnic designation for the group commonly referred to as Filipino.

REFERENCES

Bernal, M. E., & Padilla, A. M. (1982). Status of minority curricula and training in clinical psychology. *American Psychologist, 37,* 780-787.

Hsu, F. L. K. (1970). *Americans and chinese.* New York: Doubleday.

Kim, S. C. (1981). The utilization of cultural variables in the training of clinical community psychologists. *Journal of Community Psychology, 9,* 298-300.

Lefley, H. P., & Bestman, E. W. (1984). Community mental health and minorities: A multi-ethnic approach. In S. Sue & T. Moore (Eds.), *The pluralistic society: A community mental health perspective.* New York: Human Sciences Press.

Pedersen, P. B. (1977). The triad model of cross-cultural counselor training. *Personnel and Guidance Journal, 56,* 94-100.

President's Commission on Mental Health. (1978). *Report to the president.* Washington, DC: U.S. Government Printing Office.

Sue, D. W. (1981). *Counseling the culturally different: Theory and practice.* New York: Wiley.

Sue, S., & McKinney, H. (1975). Asian Americans in the community mental health care system. *American Journal of Orthopsychiatry, 45,* 111-118.

Sue, S., & Morishima, J. K. (1982). *The mental health of Asian Americans: Contemporary issues in identifying and healing mental problems.* San Francisco: Jossey-Bass.

Tanaka, M. (1981). Products of clinical-community-based training: National Asian American psychology training center. *Journal of Community Psychology, 9,* 301-305.

Wong, H. Z. (1981). Contextual factors for the development of the National Asian American Psychology Training Center. *Journal of Community Psychology, 9,* 289-292.

PART IV

CULTURALLY-SPECIALIZED INTERVENTIONS

CHAPTER 11

INTERVENTION TECHNIQUES IN THE BLACK COMMUNITY

EVALINA W. BESTMAN

INTRODUCTION

THE JOINT COMMISSION REPORT of 1961, Action for Mental Health, served as the forerunner of the Community Mental Health Center Act. The Black community nationwide suffered a paucity of mental health services prior to the community mental health, community psychology and community psychiatry movement of the 1960s. The most accessible services were the emergency room and inpatient wards of the local public and on a longer term basis, the State Hospitals.

The 1960s was a period of many movements and changes which were considered revolutionary in the history of the United States. The Civil Rights Movement, the War on Poverty and Affirmative Action legislation helped to create an air of analysis or assessment of the state of affairs in the institutions and values which govern all aspects of our daily lives. For Black-Americans it was a period of reawakening to the fact that they have a right to demand access to more than the schools, restaurants and voting booths. Blacks also began to look at the state of their health and subsequently, to mental health conditions in America.

The Community Mental Health Center Act among many other requirements required that services within a catchment area be culturally appropriate and accessible. Many Black mental health professionals believed that the requirements for community based services promulgated in the Community Mental Health Center Legislation would be a corrective factor in eliminating the enormous disparities between psychiatric treatment for Black and White Americans (Bestman, 1981). However, knowing full well that enforcement of the requirement would be questionable, the majority of the community mental health centers went about business as usual—the provision of mental health services to White middle class oriented individuals.

In most instances, the centers have not been responsive to Black and other minority groups. The Black communities nationwide have suffered a paucity of mental health services. The most accessible services continue to be crisis emergency, medication maintenance, inpatient wards of local public receiving facilities and on a longer term basis, the State Hospitals.

Researchers within the University of Miami's Department of Psychiatry under the leadership of Dr. Hazel Weidman decided to develop a model for the delivery of service which emphasized the cross cultural approaches to care. It was more than just an emphasis. The model itself was an outgrowth of research (Health Ecology Project) which was conducted on the health systems, practices and beliefs of the populations residing within the inner-city of Miami. The research results in regards to utilization rates of traditional mental health systems was consistent with the results nationwide—minority groups have a low utilization rate when compared to the utilization rates of Whites.

Dr. Weidman and her staff of social scientists, using the basic hypothesis that individuals would be more responsive to a mental health agency which embraced their cultural systems, submitted an application to the National Institute of Mental Health to fund such a center.

The Department of Psychiatry in conjunction with Jackson Memorial Hospital (JMH) prepared a Community Mental Health Program (CMHP) grant proposal, designed to serve a federal poverty designed catchment area that included the research population. The field data on cultural variations in the distribution, manifestation and conceptualization of mental health problems (Bestman, Lefley and Scott, 1976; Lefley, 1979; Lefley and Bestman, 1984) together with emergent diagnostic and therapeutic problems among ethnic patients in the hospital system strongly suggested that a CMHP established along traditional lines would neither be maximally effective nor optimally utilized. Further, while all groups suffered from multiple socioeconomic environmental stressors, the indications were that, in some cases, culturally specific therapeutic interventions might be required to deal with different ethnic groups living within the same poverty area (Weidman, 1978)

CULTURAL PROGRAM

In March 1974, the CMHP was funded to serve an inner-city area of 200,000 with a median income of $4,647 and a multiplicity of social problems. The area is predominantly Black (over 50%) and Spanish-speaking, with the balance primarily poor Anglo elderly. Distinct cultural differences between Afro-Americans and Afro-Caribbean groups, and among Cubans, Puerto Ricans and other Latinos, suggested the need for a model that would include staff with sufficient linguistic and cultural expertise to meet the needs of clients from diverse populations.

This model developed by the CMHP was specifically tailored to the ethnic communities and assessed needs of Catchment Area IV in Miami. The major characteristics of this catchment area are (a) its ubiquity of social stressors — poverty, unemployment, crime, poor housing, medical problems and the like; (b) its multilingual ethnically diverse composition; and (c) problems associated with ethnicity, e.g., a history of racial segregation and discrimination, large immigrant and exile populations; illegal alien status and differential levels of acculturative stress.

The CMHP model thus began with two primary objectives: (1) to provide highly accessible, culturally appropriate services which would encompass the range of presenting complaints; and (2) to help alleviate environmental stressors by insuring that area residents receive their fair share of adaptive resources.

The model was developed to provide services to six predominant ethnic groups within the catchment area — Anglo elderly, Black Americans, Bahamians, Cubans, Haitians and Puerto Ricans.

THE BLACK COMMUNITY

Characteristics

For the Black community, the Director of the Black American Team had the awesome task of defining the Black community and securing a location for the delivery of services. Dr. Carroo (1975) found two contrasting communities: (1) Model Cities — population 80,000 — which had received an "infusion" of federal dollars in the 1960s. The community had a "conglomeration" of social service agencies, businesses and institutions; (2) Overtown — population 15,000 — which is a community in transition.

Model Cities had large public housing developments mixed with single family and other multiple-family dwellings. Most of the major institutions, schools and churches were being built in the area to accommodate the movement from Overtown. To move to Model Cities was a move "up" and "out" of the inner-city ghetto referred to as Overtown. The population in terms of length of stay was more stable. Your professional, working and non-working classes resided in this community together.

Overtown, which is situated on prime property within the inner-city and bordering downtown development, has been and is still destined for destruction by the city planners. Urban renewal and major expressway construction were the primary methods used to destroy the community. All of the businesses, health and social services were eliminated or relocated to other parts of the greater Miami community.

> Urban renewal has created several psychologic consequences for Overtown residents. Relation and disruption have severed strong cultural and emotional ties for many families and precipitated the surfacing of many social problems. Residents have experienced profound helplessness in preserving their community and its remaining institutions, and restoring it in the aftermath of urban renewal. This sense of helplessness is coupled with a strong feeling of lack of control within an unpredictable environment, which evokes risky and fatalistic behavior. Finally, Overtown residents exhibit a profound suspiciousness of strangers, White or Black. This "cultural paranoia" is viewed by Cobbs and Grier (1968) as an adaptive survival technique among Blacks, but it seems greatly exaggerated in the Overtown community (Carroo, 1975).

As in other parts of the nation, Blacks in Dade are confronted with the full range of social and economic problems — lower incomes, higher poverty rates, more unemployment and more single parent families.

In many respects, however, Dade's Blacks differ from Blacks in other metropolitan areas. Black Miami is characterized by a diversity of cultures. There are several distinct contrasting communities differentiated by culture, national origin, language and tradition. By the latest 1980 census, one of every three Miami-area Blacks was foreign born — primarily in Caribbean countries. These range from the initial migration from the Bahamas to the more recently arrived Cubans, Haitians and Jamaicans.

TEAM ORGANIZATION

The agency sought to first develop its organizational structure. The decision was made to establish and develop ethnically identified teams. To this end, was established three teams in the Black communities — Black American, Bahamian and Haitian Teams. These teams were directed by social scientists who were specialists in the three identified cultures and had considerable expertise in the mental health field. The teams consisted of indigenous neighborhood workers, generally of the same ethnic background as the population served. Failing this criterion, the workers who were of different background than the populations served had to have extensive knowledge of and experience in the culture of the clients served. Clinical back-up staff initially consisted of a part-time psychiatrist and two social workers who provided service to each team on a rotating schedule. As the program expanded, there was a corresponding increase in clinical staff who were subsequently assigned on a full-time basis to each team. The majority of clinical staff were of the same ethnic background as the clients.

The major objectives of the CMHP were:

1. To provide highly accessible and culturally appropriate services to individuals and families encountering emotional difficulties.
2. To link individuals and families in distress with a wide range of supportive social services and resources.
3. To help prevent the onset or worsening of mental health problems through involvement and outreach in the community.
4. To sensitize the community to culturally appropriate intervention strategies and mental health care.

To implement these objectives, the teams conducted an analysis of the community data in terms of the social, psychological and economic needs and ethnic clustering to determine the best location for the clinics. The initial months were spent in developing the team concept, training and mapping of strategies for community intervention.

In keeping with the agency's philosophy of having the community take responsibility for determining its own destiny, the teams established a local advisory board which consisted of residents of the service community. The board members played a role as consultant to the Team directors in the selection of personnel and identification of key informants and needs of the community.

In addition to information secured from board members, the staff personally mapped the entire neighborhood block by block and noted the location of businesses, residences, industries, religious and educational institutions and social service and other community resources. The team members maintained high-visibility within the communities. They paved the way for entry of the agency into the various neighborhoods.

INTERVENTION TECHNIQUES

In developing services for a multi-ethnic populace within the inner-city, the staff was aware that a new course was being charted. The message within the community was that Blacks would not utilize outpatient type services. Because of neglect of the Black community by the psychiatric and mental health community for so long, the needs were tremendous. The staff designed some intervention strategies to address the pressing needs in addition to the standard services found in any psychiatric facility such as medication maintenance and therapy.

Interventions have occurred in four major areas: community organization, criminal and juvenile justice, youth services, consultation and training. Some of the examples provided below exemplify how the agency has been active as a catalyst in mobilizing community resources and initiating projects to meet community needs which may play more heavily into preventing mental illness.

Community Organization

The Black American Team was instrumental in organizing an Interagency Council (IAC) which consisted of human service provider agency representatives located within the Overtown community. Because of the limited number of agencies and services available to the residents, the team believed that all of the agencies should work cooperatively in assessing needs and coordinating services. The IAC could unify its resources in advocating for the community and monitoring the effectiveness of the provider agencies. To facilitate the formation of the IAC, the Director of the Black American Team contacted a Black State Legislator, Representative Gwen Cherry, whose legislative office was located in Overtown. Representative Cherry consented to working closely with the team in organizing the IAC. She hosted the first meeting and made her office available for meetings. The response from the other agencies was without exception positive.

A major problem confronting the community was the absence of accessible health care. More specifically, preventive medicine was needed. The urban planners noted that the county supported hospital (University of Miami-Jackson Memorial Medical Center) and the Public Health Department was located within walking distance. Thus, the request for a primary health care clinic was denied. These were the same urban planners who effectively placed geographical barriers such as major highways and expressways around the community. The Black American Team conducted a needs assessment relevant to health care. Previous research data also revealed that the population was at greater risk for major health problems including communicable diseases such as tuberculosis and venereal disease. The team with the support of IAC presented its findings to the Director of the Public Health Department and requested that the Mobile Health Team come to Overtown twice monthly. The Dade County Community Action Agency (CAA) cooperated with the team by providing parking space for the van and telephone service for the health team members. The primary service was health screening, vaccinations, physical exams and information and referral to approximately thirty individuals per day.

The Haitian Team, working within the Edison-Little River community where most Haitian Entrants reside, was confronted with a clientele with multi-faceted problems. Approximately 70% were illegal aliens with no status as refugees which rendered them ineligible for existing public benefits including work permits. The team mounted a major advocacy project for social security cards for the clients. They negotiated with Social Security to serve as a site for the filing of applications for Haitian Entrants. Over 1,200 Haitians were assisted in obtaining social security cards. The team members served as interpreters and assisted the clients in handling of immigration matters. The local Social Security Office eventually hired Creole and French-speaking staff for the processing of applications.

In response to the riots in the Model City area, the Bahamian Team formed a task force which was charged with "hanging out" on the streets, in the parks, at the local gathering places under the trees near the liquor stores, in the housing projects, at the schools, at the hospitals, etc. The objectives were to (1) identify some of the precipitating factors; (2) assist in maintaining calm within the community; (3) identify individual leaders for the formulation of a planning and coordinating group; and (4) identify individuals or families needing social service, legal and/or health assistance. A report on intervention strategies in riotous conditions was prepared for the National Institute of Mental Health. As a result of the survey and needs assessment, 1.1 million dollars was awarded to the Center for mental health services to the Black community.

Some major findings were: (1) the Criminal Justice System including Police Departments, Corrections Department and Juvenile Justice System impacted negatively on the lives of Black residents. Instances of abuse and harassment were rampant; (2) institutional racism as seen by the fact that no police officer was ever found guilty of murdering, violating civil rights, etc., of any black, was intolerable; (3) elementary school age children and adolescents were participating in the street riots. Some of them were experiencing nightmares and other signs of emotional problems; (4) relationships between ethnic groups deteriorated. More polarization occurred in schools and workplace; (5) numerous arrests occurred. Also Blacks were disproportionately incarcerated in numbers and by length of stay than White or Hispanic counterparts.

Criminal and Juvenile Justice

The agency obtained special funding (post-riot) for the Black community. One of the projects that was developed was a Courts Screening and Evaluation Unit. The staff advocated for community alternatives for incarcerated Blacks. They would conduct home studies, consult with attorneys and prepare reports for the judges. A thorough knowledge of services and resources available within the Criminal Justice System and community was essential. It was found for example that White inmates had a much greater chance of being referred to the forensic service at the jail than Black inmates. This was found to be the case even in situations where the Black had a history of mental illness. The agency would serve as a sponsor for the release for clients charged with minor crimes. This unit served 300 clients annually.

In response to the disproportionate representation of Black youth in the Juvenile Justice System, the Center established a pilot project during the past year. The aim was to prevent youngsters being sent to juvenile detention centers who were detained for a first and/or second offense. Juvenile recidivists have reported that they learned more about criminal behavior in juvenile detention facilities than on the streets. The project has one social worker for twenty five adolescents. The social worker is responsible for monitoring the client activities on a 24 hour basis. He essentially serves as a surrogate parent at the same time he works with the parents to work more effectively with their child. The project is in its second year and no client has been charged with an additional offense or been sent to a juvenile detention facility. The judges at the juvenile courts are actively pursuing additional funding for projects of this nature.

Youth Services

The Bahamian Team actively participated each summer in the Youth Employment Program. The team was limited in number of young people it could hire for the summer. During the third year of operation, the team developed a summer employment program for low-income Black teenagers. In contrast to other programs, which typically use teenagers as clean-up and recreation assistants, the focus of the team was on training the youth in a meaningful community experience. The team had developed a structured program including orientation and training in office procedures, educational films on mental health and social services, recreation, personal development sessions dealing with such topics as boy and girl relationships, good grooming, career goals and field experience (conducting needs assessments). Black professionals within the community responded positively to invitations to share their knowledge and expertise with the young people. The goals of this project were to educate the youth to: (a) become aware of and assess community needs; (b) establish community goals; (c) learn responsibility to and for the community; (d) receive training and certification as interviewers; (e) become more aware of their strengths and behaviors (Lefley and Bestman, 1984).

As an outgrowth of the Bahamian Team observation and experience with Black youth in the Model City area, a Youth Development Project (YDP) was established. The primary objectives of the project are to assist Black youngsters in becoming more knowledgeable of their history; gain a better acceptance of self; learn strategies for fighting racism; develop leadership skills. The youth attend workshops with a special focus on insight, motivation and career and vocational development. The youth through their demonstration of leadership advocated for $240,000 in funds from the county government to continue services; two of the youth have been selected to serve as congressional pages; they have been instrumental in securing funds for drug abuse services for Black youth in the Model Cities and Overtown community. The youth also formed a Crime Prevention Task Force with local merchants. This project has served over 1,000 youth since its implementation in 1982.

The Haitian Team discovered a most tragic situation regarding Haitian children and school registration as they assessed the needs of the Haitian community. They found children were not in school because of their parents' illegal status. Thus, the parents were unable to obtain student visas for their children. The team coordinated an advocacy effort which involved the Catholic Service Bureau, Legal Services of Greater Miami, Haitian American Association, Immigration and Naturalization Services and the Dade County School System. The advocacy effort resulted in a change in the admission requirements. The team established an agreement with the school system to be responsible for completing registration papers for the Haitian youngsters. The team successfully registered over 1,000 Haitian children in school. This responsibility was later transferred to a local Haitian social service organization due to budget cuts.

Consultation and Training

The Center has done extensive work in the area of consultation and training. The Team Directors who served as Culture Brokers became known within the greater community as resident experts on Black American, Bahamian and Haitian culture. The local school system utilized the culture brokers in the development of its curriculum for its desegregation center. Teachers and administrators called upon the Black Directors to interpret the behavior of students from a cultural dimension. Some of the issues that Directors were consulted about were the disproportionate representation of Black children in mentally retarded classes; the high number of suspensions that Black youth were getting when compared with White and Hispanic youth; parental involvement; academic performance; verbal skills and language — meaning of certain expressions and terminologies; lack of motivation; hygiene practices; health beliefs and practices.

Training has been conducted for the two major police departments and protective service on the cultural beliefs and practices of Blacks and Haitians. The child abuse furor is a perfect example of cultures clashing. The idiom of "spare the rod and spoil the child" is very strong within Black culture. The police could not understand the anger and rage which erupted when they would call protective services and arrest parents who were doing what they had been taught good parents should do. In other instances parents who would use alternate healers as home remedies were accused of neglecting and abusing their children. The Directors consulted with the department about specific cases.

Health practitioners at the local hospitals use the Culture Brokers to consult on hard-to-treat cases which have been cleared medically. In one case, a woman who had recovered from a heart attack and had been discharged from the hospital refused to go home. She reported that her home was possessed of evil spirits. The Director of the Bahamian Unit served as a consultant, successfully, on the case. Cross cultural training has been provided to staff and administrators of seven health establishments throughout South Florida and a College of Osteopathy.

Finally, the staff at the Center conducts workshops for other human service providers on approaches to serving Black clientele and increasing utilization rates. The agency was awarded a contract by the State to provide cross cultural training for five Deinstitutionalization Projects throughout the State of Florida. The agency participated in the development and implementation of two cross cultural training projects funded by the National Institute of Mental Health—the Cross Cultural Training Institute which trained 174 mental health professionals from 97 institutions in 22 states over a three year period. The Mental Health Human Services Training Center conducted training for paraprofessional staff throughout the State of Florida on Cuban and Haitian culture for the purpose of increasing their effectiveness in providing services to Cuban and Haitian Entrants.

In summary, the strategies discussed are but a few in a multitude of projects that the agency will pilot in its efforts to work with the community in its attempt to find answers to some of the questions and problems which prevail. Most importantly, the Black community needs to be aware that the mental health agency exists and (1) is concerned with the external and internal factors affecting the whole being; and (2) understands the impact of racism and poverty on their existence.

Thus, in addition to the provision of quality services, a major effort has to be directed toward public relations and information. The agency was wise to establish ethnic teams because the Black population identified with and responded to the Black staff. The annual meeting was a public forum which was attended by over 300 persons—it was a Citizen's Review. The agency staff including Executive Director are members of the leading Black organizations, actively participate in a church of their own choosing, make home visits, actively participate in community forums, and advocate for any person from the Black community, whether a client or not, with respect to receiving mental health services for themselves, neighbors, relatives or friends.

Essentially, all the interventions have opened the door for the Center to the community. The Center then has been able to assess the many resources which are available but not utilized by Blacks effectively. The community has likewise then entrusted the care of its chronically mentally ill and severely emotionally disturbed youth and adults to the Center.

REFERENCES

Bestman, E. W. (1981). Blacks and mental health services. In W. H. Silverman, (Ed.), *Community mental health: a sourcebook.* New York: Praeger.

Bestman, E. W., Lefley, H. P. & Scott, C. D. (1976, March). Culturally appropriate interventions: Paradigms and pitfalls. Paper presented at the 53rd annual meeting of the American Orthopsychiatric Association, Atlanta.

Carroo, A. (1975). A Black community in limbo. *Psychiatric Annals, 5,* 39-45.

Grier, W. H. & Cobbs, P. M. (1968). *Black rage.* New York: Basic Books.

Lefley, H. P. (1979). Prevalence of potential falling-out cases among the Black, Latin, and non-Latin White populations of the city of Miami. *Social Science & Medicine,* 13B, 113-114.

Lefley, H. P. & Bestman, E. W. (1984). Community mental health and minorities: A multi-ethnic approach. In S. Sue & T. Moore (Eds.), *The pluralistic society: A community mental health perspective.* New York: Human Sciences Press.

Weidman, H. H. (1978). *Miami Health Ecology Project Report: A statement on ethnicity and health.* Vol. I. Unpublished report. University of Miami.

CHAPTER 12

CHILD PSYCHIATRY AND CROSS-CULTURAL PERSPECTIVE: INDICATIONS FOR TRAINING

RAQUEL E. COHEN

Introduction

CHILD PSYCHIATRY program trainers are developing innovative approaches to educate professionals as well as to provide services to a wide variety of populations. Educators in this field affirm that in order to promote growth in this service arena, further research into the following areas needs to occur: knowledge base, manpower development, training content of educational structures, service program focus, and delivery of care (American Academy of Child Psychiatry, 1982). Over the past decade, there has been a dramatic change in social and economic realities in the United States. The structure of the nuclear family has undergone significant alterations. There has been a substantial increase in the number and proportions of single parent families, with concomitant changes in child-rearing patterns and practices. Large numbers of immigrants and refugees have permanently resettled in the United States, thereby altering population mixes and increasing ethnic diversity within the client's structure of mental health service programs.

In order to consider needs regarding the recent blend and variations in the United States' cultural values, a suitable child psychiatric training program must be designed to reassess therapeutic procedures and reconceptualize diagnostic approaches. Significant factors that will add to the existing knowledge base include child-rearing traditions and parental expectations of boy-girl behaviors within the various subcultures.

225

This chapter will focus on a specific approach by selecting the intersecting conceptual planes of a body of knowledge that incorporates cultural variables as they influence assessment, diagnosis, and treatment planning for child mental health professionals. This has been selected as a component of this chapter with the understanding that basic biological, psychodynamic and sociocultural factors in the child psychiatry curriculums need this additional component (Group for Advancement of Psychiatry, 1973). Child-rearing traditions and parental expectations of their own role and behavior as they interact with their sons and daughters need to be looked at and analyzed with the objective of selecting key areas to incorporate into our traditional curriculum. How do we blend the signs and symptoms that are catalogued in the DSM-III with signs of culturally deviant behaviors? Families continue traditional modes of child-rearing from generation to generation. Each new set of parents starts anew to bring up the next generation incorporating some novel components brought about by the settings in which they established their roots. As mental health professionals we need to find answers to many of the following questions so as to enhance our understanding of the forces interacting between parents and children. Do cultural patterns inherently unique to the family offer minimal, partial or fully supportive assistance through different developmental stages? What solutions do they provide for mastery with regard to the child's successful developmental tasks? What are the cultural processes at work that are significant determinants of the child's value system? How do specific parental role patterns contribute to the lifestyle of the child? How do psychobiological and psychosocial forces unite to promote developmental tasks? As we sort out the variables obtained from our increased focus on these issues, we will be able to develop a psychosocial profile that singles out the characteristics of the child within his culture and alerts us to the degree of deviancy, if it exists.

Parenting Roles and Child Development

The following component will attempt to incorporate some important sociological-cultural concepts into the child psychiatry clinical body of knowledge necessary to consider cultural factors. That is, to be able to use findings and principles from the field of sociology, some bridges need to be built to take those factors and place them in the context of child psychiatry training. One of the concepts that has been found to be helpful is to conceptualize the parental role as a set of important influences in the child's sense of self and guidelines for behavior. The parental role patterns are one of the developmental behavior configurations that couples begin to exercise with the birth of a child. Each member of the couple brings to the parental role previous behavior that influenced her or his identity configuration of woman and man. To understand how influential these emerging roles of parenting are, we have to consider the influences that mold culturally the child's perception of self and his unique world. To be able to sort out deviant, pathological child development signs and symptoms, we need to take into consideration the parental roles, their culture, and their child-rearing approaches.

The role of the parent can be defined as a set of specific behaviors that serve the function by which individuals fulfill physiological, psychological, and social goals. Role behaviors and their various aspects can be conceptualized as dynamic properties of that role. Parents' roles then, are socially defined within a culture by the normative expectations of that society about the responsibilities, approaches and methodologies that are exercised within certain boundaries of a set of functions performed by individuals who are ascribed the role of parent in the social system. These powerful expectations provide assurance that the sense of parental functions of nurturance, care and discipline, will be fulfilled and will mesh with roles and functional activities of other individuals (Mendel & Habenstein, 1976). There is a tendency in mental health practice to generalize cultural expectations of behavior and reactions to life events. We need to consider subcultural variations among different social classes, ethnic groups, age groups and areas of geographical setting which often alter these role expectations. This is important to realize so as not to stereotype approaches of parents toward their children's behavior across large groups identified as "Hispanics" or "Blacks." To support this statement one need only to look at the bibliography that is accumulating in the research area of Mexican Americans, Puerto Ricans, Latin American, Cubans. The same can be said about the Blacks in terms of the North, the South, or foreign-born, e.g., Haitians or South Africans. At the same time it is also important to consider the individual dynamics by which each member of a couple influences the other, by understanding the fact that these two individuals may come from two different backgrounds and present different approaches to parenthood behavior. The manner in which the behavior of each partner affects and influences the other must be examined. This is one of the major areas of further research needed in the

United States studies with regard to the role of the father. As gathered from the signaling of the multiple variables that enter into our understanding of cultural factors it shows the multifaceted sources of values, guidelines and traditions that enter into the manner in which each partner discharges his or her parental functions and so influences the child's development.

Role Characteristics of Parenting

We have to conceptualize the many functions that an individual performs within the different behavioral and role components of being a parent as the child grows up through the many developmental stages — babyhood, toddler, preadolescent and adolescent. For example, the child-rearing function of the mother is only one of her roles, in addition to the role of wife, partner and friend. This means then that an important area of knowledge that generally does not appear within a cultural context in our history-taking process and documentation, is an individual role characteristic of the mother or father of our patient. We tend to take very little notice of these aspects of the parents and have few frameworks in which we can incorporate them to make the dynamic factors influencing child-rearing become consonant with our theories.

Individual differences, personal preferences, cultural styles and subjective fulfillment can often influence the manner in which the roles are discharged in child-rearing practices. Again, many blind areas in child psychiatry history taking is found when not enough exploration of the psychological makeup and the cultural background and specific data-gathering of parent thinking, feelings, and fantasy are investigated. The behavior of parents within the cultural society in which they live is influenced by important members of extended families. As an example, we always need to consider the grandparents' "shadowy powers" that exert dynamic hidden influences and do not appear in our diagnostic workup documentation.

Psychosocial Adaptation of Parental Role vis a vis Cultural Settings

The analysis of issues of adaptation of an individual within a human setting is a process by which stress and strain accompany these types of behaviors so as to gauge whether there is congruence or discrepancy between the behavior role of the parent and the society in which a parent lives. This is a core concept in cross cultural evaluation of a family's level of mental health. It becomes quite dramatic when working with families who are immigrants or refugees. The areas of submerged tensions, mixed loyalties, sense of guilt and unresolved conflicts influences the quality of child-rearing within new settings and needs to be incorporated into our theoretical frame of reference (Brussel, 1971). We have to analyze whether there is congruity between individual objectives and socially normative approaches as well as whether the child-rearing role appears desirable and is shared by both parents. In every one of these issues the cultural influence plays a significant role and needs to be part of our hypothesis. Several dynamic forces tend to coproduce modification in role definition and behavior and they can be conscious or unconscious. Added to this the physical, social, cultural and economic realities define the option and constraints of daily life, superimposed on a socialization process that prepares the couple for the next stage of child development. This is highlighted in many of the couples with young children who have moved from the South to the North for job acquisition. It also can be seen in many of the settings of Mexican families who have moved across the border from Mexico to Southern California. In a few hours these families are submerged in a completely new world with different settings in their homes, schools and neighborhoods that have an influence on parental role configurations (DeVos, 1982).

Key Mental Health Issues and Value Systems

The family setting provides training patterns or models for a child's testing of behavior. Over time, the family's influence on these behaviors becomes inversely proportional in strength and reinforcement to that of other social institutions. That is, in the early years the parental systems of influence are intense and mold the child in a specific approach which is then shared. The family system is the major social unit in which the child develops from birth up to school entrance. It is therefore an important molding and powerful influence that holds a unique place as the child's training climate. Social institutions available outside the family serve mainly to reinforce and establish cultural sanctions or constraints to training approaches (Lampkin, 1971). The fact that schools are set within neighborhoods promotes this experience. A therapist who wants to consider the highly individual cultural patterns of a particular family has to be familiar with both the neighborhood and the geographical locale where the family lives and works

(Pearce, 1982). It is not enough to know where the family came from nor the traditions that they left behind. The interactive effects of new settings have to be conceptualized as one looks at immigrant families (Szapoczni, Kurtines, & Hanna, 1979). The therapist will need this knowledge to evaluate adequately the child whose growth patterns are affected by customs and traditions. Only through including in the assessment an understanding of how children grow in this new geographical region that is new to the family, can the clinician gain a sense and perspective of how some cultural practices may support childhood symptoms and psychopathology while other expectations influence the child to function in more adaptive ways. The following clinical vignette will highlight this point:

> A Vietamese family of six settled near New Orleans, to work in a shrimpboat fishing operation. Although the family settled in a physical location where other similar families lived and worked, their 15-year-old son had to be bussed to a high school many miles away. The teacher had difficulty in understanding the behavior cues of the adolescent and tended to misinterpret his passive acceptance of criticism or constructive encouragement that the teachers provided. Slowly they gave up on him and eventually labeled him as belonging in the retarded range of intellectual achievement.

An intergenerational heritage of different values, guidelines, attitudes and coping methods are generally practiced among families of different cultural backgrounds even though realities of socioeconomic status, education and job opportunity will offer similar lifestyles to the families living in the same geographical area. This combination of important social variables has inherent in it a potential to exert influences that both strengthen and weaken the support of family functions. The combination may or may not enhance parental attitudes that are adequate to direct the daily lives of children. Consider the following case:

> A family of upwardly mobile Haitians had moved to a middle class suburb where they had no difficulty in guiding their three children through their church and school activities. They were faced with a crisis situation when publicity about the "carrier groups" of the disease AIDS appeared in the media. The children were at a loss as to how to handle peer rejection, and the parents retreated into their traditional methods of family problem-solving which cut them off from an assertive, Anglo-American approach to help their children deal with the school bureaucratic situation. Even though this placed a strain on the children as they dealt with the public systems, on the other hand the children felt supported and understood at home by the traditional closing in of all the family members.

Groups of families or cultural groups can be identified, for example, as having traits of individualism, traditionalism, fatalism, action orientation, stoicism, and pride and self-reliance (Looff, 1979). Many of these traits are woven into the family tradition and culture that has enabled the family to adapt to stresses and deal successfully with the impact of crisis events. It is doubly difficult when these patterns prove ineffective in a new cultural setting. For example: Juan, age five years old, was brought to the clinic because he was difficult to manage. The mother, a 25-year-old woman from Nicaragua, who had arrived in the U.S. without her husband, reported that Juan "put up a fight" every time she had to ask him to do things like going to bed, bathe, or obey her. She could not understand the fact that he would not follow all her traditional ways of behaving and accepting some of the situations that they had to face. She expressed with strong affect her "difficulty of being a mother in this new country with all the new ways" and her longing to have her older relatives back home help her with the daily problems and solving the issues in the way that she was accustomed to in the past.

Child Development and Traditional Family Childrearing Practices

It is essential for child mental health professionals to be knowledgeable about and to differentiate between the social and pathological characteristics of the family setting in which a child is being reared. The need to explore the quality of family traditions, their interactions as they overlap and influence one another is absolute, prior to involvement with the clinical problems presented by troubled children. Such explorations seek to define the expected developmental milestones in a particular cultural group. Determination of symptoms which represent pathological development, deviations, or normality in children, are suggested only after such a baseline is conceptualized. Whether a clinician views child psychopathology as evolving aberrant ways in which the individual internalizes the communication, feeling and behavioral characteristics of significant parental figures in his upbringing, it is evident that the strength of parental external forces will be incorporated into the inner psychological world of the child. These internalized cultural traits of a family will characterize some of the interpersonal relationships between parents and children. Questions for consideration include:

1. What are the dynamic characteristics of the interaction between members of the family?
   a. Are they closely interdependent in their self-reliance behaviors?

b. Do they show strong expectations of behavior with an overriding sense of obligation to extended family members, or do they isolate themselves with no meaningful communications with relatives living within commuting distance?

2. Does the family system communicate in both verbal and non-verbal ways to express the family traditions? What are the cues that the therapist can pick up?

a. Is the individual family member's personal-social maturation in conflict with expected obedience to family tradition?

In such a context it is expected that the individual's own growth and development are clearly subordinate to the prime task of maintaining the family as a unit. This characteristic can be labeled as pathology or as mature, social loyalty depending on the therapist's perspective.

3. What are the parental patterns in terms of reactions to children's autonomy, initiative, curiosity, exploration and adequate sexual differentiation? Do they control it? Do they reward and support it, or do they shame it?

4. How do the parents display a sense of protection of childhood pursuits in terms of their own behavior? Do they use an indulgent permissive approach, or do they expect clear definitions of schedules, organized time for recreation, and duty-making discipline as a core value system?

A Cuban couple brought in their 16-year-old daughter to the clinic with a complaint that she was "rebellious," depressed. The history of these parents reveal that they had been sent along to the U.S. at the age of 16 and placed in camps for "unaccompanied Cuban youth." They met and soon after married. They have three children, the patient being the oldest. They tried to keep the family in a close-knit setting, allowing very little room for individuation. When the 16-year-old daughter began to make serious efforts of independence, she was criticized and shamed about her lack of "affection" for her parents. After, the parents were helped to see how their own unresolved conflicts at leaving home had been defended and were now projected onto their 16-year-old adolescent. They were then able to "let go" and allow the patient to develop her own independent behavior within her bicultural world.

Children's responses to the above issues will show some tendency to match the expectations of the parents' cultural norms in terms of either displaying independent behavior, following impulses with poor controls when separated from adults, or becoming infantile, clinging, demanding, and enjoying the latent pleasure of being controlled and babied. An important area in sorting out cross-cultural assessment is to ascertain the expectations of the parents that produce conflicts in the context of their approaches to sexual upbringing emerging from cultural differences about sexual development, mature behavior, and adult functioning. For example, due to overcrowded housing conditions in the low socioeconomic groups, the opportunity to create psychophysiologial tension, sexual, as well as non-sexual, exists. Many of the child-rearing techniques used by parents living in these physical conditions may reinforce their traditional attitudes and act as a powerful shaping force in the sexual development of the child. These techniques, which are expressed emotionally and cognitively at different levels of child development, may influence, at specific times, the developing capacity of the child to deal with these types of impulses. That is, behaviors exercised in bathroom or bedroom settings dealing with nudity, "horse-play," experimentation in touching body parts, exhibitionism, can convey to the child the "cultural" guidelines to deal with arousal and socially-approved or disapproved methods of dealing with them.

Clinicians should assess how families influence their children as well as what they reinforce and teach them, in order for the child to be able to cope with the developmental tasks and crises in their lives. Examples of deviations in developmental tasks which may be manifested by a variety of symptoms need careful assessment to sort out cultural conflicts. Some of the following are examples found in clinical practice:

1. Acute and chronic school phobia reactions. This clinical phenomenon has to be differentiated from situational factors found among many children who do not go to school for cultural reasons. Among these we may find the expectation that the oldest child has to stay home to take care of the smaller babies. In some cases the child is reflecting some of the fears that parents may have in new settings that they consider dangerous and unfamiliar.
2. Deviation and social development such as infantilization of overprotected children or children that have difficulty with impulse control. This can be found in some of the child-rearing methods that expect children to "not be seen and not be heard." These methods do not offer children the opportunity to exert a trial and error approach to problem-solving in an independent fashion.

3. Problems of interactional symbiotic relations between child and parent. For example, in some Hispanic refugee families in the United States, we can find specific family interactional patterns. Many of these families encourage their children in obligatory closeness, coupled with rigorous traditional training and avoidance of any separation that would disrupt the close family system. These attachments represent an intense need for closeness that appears both protective and also anxiety-provoking to the child. In some cases there is a possibility that later psychopathological disorders in the child appear which are based on these conflicting dependency themes and related to separation anxiety. This approach by the family appears to prevent a formation of specific coping abilities and denies the child the opportunity to practice appropriate social skills.

Many of these cultural child-rearing methods based on family traditions reinforce healthy aspects of the personality functions at the same time. The trust and belief in the family unit and available support are basic to ego strengths with which children solve their problems and overcome their difficulties. When the family has a coherent structure and provides a model for support functioning, it strengthens the steady state and emotional modulation of a child's tension as it faces difficulties in the social world. Even though the families that present themselves to the mental health system have some disorganizing tendencies and manifold problems, as members of parental systems they may interact with the child in a different modality and in many fundamental aspects may be supportive and sensitive to the child's needs.

In some affectionate but culturally-conflicted and disorganized families, many of the children are observed to have developed basic trust but they were not equally equipped to acquire controls over their aggressive impulses. Whether this is an outcome of traditional cultural child-rearing methods, or whether it is an expression of a child's conflicts, needs to be ascertained. Appropriate developmental support involving a balanced gratification of need and capacity to delay, along with the achievement of limits and controls, are not readily maintained by some cultural traditional methods of child-rearing beyond infancy. This attitude toward child-rearing results in children who adjust satifactorily within the culture of origin but will have difficulty when moving to a foreign culture which exerts and expects earlier controls in social behavior. Overt psychopathological symptoms might never appear until after a transition to a culture setting which demands new behaviors which the children have no capability for developing at that point. The family influence becomes ineffective because the key members, that is the parents, themselves experience difficulty adjusting to the new settings and in turn cannot give controls from outside. This was exemplified by one of the families coming to the clinic with a history similar to many of the Cuban refugee families that entered the United States through the Mariel lift. The mother brought her 7-year-old son to the clinic because of his difficulty in adapting to school norms and coping with the many issues presented by the children in his neighborhood. The mother did not speak English and had difficulty in communicating with the school personnel, and the father was unemployed. They were living with relatives who themselves were beginning to adapt to the new culture. The mother shared with us some history of the difficulties in exerting family influences in the new political climate of the city in which they lived in Cuba, and acknowledging having lost some controls over the upbringing of the children. This was compounded as they came to a new setting in the U.S., where many of the skills of both the children and families were not adaptive to the expectation of the Anglo world.

Various cultural processes act to influence child-rearing patterns very early in the life cycle of the family. Cultural patterns inherent in geographical areas and neighborhoods, stages of development of the child and the shifts of socio-economic status of the family, may all exert specific influence on a historical basis which are manifested at later stages of the child's development. These need to be taken into consideration, because in some stages children may not show dynamic conflicts which are manifested at a later stage of development.

Clinical Application of Cultural Child-Rearing Processes: Diagnosis and Treatment

The focus of this component of the chapter will be to present certain dynamic factors that affect the interactions between child psychiatrist and the family with a child patient. The aim is to conceptualize signs and symptoms of psychopathology within the transcultural framework of psychiatric diagnosis and treatment (see Szopocznik, Scopetta, & King, 1978). The transcultural framework provides a method of highlighting the cultural differences between the child patient and the therapist, including different aspects of ethnic cultures, ecnomic status and racial roots. The word "culture" will be used in this component to denote a "number of socially-transmitted behavior patterns, beliefs and other

products of human thought characteristic and peculiar of special groups"
(see Cohen, 1974). Both the definition of the child mental health syndromes and the expression of the developmentally-dysfunctional behavior
have a bearing on the interaction between the therapist and the family
and both are affected by their own cultural backgrounds.

In most instances, the therapist takes the initiative for the organization, classification, and meaning of the symptoms as they are valid
within his cultural system; this is his frame of reference in the United
States.

This approach is based on findings from research studies and professional experiences that present many conceptual problems and issues of
cross-cultural equivalents due to the fact that premises used to form the
theories and hypotheses are culturally-biased. The psychodynamic
therapist relies on a theoretical body of knowledge based in intrapsychic
factors, conflicts, defenses, and general theoretical schools of thought,
which he uses to develop a framework vis a vis the study of human behavior in the family. If he only relies on his own culture's framework,
and does this only from the vantage point of his conceptual knowledge
and his experiences, he may have a high probability of error in his
diagnostic approach. This potential for error may be compounded if he
conceptualizes the developmental patterns and psychic health structures
within psychodynamic theoretical terms as well as through his own personality and value systems. That is, he must take into consideration
both the cultural, traditional, ethnic background of his patient and the
psychological reactions and feelings he has for that culture. The conceptual guidelines that would influence the therapist's relationship with the
family in addition to his experiential development with his own family,
need to be included as part of the knowledge base that integrates the influences of familial cultural factors on problems in child pathology.

Cultural Factors and Diagnosis

There appears to be universal agreement that types of symptomatology do not differ significantly from one culture to another. The greater
differences exist in (a) the culturally-determined influences, (b) the
culturally-acceptable labeling and categorizing of emotional disturbance
of deviant behavior, and (c) the symbolic and traditional behavioral
modes of expressing feelings and emotions of the patient's culture
(Kleinman, 1977).

During diagnosis and treatment, mental health professionals do not
appear to exert remarkable systematic attention to the child's ethnicity,

race, cultural identity conflicts and/or bilingualism. There may be a conscious avoidance of the reality of ethnic differences based on a hypersensitivity and pseudoliberal concern not to be "discriminating" or to "show prejudice" in the clinical setting. It appears as if noting the differences in family cultural backgrounds, especially in the minority family, means to denigrate and/or judge inferior rather than unique and different (Karno, 1966).

Another problem in clinical activities is the pervasive use and reliance upon a model for the child psychiatric interviews which derives directly from the classical organic medical history with definite boundaries and specific phenomenology. This appears to ignore some of the variations of behavior influenced by cultural traditions which should be diagnosed and accepted as within normal limits. Many children who are influenced by strong belief systems of some of the religions practiced by the parents as Santeria, Vodou, and other traditional cultural sets of beliefs will present some strange descriptions of things they see or hear. This needs to be differentiated from hallucinations or delusions.

Transcultural Factors Affecting the Child Diagnostic Procedures

The conceptual and clinical process in child psychiatry which identifies the impact of the child on his world — which generally is presented as the chief complaint that brings the parents to the clinic — has to incorporate cultural factors in the definitions. The problems categorized as originating either from the behavior of the child or the perception of the family about the child, starts the process of fact-finding and needs to rely heavily on sorting out cultural vs. pathological factors. The perceptions, reactive adult emotions, and anxiety on the part of the adult world about a child's "symptoms" needs to be put into the context of the interrelated and interacting dynamic and cultural issues facing the child, and the family, within their human environment. All these factors have a continuous influence on each other in a circular, feedback mechanism.

The therapist's diagnostic methodology is guided by an **a priori** set of conceptualized principles ascribed through:

1. Personal life experiences, sex, age.
2. Types of patients seen in the therapist's clinical practice.
3. Theoretical framework developed and practiced while training and being indoctrinated within the therapist's professional training program.

The above factors may produce the following consequences:

1. Influence of life experiences on value systems of the therapist will influence his evaluation judgement.
2. Influence of training on the therapist.
3. Methods of obtaining the data to understand the child's problems:
   a) How to identify the characteristics of psychopathological symptoms in the child.
   b) How to interpret psychodynamic behavior patterns in the family.
   c) How to plan modes of therapeutic intervention.

The organization of a theoretical, culturally-sensitive framework in which the therapist arranges factors to describe the behavioral manifestation of his child-patient as well as the emotional and verbal communication of the family as they express and share their child-rearing patterns will assist the therapist in developing a set of theories to conceptualize both the effects of cultural influences and psychodynamic conflicts. The therapist's findings will be integrated and organized before he formulates an intervention program with specific goals and objectives. If the therapist is able to develop this conceptual framework he will be assisted in interpreting the meaning of the multi-variate factors that are acquired through observation, history-taking, and tests. He can then arrange this acquired knowledge in a multi-dimensional perspective according to the age of the child and the type of the family structure within their own cultural setting.

There appears to be a greater potentiality for successful therapy when there is a higher positive correlation between the theories considered, the culture of the therapist and the culture of the patient. In addition, the therapist must be knowledgeable of his own culture, comfortable in his biculturalism, and possess and integrate biopsychocultural frames of reference with which he can organize the acquired data. When the therapist is not exposed to a training program that incorporates different sociocultural backgrounds, he will have had less opportunity to integrate in his thinking and feelings the factors brought about by the following:

1. Different cultural meaning of symbolism as expressed in behavior patterns and use of speech of his patient.
2. Different meanings of translated verbal interactions as expressed by disorganized or pathological behavior within different families of foreign cultures.

3. Lack of self-awareness.
   a) Personal reactions to patients' verbalizations and non-verbal expression.
   b) A personal sense of dissonance and discomfort in the presence of the family.
   c) Patterns of defenses to guard against a sense of professional incompetence because he does not understand, cannot integrate, and/or cannot interpret unfamiliar cues and signals given by patient and family.

If unsuccessful, the therapist may become uncomfortable, controlling, and rely on the need to project the cause for the lack of success of the therapeutic intervention on the child and family. This is an underlying rationalization that views the child as unmotivated and the conclusion is reached that the child cannot benefit from his specific type of therapy. This viewpoint generally highlights the frustration of the therapist who cannot become invested in culturally different types of families because he is not receiving a feedback message that this family and child are progressing and processing their emotional conflicts toward a resolution which is hoped for by the therapist.

Diagnostic Issues Within a Transcultural Frame of Reference

Categorizing symptoms of emotional syndromes of children can be guided by theoretical and conceptual frameworks. The therapist in the United States recognizes disorders of mood, thought and behavior, within certain theoretical norms (DSM III). If we assume that the therapist is basing his approaches on observed and documented modes of behavior that express disorganized psychological functioning, he will have to take into consideration the superimposed cultural content of the observed responses. This will enable him to understand why the type of psychiatric symptoms appear in the specific cluster within a specific developmental stage, and within this specific family. To the meaning of these symptoms, he also has to attach a culturally determined and psychologically specific type of family defense or adaptive pattern which will have an impact on child-rearing behaviors. If we assume that the symptoms are influenced by sociocultural factors, then it follows that unless there is understanding of the cultural background, it will be difficult to comprehend the meaning of the symptoms, as for example the behavior in a girl as reported by a mother who believed this girl was hyperactive. What the therapist had to realize was that in the mother's cultural expectations, girls are behaviorally self-controlled and "ladylike."

Culture plays a crucial role in diagnosis for it is culture that influences both a natural expression and direction of behavior manifested by the child in expression of conflicts, and the way that the therapist interprets, organizes, and identifies it.

Issues of severity and future prognosis of psychopathological conditions are correlated to the diagnostic capabilities of the therapist, who uses a method of trying to relate cause and effect among the interrelationships of stressors, stress responses, coping and adaptation. By ordering and organizing these pieces of data, the therapist will be able to sort out the behavioral deviances that signal the problem of his child patient. His own understanding (according to his own experiences and training) of what may be stressful to the child and which behaviors might be induced by emotions of fear, guilt, jealousy, anger and other emotions balanced by efforts to control them according to the child's developmental ability of coping, may be judged either adaptive or maladaptive for the therapeutic process. This points to the importance of incorporating the cultural value system and attitudes of the therapist toward a particular family system, patterns of behavior as expressed by the family, and the way they manage the behavioral dysfunction of the child. This self-awareness will influence whether the therapist labels a child as severely or moderately ill, dangerous or not, in need of hospitalization, or demonstrating pathological developmental behavior carrying a poor prognosis.

Transcultural Factors Within the Treatment Process

In the treatment of families from different cultures or different racial backgrounds, the therapist becomes less of a neutral figure to the family members. They will develop emotional reactions influenced by their own stereotypes about individuals belonging to the therapist's cultural background. If the therapist accepts these stereotypes without questioning them, he may in turn overlook symptoms and resistances of the family or the child as he initiates treatment. This area—working through the conflicts and psychological defenses and separating them from social cultural processes in the interactive method of psychotherapy—becomes a major therapeutic goal of treatment. This process has to precede any "working-through" of the intrapsychic conflicts of the child. As treatment proceeds, there is an ongoing need to continually sort out the factors that appear culturally determined from the psychological, developmental conflicts of childhood. Each stage of therapy, including initiation and conclusion of therapeutic intervention, will carry the overlay of both therapist and family cultural values and beliefs as they influence the therapeutic process. This means then, that the therapist needs an ongoing and continual surveillance of both the cultural systems of the family as they evolve in therapy, and his own continuous and evolving attitudes and reactive emotions as he moves through the therapeutic process. For most therapists treating families that come from an unfamiliar culture, the need for double level supervision or consultation with colleagues is necessary. The therapist needs to be sensitized on a continuous basis to sort out the cultural factors from the intrapsychic psychodynamics, if he happens to be a psychodynamic therapist, or behavioral phenomenology if this is his school of thought. Attention to the meaning of words if he is talking in the same language as the family, or the translated conceptual meaning if he is using a language foreign to the family, is another area of ongoing attention. The many forms of expressing emotions or dealing with intimate, personal items, specially in families who keep some of the intimate activities as a family secret, will have to be dealt with in a sensitive manner. Different cultures have traditional methods of moving from a less to a more intimate theme and the "permission taking" needs to be incorporated into the therapeutic manner. Another sensitive area of treatment appears in the effort to exert some changes in the distance and independence between child and parent within the Anglo, United States environment. Due to the fact that many of the children of different cultures go to schools that are designed by U.S. models, the independent expectation of self decision-making and the peer pressure toward this style need to be worked through with families who cannot accept it. These are but a few examples of the multiple themes that will appear in treatment and will be part of the working-through process.

These questions appear constantly in many training programs where there is no integrated curriculum that includes the interactive influences of cultural variables within a psychodynamic framework, or whatever theoretical school of thought the training program uses. Some efforts are appearing in developing textbooks and training documents bringing closer the two streams of knowledge (Becerra, Karno, & Escobar, 1982; Gaw, 1982). As of the present, the main responsibility will be with the director of training programs and trainers in child psychiatry who will have to integrate this material in their daily interaction with child psychiatry trainees. That is, they will have to bring into the areas of diagnostic and therapeutic clinical examples, the multi-variables that are necessary to understand families of different cultures, and place the factors arising from traditional modes of child-rearing into the context of diagnosis and therapy. The basic descriptions of the DSM-III as they appear to categorize behavior indicative of psychopathology need to be modified according to the culture of the family studied and programmed for treatment. The field of child psychiatry is embarking on a vigorous biological research program which will need to reach out to the behavioral sciences, including sociology and anthropology, to understand the individual patient.

REFERENCES

American Academy of Child Psychiatry. (1983). *Child psychiatry: A plan for the coming decades.* Washington, DC: Author.

Becerra, R. N., Karno, M., & Escobar, I. J. (1982). *Mental health and Hispanic Americans: Clinical perspectives.* (Seminars in psychiatry). New York: Grune & Stratton.

Brussel, C. B. (1971). Social characteristics and problems of the Spanish-speaking society. In J. C. Stone & D. P. Denevi (Eds.), *Teaching multicultural populations.* New York: Van Nostrand.

Cohen, R. E. (1974). Borderline conditions: A transcultural perspective. *Psychiatric Annals, 4*(9), 7-20.

DeVos, G. A. (1982). Adaptive strategies in U.S. minorities. In E. E. Jones & S. J. Korchin (Eds.), *Minority mental health* (pp. 74-117). New York: Praeger Scientific.

Gaw, A. (Ed.). (1982). *Cross-cultural psychiatry.* Boston: John Wright PSG, Inc.

Group for the Advance of Psychiatry. (1973). *From diagnosis to treatment: An approach to treatment planning for the emotionally disturbed child* (Report No. 87, Vol. 3). New York: Brunner/Mazel.

Karno, M. (1966). The enigma of ethnicity in a psychiatric clinic. *Archives of General Psychiatry, 14*(5), 516-520.

Kleinman, A. (1977). Rethinking the social and cultural context of psychopathology and psychiatric care. In T. Manschseck & A. Kleinman (Eds.), *Renewal in psychiatry: A critical rational perspective* (pp. 97-138). Washington, DC: Hemisphere Publishing Co.

Lampkin, L. C. (1971). Alienation as a coping mechanism: "Out where the action is." In E. Pavenstedt (Ed.), *Crisis of family disorganization* (pp. 43-40). New York: Behavioral Publications.

Looff, D. (1979). Sociocultural factors in etiology. In J. D. Noshpitz (Ed.), *Basic handbook of child psychiatry* (pp. 87-99). New York: Basic Books.

Mendel, C., & Habenstein, R. (1976). *Ethnic families in America.* New York: Elsevier Press.

Pearce, J. (1982). Ethnicity and normal families. In F. Walsh (Ed.), *Normal family processes.* New York: Guilford Press.

Szapocznik, J., Kurtines, W., & Hanna, N. (1979). Comparison of Cuban and Anglo American cultural values in a clinical population. *Journal of Consulting and Clinical Psychology, 47*(3), 623-624.

Szapocznik, J., Scopetta, M. A., & King, O. (1978). Theory and practice in matching treatment to the special characteristics and problems of Cuban immigrants. *Journal of Community Psychology, 6,* 112-122.

CHAPTER 13

FAMILY EFFECTIVENESS TRAINING (FET) FOR HISPANIC FAMILIES

JOSE SZAPOCZNIK, ARTURO RIO, ANGEL PEREZ-VIDAL,
WILLIAMS KURTINES, and DAVID SANTISTEBAN

Introduction

FET IS AN EARLY intervention/prevention modality that was developed within a Strategic Structural Systems framework. Such an
approach views individual behavior problems within the context of the
family system. From this perspective, early prevention requires the use
of interventions designed to strengthen the family system against the potential for future drug abuse and acting out behaviors, i.e., the behavior
problem syndrome.

Families with pre-adolescents (8-12 years) are hypothesized to be at
risk for the behavior problem syndrome when current family functioning displays maladaptive interactional patterns. The critical structural
dimensions identified as potential antecedents of the behavior problems
syndrome are: family structure, flexibility, resonance, developmental
stages, identified patienthood, and conflict resolution (c.f., Szapocznik,
Kurtines, Foote, & Perez-Vidal, 1983). Specific patterns of these dimensions that have emerged in our work have included an enmeshed or
overinvolved mother-son relationship and a distant father who tends to
be excluded from the enmeshed relationship, and resonance (i.e., the
family dimension). In addition, we have also found that such families
display the inability to resolve conflicts (i.e., the conflict resolution dimension) and inadequate structure (i.e., the family structure dimension) such as a mother and son alliance that renders the father peripheral

to the family. When pathology occurs along these interrelated dimensions of family functioning in families with pre-adolescents, these families are hypothesized to be predisposed for future serious family dysfunctions that may become manifest in behavior problems during adolescence.

In particular, when families make the transition from childhood to adolescence all families are exposed to intergenerational/intercultural conflict (also described below). When families with pre-adolescent children exhibit family dysfunction along the six dimensions outlined above, these families are singularly incapable of successfully overcoming the added demand and stresses associated with the intergenerational/intercultural conflict that come into play as the family approaches the developmental stage of adolescence. **Thus, family structural dysfunctions represent the necessary conditions and family intergenerational and intercultural conflict the added stressors which when combined tend to give rise to high rates of Behavior Problem syndromes in adolescents.** Such syndromes typically include drug abuse. Level of current family functioning (or dysfunction) is thus hypothesized to serve as a moderator of potential future family stressors that come into play as the pre-adolescent approaches adolescence. As a moderator, it functions to minimize or exacerbate the effects of these sources of stress. Current family dysfunction is thus viewed as one of the factors that define a family as "at risk" for the behavior problem syndrome. Hispanic families with pre-adolescents are also subject to at least two other major sources of potential future stress: intergenerational conflict that arise from within the family and intercultural conflict that arises from sources outside the family.

Intergenerational Conflict

Intergenerational conflict is exacerbated by family developmental transitions such as the transition to adolescence. As Stanton (1979) notes, it is helpful to view the family in terms of its place in the family developmental life cycle. Most families encounter a number of similar stages as they progress through life, such as birth of first child, adolescence, and separation. These are natural developmental crisis points which are usually weathered by the family system without inordinate difficulty. On the other hand, families with dysfunctional structures such as those exhibiting the high risk syndrome develop problems/symptoms because they are not able to adjust to the transition. They become "stuck" at a particular point or stage of development because the family continues to behave in its prior habitual ways and fails to change its ways of interacting to adapt to the changing needs of the child, now become adolescent. Intergenerational conflict is thus a potential source of stress for all families with pre-adolescents and is in itself not a sufficient condition for the behavior problem syndrome. However, it does become an additional source of stress for families whose current level of functioning is inadequate, and thus serves to exacerbate the already existing dysfunction.

Intercultural Conflict

A major potential future source of conflict for families with preadolescents is conflict which emerges when the extra-familial world introduces different and new stressors through some family members which are not shared or acceptable to the other members, thereby stressing the relationships and creating rigid boundaries between members which impeded needed transactions. In the case of the Hispanic population used in this study, acculturational differences between generations can become major sources of conflict. One of the most consistent and significant findings of the research at the Spanish Family Guidance Center (e.g., Szapocznik & Kurtines, 1980) has been that acculturation presents the migrant family with special problems and difficulties. Our observations and data reveal that since youngsters acculturate more rapidly than their parents, the substantial intergenerational differences in acculturation that develop in the family may either precipitate or exacerbate existing familial and particularly intergenerational familial disruption (Szapocznik & Truss, 1978).

As part of the Center's ongoing research program, a psychosocial model of acculturation was developed (Szapocznik, Scopetta, Aranalde & Kurtines, 1978) to account for the occurrence of intergenerational/acculturational differences and the consequent family disruption. According to this initial theoretical model, intergenerational differences in behavioral acculturation develop over time because younger members of the family acculturate more rapidly than older family members.

This initial model of acculturation was based on traditional views of acculturation which held that acculturation is a linear and unidimensional process involving an accomodation on the part of a migrant culture to a host culture (Berry, & Annis, 1964; Szapocznik, Scopetta, Aranalde & Kurtines, 1978). More recent views, however, suggest that acculturation may not necessarily be an unidimensional process, but rather may occur separately along host and culture-of-origin dimensions (Lasaga, Szapocznik & Kurtines, 1980). Building on these perspectives, a second theoretical model of acculturation was developed which views acculturation as a complex process of accomodation to a total cultural context that may be either unidimensional or two dimensional, depending upon the type of cultural context involved.

The acculturation/biculturation model hypothesizes that acculturation is a multi-dimensional process that functions differently depending upon the cultural context. Under certain conditions (i.e., a mono-cultural context), the model holds that acculturation will be basically a unidimensional and linear process moving **from** the culture of origin **to** the host culture. Under other conditions (i.e., a bicultural context), the biculturation model holds that "acculturation" will be two dimensional, involving an accomodation to the host culture as well as retention of the culture of origin. Furthermore, the model explicitly recognizes a normative component of the accultuation process which is closely related to the amount of exposure to the host culture, and a pathological component which deviates from the normative component and is reflected in excessive over or under acculturation. It is our hypothesis that **what makes this deviation from the normative component maladjustive in bicultural settings is that it renders the individual inappropriately monocultural in a bicultural context.**

The most important implication for family functioning is that in families where members are characterized by culturally related differences, the typical intergenerational differences found with families of adolescents are exacerbated by cultural differences. Thus, cultural differences across generations compound the typical source of stress resulting from the developmental transition to adolescence.

PREVENTION-INTERVENTION STRATEGIES

As a prevention intervention modality, FET is targetted at both current family dysfunction and the prevention of potential future family dysfunction. The FET modality thus includes intervention strategies that are aimed at current or existing structural family dysfunctions and prevention strategies that are designed to strengthen the family to deal with potential future stressors such as intergenerational and inter-cultural conflicts that tend to weaken and disrupt healthy family functioning. FET thus involves both intervention and prevention strategies designed to minimize the likelihood of emergence of the behavior problem syndrome in adolescents. Figure 13-1 displays the three complementary intervention strategies (Brief Strategic Family Therapy, Bicultural Effectiveness Training, and Family Development) included in FET and the dysfunctions targetted by each strategy. These intervention strategies are explained more fully below under the description of the FET modality.

Figure 13-1

FAMILY EFFECTIVENESS TRAINING:

TARGETTED DYSFUNCTIONS AND INTERVENTION STRATEGIES

Current Dysfunction	**Intervention Strategy**
Dimensions of Family Dysfunction	Brief Strategic Family Therapy
1) structure	Techniques
2) flexibility	
3) resonance	
4) developmental	
5) identified patienthood	
6) conflict resolution	
Future Stressors	**Prevention Strategy**
Intergenerational Conflict (developmental transition to adolescence)	Family Development Techniques
Intercultural Conflict (acculturation gap)	Bicultural Effectiveness Training Techniques

---

Figure 13-2 below depicts the relationship between the high risk (HR) syndrome, the behavior problem (BP) syndrome, and the FET prevention intervention modality as conceptualized within the context of the Strategic Structural Systems approach. The reader should compare Figure 13-1 and Figure 13-2 which further clarifies the role of FET as a moderator variable. As Figure 13-2 indicates, within the Strategic Structural Systems model, FET is conceptualized as an intervening or moderator variable that operates to moderate the effects of high risk antecedents conditions which place preadolescents at risk for future (adolescent) behavior problems.

Figure 13-2

A STRUCTURAL SYSTEMS PREVENTION INTERVENTION MODEL

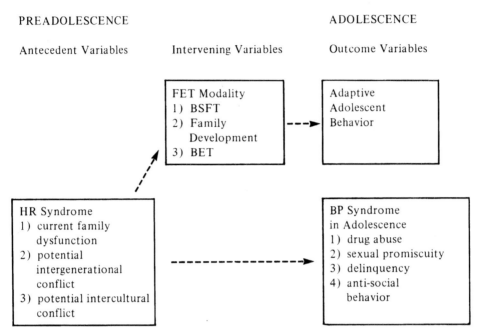

PREADOLESCENCE   ADOLESCENCE

Antecedent Variables   Intervening Variables   Outcome Variables

The FET Modality

FET consists of three basic components: Brief Strategic Family Therapy (BSFT) intervention strategies, Family Development (FD) prevention strategies, and Bicultural Effectiveness Training (BET) prevention strategies. Each component is targetted at a specific constellation of factors hypothesized to be potential antecedents of future behavior problems in adolescents.

In its application, FET consists of didactic and experiential material presented in a classroom-like atmosphere to the entire family in a series of thirteen weekly sessions. The sessions are conducted by a facilitator who takes a leadership role vis a vis the family. The FET lessons are simultaneously conducted at both a treatment/intervention level and a prevention intervention level. The facilitator uses the FET (i.e., Family Development and Bicultural Effectiveness Training) lessons as the context within which to conduct BSFT (explained more fully in the following section). At another level the facilitator uses the psychoeducational component of the FET lessons (Family Development and Bicultural Effectiveness Training) to strengthen the family against potential stressors arising from future intergenerational and intercultural conflicts respectively. These psychoeducational components rely heavily on content oriented presentations. In contrast to FD and FET, the BSFT component aims at improving current family dysfunctions.

Both the treatment intervention and the psychoeducational prevention components of FET are operationalized within a Strategic Structural Systems approach. The Strategic Structural Systems approach is built on the pioneer structural family systems work of Salvador Minuchin (1974, 1976), and the strategic concepts of Jay Haley (1976) and Cloe Madanes (1981) and the later contributions of Szapocznik, Kurtines, Foote, & Perez-Vidal (1983) and Szapocznik, Kurtines, Hervis, & Spencer (1984). The Strategic Structural Systems approach is strategic in that prevention intervention techniques are explicitly designed to bring about particular structural (interactional) changes. Thus, each intervention is focused on achieving planned goals utilizing a deliberately planned strategy to promote new and more functional ways of interacting.

From a structural systems perspective, families in which dysfunctional behaviors are expressed tend to identify one member (e.g., the pre-adolescent) as the patient. Within the structural family framework, this person is referred to as the family's Identified Patient. When a family enters the program, the family's typical expectation is that the identified patient needs to be changed. FET, however, recognizes that although one of the members may be manifesting symptoms, the whole family systems needs to be changed because the symptomatic behavior of the Identified Patient merely signals that the family's usual (habitual) patterns of transaction either promote the symptomatic behavior or at least maintain it such as the case when the family's executive functioning (e.g., parenting techniques) have failed to change to meet the system's needs. In this sense, we would say that the family system is manifested or has developed dysfunctional or maladaptive interactions. That is, patterns of interactions which fail to achieve what the family purportedly would like to achieve: the elimination or prevention of the symptomatic behavior. The FET modality is designed to use the family's concern over the symptomatic behavior to keep the family engaged in the program. Thus, while the FET modality uses the content by strategically focusing on the Identified Patient's problem to engage, maintain and mobilize the family for change, the prevention intervention strategies (i.e., BSFT, FD, and BET) target the entire family's system functioning, including the interactional patterns. Therefore, FET focuses on the Identified Patient's symptoms as a strategic maneuver to engage the whole family system into treatment and as a focal point around which to restructure the family as a whole. In our work with conduct problem youngsters, for example, the Identified Patient's transgressional behavior is used to mobilize the family to participate in therapy. Identified Patient symptomatology is used as a content (a working topic) around which to encourage and direct changes in family interactional patterns. Thus, while the identified patient's symptomatic behavior is perceived as the signal or symptom of dysfunction in the interactions among family members, in the Strategic Structural Systems approach it is used as the source of motivation to mobilize the family to change its interactional patterns. Since the system is typically organized around the presenting complaint, it is useful to strategically focus on the presenting problem as a maneuver around which to restructure the system. It is thus a strategic maneuver to use the current symptomatic complaint of the family as a vehicle around which to motivate the family to change its way of relating to the youth. The goal of FET, however, is not only to use strategic interventions (i.e., BSFT) to bring about immediate symptomatic relief, FET also has built into the psychoeducational components (i.e., FD and BET) strategic restructuring interventions that prepare and strengthen the family to confront future stressors.

Thus, all of the FET components are aimed at either changing current transactions or preventing certain pathological transaction from occurring. A general overview of each component follows.

1. The BSFT Component

The BSFT component focuses on intervention strategies designed to bring about structural (interactional) change thereby eliminating current family dysfunction. BSFT is administered flexibly and focuses on current dysfunction manifested as behavior problems in preadolescents, family conflict or marital discord. BSFT is designed to bring about immediate relief for symptomatic complaints that bring the families into the project as well as correcting the structural problems that give rise to the symptom, thereby preventing its re-occurrence in the future. Because the BSFT component is tailored to each family, it is not incorporated in a systematic fashion into the didactic component of the FET lessons. Consequently, some familiarity with BSFT is assumed on the part of the facilitator.

The BSFT component of FET is derived from Brief Strategic Family Therapy (Szapocznik, Kurtines, Foote & Perez-Vidal, 1983). The goal of BSFT is to diagnose or identify the family's habitual and repetitive interactional patterns that are maladaptive (in the sense that they encourage or maintain dysfunctional behaviors in family members) and to manipulate family interactions (through the use of strategic interventions) in order to create the opportunity for new interactions to emerge that are more functional.

The dimensions of family interaction on which BSFT focuses are: family structure, flexibility, resonance, developmental stage, identified patienthood, and conflict resolution. The major techniques used in BSFT fall into two primary structural family therapy categories: joining techniques and restructuring techniques (Minuchin, 1984).

Joining. The facilitator joins by initially supporting the family structure, by tracking its patterns of communication (i.e., initially following the content and patterns of communication set up by the family) and by mimesis of the family's style, affect, activity and mood. These techniques help the facilitator to enter the family system and be accepted as well as to encourage the family to interact in its usual fashion. In structural therapy this is called enactment. Enactment refers to permitting the family to interact in its characteristic fashion. In joining it is essential that the facilitator accept and maintain the family organization rather than challenge it so as to eliminate the possibility of perceiving an artificial system or be rejected by the family. In order to encourage enactment, the facilitator systematically redirects communication so that interaction will occur between family members rather than between the family and the therapist. It is through joining that the family makes a commitment to the therapeutic system (i.e., a system that includes the family and the facilitator into their fold), thus minimizing the chances of dropping-out or resisting change. Finally, it is in the process of joining that the facilitator establishes her/himself as a leader of the therapeutic system. A leadership position is essential in order to facilitate the family's acceptance of the changes that the facilitator will be introducing into the family system.

Restructuring. The facilitator restructures by promoting, facilitating, suggesting, and actually directing alternate organizations and interactional patterns. It is here that the facilitator challenges the familial status quo and their existential reality by reframing the family's perceptions and creating new frames which permit more functional alternatives to emerge. There are a variety of ways in which change-producing interventions can be made. These techniques include shifting of alliances or changing boundaries within the family system. For example, the facilitator can block inappropriate communication patterns while directing the family to open new channels of communication. Joining and restructuring takes place simultaneously and are only separated as concepts for the sake of explanation. In particular the facilitator needs to be supportive in order to prevent the family from withdrawing from the challenge of growth and change because it feels overly stressed. Thus, even though it is sometimes necessary for the facilitator to promote stressful situations, there are times when the facilitator is supportive as a technique to keep the stress within a tolerable range and to maintain the family's willingness to remain in treatment.

A number of techniques can be used to restructure and shift family interactional patterns. Some of the more frequently used techniques include reframing, reversals, detriangulation, opening up closed systems and homework tasks. These are discussed more fully in Szapocznik, Kurtines, Foote, & Perez-Vidal (1983) and Szapocznik, Kurtines, Hervis, & Spencer (1984).

2. Family Development Component

The Family Development component of the FET focuses on prevention strategies designed to eliminate or minimize future potential family stressors that arise out of intergenerational conflict that will result from family developmental transition from childhood to adolescence. The Family Development component is built into the FET lessons. The Family Development component is designed to help prepare the family to move effectively from being a family with a child to being a family with an adolescent while minimizing intergenerational conflict. The content of the Family Development lessons is also used strategically as a context for confronting already existing family dysfunctions.

The focus of the Family Development strategies, as with all the FET components, is on changing transactions. The structural changes which the Family Development component focuses are built into the FET lessons and include the development of communication skills, the concept of healthy family, taking responsibility and sharing.

In order to help the family make the transition from the family of a child to that of an adolescent more smoothly, parents are taught interactive skills in which they are more likely to treat the youngster as an equal. Thus for example, parents are taught to listen to their youth, to take responsibility for their own behaviors while simultaneously teaching the youth to take responsibility for his or her own behavior, to allow the youth increased decision making, thereby encouraging a transition from a lineal to a democratic relationship. These new skills on the part of the parents allow the parents to smoothly shift away from the habitual interactive patterns of being more directive (which may have been more appropriate with the young child) to new interactive patterns where the parents learn to join and track the youngster and thus through skill, rather than force, becomes a leader (which is more appropriate with an adolescent). Within a skillfully framed leadership position, the parent is now able to continue to guide and direct the youth. Guidance is critically necessary in adolescence since the adolescent without direction tends to lose control. Yet **by using leadership skills rather than forced authority to provide direction the parent minimizes the likelihood of arousing rebelliousness which along with lack of proper limits seems to be at the crux of the behavior problem syndrome.** With respect to limits, it should be noted that parents are taught in the Family Development lessons to make a critical shift from imposing external limits in the youth, thereby encouraging the internalization of parental values and the development of judicious decision making.

A drug education section is included in the Family Development component because it is our belief that youth should learn from their parents about the dangers they may confront in adolescence. It is our position that it is critical for parents to be well informed and that the youth perceive the parents as capable leaders who can guide them in the drug use area. From a structural point of view, it is desirable for the parents to become leaders who provide guidance to the family, and that such leadership include drug abuse concerns. For the parents to be effective leaders on drug abuse issues they must be well informed.

3. The Bicultural Effectiveness Training Component

Hispanic families face special problems of adjustment due to their exposure and reaction to the acculturation process. Research at the Spanish Family Guidance Center has demonstrated that behavior and conduct problems of the behavior problem variety, including drug abuse, may be associated with the lack of biculturalism on the part of parents and adolescents (Szapocznik & Kurtines, 1980). Family dysfunction due to acculturation stress includes breakdown of communication between parents, and between parents and children (which can develop into behavior problem syndromes including drug abusing behavior at later ages).

The Bicultural Effectiveness Training component of FET aims at eliminating or minimizing potential for future **intergenerational culture conflict** that will emerge when the child reaches adolescence by teaching the family bicultural skills and a transcultural perspective. The Bicultural Effectiveness Training component, in this way, overlaps with the Family Development component to the extent that it aims to avoid potential future intergenerational conflict, but it differs from the Family Development component in that it specifically aims at those elements of conflict that are most culturally related.

The Bicultural Effectiveness Training component is designed to minimize potential future intergenerational/cultural values conflicts. It is designed to reduce these conflicts by bringing about structural changes within the family system. Structural change is brought about at the content and application level by focusing primarily on cultural content, with particular emphasis on the disruptive effects of intergenerational cultural conflict.

The Bicultural Effectiveness Training component of FET includes five Bicultural Effectiveness Training lessons and focus on establishing a transcultural, shared world view as a means for moderating the effects of future potential intergenerational/intercultural conflict (Szapocznik, Santisteban, Kurtines, Perez-Vidal, & Hervis (1984).

The FET Curriculum and Specific Implementation Strategies

The FET lessons described in this section provide an intervention/prevention **tool** for moderating the potential future emergence of the behavior problem syndrome in families exhibiting the high risk syndrome. Based on clinical observations and assessments of the families who were undergoing FET, it became apparent that there is a need for a flexible lesson package in which the program can be delivered to the family in a minimum of 9 sessions and a maximum of 13. This decision is based on the fact that families differ in terms of their needs and their ability to process information. It was our experience that for some families the delivery of the FET curriculum could be accelerated without compromising effectiveness.

The FET Lessons

The FET lessons can be applied by family therapists skilled in BSFT. In addition, the facilitator should also be knowledgeable and comfortable with the cultures involved (in this project, Hispanic and American),

FET consists of 13 lessons presented to the conjoint family, whenever possible, which is made up of all family members above the age of 7 that live with the family. Each of the 13 sessions takes approximately 1.5 to 2 hours. The sessions are organized around the lessons which are designed to permit the achievement of two general sets of goals. The first is preventive, that is, to provide the family with knowledge and skills that will strengthen its present functioning and prepare them for coping with future stressors. The second goal of sessions is to provide treatment for current dysfunctions. The lessons provide a vehicle for the enactment of family dysfunctions in order to carry out the BSFT treatment interventions.

The 13 FET lessons are grouped into four general phases. The phases presented below are the recommended sequence although in actual application they may be varied to suit the needs and problems of particular families.

Phase I

(Lessons 1-2), **Effective Parenting Skills** is part of the Family Development component and is oriented toward providing the family with a broad understanding of the structure and functioning of families from a structural systems perspective and the type of problem familes encounter. Areas covered include the functioning of the parental sub-system, family rights and responsibilities, and the need for flexibility in families.

Phase I
Lesson 1. Orientation/Role Induction/Effective Parenting Skills
Lesson 2. Effective Parenting Skills (continued)

Phase II

(Lessons 3-6), **Bicultural Effectiveness Training** is a part of the Bicultural Effectiveness Training component and is oriented toward providing the family with a broad understanding of cultural/developmental factors that impose upon Hispanic families living the the United States as well as to create certain structural arrangements that will prevent intergenerational culture conflict. The Bicultural Effectiveness Training lessons begin with an introduction to biculturalism, culture conflict and family development. These very difficult concepts are presented in **very simple form** and in a language that is familiar to the family. The first lesson is essentially oriented toward establishing the basis for a transcultural, shared world view. The next three lessons target for intervention those specific areas in which culture conflicts intersect family interactions. For the FET modality, three such areas are targetted: family composition style, family interactions style and interpersonal boundaries. For each of the three content areas, a common worldview is established. The purpose of the sequence of Bicultural Effectiveness Training lessons is to teach the family how a transcultural perspective can be applied to all areas of family functioning.

Phase II

Lesson 3. Family Change and Development; Cultural Change and Conflict

Lesson 4. Family Composition Styles

Lesson 5. Family Interactional Styles

Lesson 6. Interpersonal Boundaries

Phase III

(Lessons 7-9), **Conflict and Communication** is another part of the Family Development component and is oriented toward providing the family with the family developmental skills necessary for coping effectively with conflict and keeping the lines of communication open in families. Areas covered include conflict resolution patterns and family communication.

Phase III

Lesson 7. Conflict Resolution Patterns

Lesson 8. Family Communication

Lesson 9. Family Communication (continued)

Phase IV

(Lessons 10-13), **Drug Use within the Context of Family Functioning** is oriented toward providing parents with the information about drugs which they will need to enable them to maintain their leadership role (i.e., effective executive functioning) within the family. Areas covered didactically include information about drugs and drug use patterns, the role of peers and family in drug prevention, and alternatives to drugs.

The final phase of FET makes greater use of BSFT interventions within the context of the provision of information of drug use and abuse. Although BSFT is used throughout FET, it is used more intensely and systematically in the final phase in the process of preparing the family for termination. **BSFT techniques are used to facilitate changes in the**

habitual patterns of interactions that block parental leadership on drug use and abuse topics, and promotes establishing parents as effective leaders, particularly with regard to their children's future drug using behavior.

Phase IV

Lesson 10. Drug Information
Lesson 11. American vs. Hispanic Patterns of Drug and Medicine Use
Lesson 12. How to Deal with Peers and the Role of the Family in Prevention
Lesson 13. Prevention Alternatives to Drugs

BSFT as a Component of the FET Lessons

The BSFT component of FET is interwoven throughout the FET lessons. The BSFT techniques that were discussed earlier are used to facilitate changes in the dysfunctional habitual patterns of interaction (i.e., structures) that are current sources of family distress or may become future sources of family dysfunction.

There are four strategies that are useful in weaving in the BSFT techniques into FET's didactic presentation. These strategies build on each other and help to move the family from a student or recipient role to the more active participant role that characterizes BSFT work. The four strategies can be summarized as follows:

a. The facilitator encourages the family to express any opinions or feelings that might emerge in response to the information presented.

b. The facilitator encourages family members to bring in examples of their own to illustrate didactic material being presented by the facilitator.

c. The facilitator strategically uses the examples brought in by the family to encourage the family to enact their usual way of interacting around the topics and issues being presented. The facilitator uses these enactments as opportunities for implementing restructuring strategies; that is, to bring about more functional ways of interacting with regard to the topics and issues being discussed.

d. The facilitator can use the interactions generated by the exercises to carry out BSFT intervention. It is important to note, however, **that whatever interventions are made by the facilitator, they must be oriented toward restructuring current family interactional dysfunctions that are responsible for presenting com-**

plaints as well as those interactional dysfunctions that have the potential for creating behavior problems and particularly drug abuse as the child moves into adolescence.

The Logic for the Internal Organization of the Sessions

At the beginning of the sessions emphasis is given to joining. Joining actually occurs throughout all sessions although typically emphasized at the beginning of the program and at the beginning of each session.

The second step in each session is to present the didactic lesson. The didactic material is actually intended to initiate a process of reframing how the family perceives, handles, and responds to the various topics covered.

After the didactic presentation, the facilitator encourages the family to enact their usual way of interacting but initially with a focus on the topic discussed in the didactic presentation (note that while the content of the didactic presentation is used as the launching pad for enactment, the enactment may be allowed to flow into other contents that facilitate the enactment process).

Finally, the facilitator intervenes by giving the family tasks within the sessions that will cause the family to change their interactions and, where appropriate, tasks are given to take home to reinforce in the life context new interactions rehearsed in the session.

Since the topics of the lessons are considered central to behavior problem and drug prevention, interactional dynamics around these topics are definitely addressed, and whenever appropriate interactions around other contents central to the family are also restructured.

NOTE

The Family Effectiveness Training Program was funded by the National Institute on Drug Abuse, grant number 5R01DA2694 to the University of Miami, Jose Szapocznik, Ph.D., Principal Investigator. The authors would like to express their appreciation to Anthony Wagner, Maria Elena Lopez, and Ana Maria Faracci, who worked as therapists in the project and to Olga Hervis for clinical conceptual consultation.

REFERENCES

Berry, J. W. & Annis R. (1974). Acculturative stress: The role of ecology, culture and psychological differentiation. *Journal of Cross-Cultural Psychology, 5,* 382-406.

Haley, J. (1976). *Problem-solving therapy.* San Francisco: Jossey-Bass.

Lasaga, J. I., Szapocznik, J., & Kurtines, W. (1980). *Cultural integration or acculturation.* Unpublished manuscript, Spanish Family Guidance Center, University of Miami.

Madanes, C. (1981). *Strategic family therapy.* San Francisco: Jossey-Bass.

Minuchin, S. (1974). *Families and family therapy.* Cambridge, MA: Harvard University Press.

Minuchin, S. (1976). Structural family therapy. In G. Caplan (Ed.), *Child and adolescent psychiatry, sociocultural and community psychiatry.* American Handbook of Psychiatry, Vol. II. New York: Basic Books.

Stanton, M. D. (1979). Drugs and the family. *Marriage & Family Review, 2,* 1-10.

Szapocznik, J. & Kurtines, W. (1980). Acculturation, biculturalism and adjustment among Cuban-Americans. In A. Padilla (ed.), *Recent advances in acculturation research: Theory, models, and some new findings.* Boulder, CO: Westview Press.

Szapocznik, J., Kurtines, W., Foote, F., & Perez-Vidal, A. (1983). Conjoint versus one-person family therapy: Some evidence for the effectiveness of conducting family therapy with one person. *Journal of Consulting and Clinical Psychology, 51,* 889-899.

Szapocznik, J., Kurtines, W., Hervis, O., & Spencer, F. (1984). One-person family therapy. In W. A. O'Connor & B. Lubin (Eds.), *Ecological approaches to clinical and community psychology* (pp. 335-355). New York: Wiley.

Szapocznik, J., Santisteban, D., Kurtines, W., Perez-Vidal, A., & Hervis, O. (1984). Bicultural effectiveness training: A treatment intervention for enhancing intercultural adjustment in Cuban American families. *Hispanic Journal of Behavioral Sciences, 6,* 317-344.

Szapocznik, J., Scopetta, M. A., Aranalde, M. A. & Kurtines, W. (1978). Cuban value structure: Clinical implications. *Journal of Consulting and Clinical Psychology, 46,* 961-970.

Szapocznik, J. & Truss, C. (1978). Intergenerational sources of role conflict in Cuban mothers. In M. Montiel (Ed.), *Hispanic families,* Washington, DC: COS SMHO.

PART V

EFFECTIVENESS OF CROSS-CULTURAL TRAINING

CHAPTER 14

EVALUATING THE EFFECTS OF CROSS-CULTURAL TRAINING: SOME RESEARCH RESULTS

HARRIET P. LEFLEY

UNTIL FAIRLY RECENTLY, evaluation materials for cross-cultural training have typically been limited to specific uses such as preparation for the Peace Corps, diplomatic services, overseas business ventures, and the like. Many of these sourcebooks have interesting cross-cultural exercises, but limited potential for adaptation in other settings. Some valuable theoretical (Triandis, 1977) and applied (Renwick, 1981) models have been developed for evaluating effectiveness of any type of cross-cultural training, with some generalizability to training in mental health.

Specifically focusing on issues in culture and mental health service provision are contributions by D. Sue (1981) and Lambert (1981) on the respective evaluation of process and outcome variables in cross-cultural counseling and psychotherapy, and by Sundberg (1981) on developing appropriate research hypotheses. D. Sue (1981) in particular has pointed out the grave methodological problems inherent in evaluating cross-cultural helper effectiveness, citing the inappropriate rating systems currently available for measurement of such attributes as counselor empathy, warmth, and genuineness. Moreover, targeting specific verbal behaviors and skills requires utilization of response taxonomies that ignore the possibility of cultural inappropriateness of helper behaviors. Sue cites Ivey & Authier's (1978) system as a valuable exception, since their model attends to a range of cultural influences and foci in the counseling process.

Unfortunately, none of these contributions provides a paradigm for evaluating the effects of cross-cultural counselor training in changing process and outcome in the therapeutic encounter. Rather, they raise more questions than can presently be answered definitively, given our limited technology is evaluating the effects of any type of clinical education.

In a book devoted exclusively to evaluation of professional training in mental health, Guttentag, Kiresuk, Oglesby, & Cahn (1975) note that assessment of such programs is typically piecemeal, focusing on discrete structural and process variables rather than on outcome. The focus may be on the stated objectives of the program or the teaching method employed; the trainees' knowledge and attitudes; qualifications and capacities of the trainees; or the quality of positions attained following training. Rarely is evaluation focused on the effects of training on the patients served, i.e., on the transfer of training to actual practice.

One of the reasons for this may be the still problematic nature of the research methodologies for evaluating psychological therapies (APA Commission on Psychotherapies, 1982; Spitzer & Klein, 1976). The issue is compounded in evaluating outcome of continuing education efforts. Even with carefully controlled experimental paradigms, there is still a large domain of patient-therapist characteristics that may interact or be confounded with the effects of the new content and/or techniques learned.

The evaluation design developed for the University of Miami's Cross-Cultural Training Institute for Mental Health Professionals (CCTI) involved the full range of questions relating to structural, process, and outcome components of the training. This program, too, was interested in attainment of curriculum objectives, trainer competencies, trainee change, transfer of training, and long-range effects on service delivery. The evaluation model attempted to integrate these various components in an overall research design with interrelated parts and its own internal logic. It was believed that short-term impact on trainees following the workshop experience should generalize to long-range impact on the patient or client population in order to support an inference of effectiveness of training.

The CCTI Evaluation Model

In our overall research design, six major modalities were used in evaluating the CCTI. Two modalities, involving subjective assessment, have been discussed in the previous chapter and are not included here. These included participant feedback in evaluating the workshops, and a follow-up report of the long-range impact of the training on the participant's own work, self-concept in various specified dimensions, analytic perceptions of one's own professional education, and views of good mental health care.

The objective modalities similarly focused on both short-range and long-range evaluation, the latter occurring six months to two years following CCTI attendance.

Short-Range Evaluation

This evaluation focused on the conceptual and experiential impact of the CCTI training on the participants, assessed in a series of paper and pencil measures and a videotaped exercise on a pretest-posttest basis. Trainees completed the battery prior to the first day's training, and again on the final day of the workshop.

We had developed a set of primary research questions to assess the short-term impact on trainees, and had operationalized them in a series of dependent measures. The questions were as follows:

1. Has the trainee gained new knowledge about the client's culture? Is there a significant improvement in level of knowledge from the baseline levels, i.e., a reduction of cognitive distance?
2. Is there a significant reduction in social/affective distance, i.e., in willingness to accept a person from another culture and/or SES group at varying degrees of closeness of intimacy in one's personal life?
3. Is there a reduction in attitudinal distance and in stereotyping?
4. Is there a change in value distance (difference between one's own values and values attributed to one's own culture and two contrast cultures)?
5. Can the trainees demonstrate, behaviorally, greater therapeutic effectiveness after training, as rated by knowledgeable members of a different ethnic group (professionals and potential clients)?

Long-Range Evaluation

(a) **Effects on Clinical and Administrative Practice.** These were primarily based on action plans and the attainment of operationalized objectives, related to clinical or agency practice, which were developed by each trainee at the end of each training session. Objectives were established on Kiresuk-Sherman (1968) Goal Attainment Scaling (G.A.S.) grids for managerial goals. These objectives typically involved the joint effort of two or more participants of a particular agency. CMHC staff were assigned to facilitate the completion of the G.A.S. grid, since many of the participants were not familiar with the procedure. Each trainee or cluster of trainees was assisted in setting up realistic, attainable goals within a reasonable time frame. Operationalizing the objectives at each of five levels of expectation was completed through joint discussion of trainees and CMHC facilitators.

(b) **Agency Changes and Spinoff Effects.** These referred to structural changes in agency practice and spinoff effects that ensued as a result of CCTI participation but were not anticipated in the action plan phase.

(c) **Impact on Clients: Minority Utilization and Dropout Rates.** These objective measures were considered among the most powerful indicators of long-range impact of training. Specifically, it was hypothesized that if training were successful, the results would be manifested in more culturally sensitive services, both in clinical and administrative practice. The prediction was that these changes would generate (1) an increase in minority utilization, and (2) a significant reduction in dropout rates. Because CCTI content had focused heavily on Black and Hispanic populations, it was expected that a dropout reduction would be seen in these specific populations. However, if the training actually resulted in more sensitive service provision, it was further expected that this sensitivity would generalize to all clients, minority and nonminority alike, for both clinician-participants and agencies as a whole.

In the following section, each one of the above-mentioned evaluation modalities is presented separately, with its methodology, findings, and brief discussion and conclusions, if warranted, together with a final integrative summary at the end. In most of the analyses, it was possible to do intragroup comparisons of black and white participants to determine possible interactions with trainee ethnicity. Unfortunately, there were insufficient Hispanics for a tri-ethnic comparison. Major findings are presented here, with more detailed tabular data available elsewhere.[1]

I. SHORT-RANGE EVALUATION: CONCEPTUAL AND EXPERIENTIAL IMPACT ON TRAINEES

Cognitive Measures

In addition to a didactic test, specific to each workshop, two major instruments were used for all Ss: the **Chitlin' Test,** and **Personalities.** The Chitlin' Test has been characterized as follows:

> The Chitlin' Test is a "classic" instrument of unknown origin that has two major uses: (1) to teach that cultural deprivation in situation-specific — the members of the dominant majority may be ignorant of the culture of others; and (2) to motivate participants early in training to explore their attitudes about minority-group cultures (Fromkin & Sherwood, 1976, p. 144)

Essentially, the Chitlin' Test is a three-part instrument. Part I is a 10-item multiple choice test of knowledge of Black language and life-style; Part II requests fill-ins for initials of Black organizations, such as N.A.A.C.P., S.N.C.C., etc.; while Part III consists of matching names with descriptions. Part II of the test, which contained some items considered obselete, was not used.

Part III was adapted and expanded into the **Personalities** Test. From a 13-item instrument dealing only with Black public figures, we expanded the list to a 22-item instrument which included persons of Afro-American, Afro-Caribbean, Haitian, Hispanic, and American Indian heritage of historical or contemporary political significance.

One of the most significant aspects of this cognitive testing is that the measures were designed to test motivation rather than mere retention of content. The motivational aspect, mentioned by Fromkin and Sherwood's prior description, was utilized in this investigation to tap whether, indeed, the trainees would be interested enough to add to their knowledge of minority cultures on their own. There was no attempt purposively to insert the information on personalities or linguistic specifics in the formal lectures. Rather, the tests were intended to tap individuals' interest in actively obtaining the missing information from staff, other trainees, books, and the like, or by specifically asking lecturers about material they did not know.

Method

A 2 x 2 ANOVA was performed on both Personalities and the Chitlin' Test. Ethnicity was the grouping variable and pretest-posttest was a repeated measure.

Results

Personalities: The participants were able to identify significantly more Black, Hispanic, Haitian, and American Indian historical and contemporary personalities in the posttest than in the pretest $(F(1,128) = 60.73, p < .001)$. There were no significant effects due to ethnicity or ethnicity x trial interaction.

Chitlin' Test: All trainees showed significantly higher knowledge of Black language terms and lifestyle terms in the posttest $(F(1,128) = 27.49, p < .001)$. Expectedly, Black trainees were more knowledgeable than Whites, so that main effects due to both ethnicity and time were significant at the .001 level. However, it is noteworthy that they, too, added significantly to their knowledge, with scores increasing over time. Interaction effects were not significant.

Attitudinal Distance

In tapping attitudinal distance, we decided to adapt a teaching device which had been developed by David Landy called "Controversial Statements" (Fromkin and Sherwood, 1976, pp. 60-61). This was a 24-item instrument originally developed for group discussion of selected statements in a structured experience on minority relations. In our usage, we modified and expanded the sheet to a 27-item instrument, with the input of minority professionals. The statements primarily were commonly heard prejudices and stereotypic complaints, such as too rapid progress made by minorities in terms of economic advancement, affirmative action and other preferential treatment, political power and "welfare coddling," rights to exclude others from private clubs, and the like. Some positively phrased items were also included, although most were unidirectional. Respondents were requested to agree or disagree on a five-point Likert scale.

Method

The 27 items on controversial statements were subject to a principal components factor analysis with iteration and varimax rotation. The first 8 factors were used for subsequent analysis. These factors had eigen values greater than one and cumulatively accounted for 62.9% of the variance in the data.

Factor scores were computed for each subject by summing the responses on all the items within each factor. Scores on items with negative loadings were reversed. A 2 x 2 repeated measures ANOVA was performed on each of the 8 factors. Ethnicity was the grouping variable and time (pretest-posttest) was the repeated measure.

Results

Since almost all items were unidirectional, with most reflecting common stereotypic statements about minorities, almost all responses of Black and White trainees alike, were in the "disagree" end of the continuum. With the positively phrased items reversed, the factor scores reflect disagreement with the indicated categories of stereotypes. On some factors, however, the responses of Black trainees reflected significantly more disagreement than the responses of White trainees. The following differences were all significant at the .001 level.

Factor 1 - "Making It." Blacks disagreed significantly more strongly than Whites that minorities had made progress or could work their way up as easily as Whites. They did not believe courts were too lenient on offenders.

Factor 2 - Preferential Treatment. Blacks disagreed significantly more than Whites that it is unfair to give preferential treatment to minorities. But Whites disagreed more over time and Black disagreed less over time, (p < .025).

Factor 3 - Integration/Busing. Blacks disagreed significantly more strongly than Whites that integration and busing may have adverse effects.

Factor 4 - Intrinsic Prejudice. Whites disagreed significantly more strongly than Blacks that Whites feel intrinsically superior.

Factors 5, 6, 7, 8 - No significant differences. These factors were Political Power; Self Help; Confrontation; and Welfare.

Summary: Overall, Black and White trainees tended to disagree with common stereotypic statements about minorities that refer to rapid progress economically, in affirmative action, integration, and political power; but Blacks disagreed significantly more strongly than Whites. On one item, however, significant changes over time might be attrib-

uted to the training. That is, the White trainees showed greater acceptance of the need for preferential treatment of minorities. Black trainees,
on the other hand, indicated less strong affirmation of this need.

Social Distance

Method

The Social Distance Scale developed for this research is an adaptation of the Westie Summated Differences Scale (Westie, 1953), which
was specifically developed as a measure of racial attitudes. The Westie
format consists, essentially, of four separate social distance measures
within four interactional contexts: A. Residential; B. Physical; C. Interpersonal; and D. Positional. Residential, Physical, and Interpersonal
scales measure the degree of closeness or proximity which the respondent is willing to grant while the Positional scale is supposed to measure
the extent to which the respondent is willing to have the attitude-object
person occupy positions of power and prestige in the community.

The summated difference scores is calculated by comparing a person's distance responses to White and Blacks in the same occupations. In
our adaptation, however, we essentially developed a new instrument by
modifying the stimulus items and adding one ethnicity and three SES
levels. These were designed by the stimulus pull of three occupational
levels: professional, storekeeper, laborer.

Our Social Distance Scale thus includes four dimensions of social distance (residential, physical, interpersonal, positional) for three ethnic
groups (Black, Anglo, Hispanic) each at three SES levels (high, middle,
low). Trainees completed a grid in which they indicated the extent of
their comfort with selected situations of closeness.

Results

Two by two ANOVAs were performed on the nine social distance
subscores and the three summary scores with rater ethnicity and time
the independent variables. The effect of ethnicity was significant on five
of the subscores and two of the summary scores. Blacks indicated significantly more social distance than Whites to White storekeepers and professionals ($p < .001$), and to Hispanic professionals ($p < .001$). Whites
indicated significantly more social distance than Blacks to Black laborers
($p < .01$) and to Black storekeepers ($p < .05$). On the summary scores
Whites showed significantly more social distance to Blacks overall

(p < .01) and Blacks showed more social distance to Whites overall (p < .001).

There were few main effects due to time independently of ethnicity. This seems to be due to the fact that on almost all of the dependent variables the Whites showed a decrease in social distance scores and Blacks showed an increase (see Figure 14-1). The only significant Black increase due to time is to Black professionals (p < .05). The Whites, however, had significant decreases over time in social distance toward Hispanic professionals, Black storekeepers, White storekeepers, Hispanic storekeepers and Blacks overall (p < .05).[1]

Figure 14-1

SUMMED OVER CLASSES: PRE AND POST

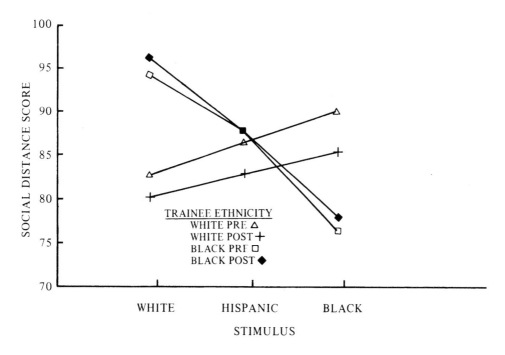

The pre-post *r* for all stimulus figures was analyzed to assess whether there was response stability across time for both Black and White respondents. All *r*s were significant at the .001 level for both Black and White trainees (R = .67).

Discussion

The Social Distance Scale yielded the first finding of what subsequently emerged as a pattern of differential response to the training on the part of Black and White mental health professionals. Overall, Blacks and Whites performed in a culturally predictable manner; they preferred their own groups. This response, as well as all the others, tended to suggest that we were tapping honest responses rather than an acquiescence factor. However, only the White trainees performed in the hypothesized direction; on almost all dependent variables they showed a significant decrease in social distance. The trend was quite opposite for the Black trainees, as may be seen in Figure 14-1.

Black trainees thus showed: (a) overall, a rise in social distance to professionals of all cultures, as opposed to other SES stimulus figures; (b) a significant rise in social distance to peers of their own culture-Black professionals. Black mental health professionals were in effect distancing themselves from themselves. This was supported behaviorally by the open verbalization of role conflict during the processing of the experiential and didactic materials that related to the Black experience in the Americas. In these discussions, Black trainees appeared to have problems with their identity as mental health professionals. These stemmed primarily from three factors: (a) they were typically a minority— sometimes a "token" in a largely White agency; (b) they were uncertain that their professional education had given them all of the appropriate tools to help their own people, and (c) interrelated with (a) and (b), they felt marginal within the mental health establishment, simultaneously alienated from the White power structure and from their own roots. The street and church experience, in particular, led many Black trainees to make statements such as: "I felt as if this is the first time I've gone home in ten years." And this was in a strange city and an unknown neighborhood.

As "tokens," Black trainees verbalized their loneliness in White agencies and their powerlessness to affect policy or make changes they felt were needed to provide better services to minorities. As clinicians, they felt that much of the technology they had learned was inappropriate for their clients, or directed toward the wrong target—such as insight into intrapsychic conflict, when massive environmental interventions were needed for survival.

It is not surprising, then, that the consciousness raising aspects of the cross-cultural training generated the rises in social distance indicated above—crystallized in the trainees distancing themselves from their own identity as Black professionals. The following represents our thinking on this finding:

We feel, in retrospect, that the initial hypothesis of a linear reduction in social distance was far too simplistic, given the consciousness-raising aspects of the cultural training. It should be emphasized that at no time did the training take on confrontation overtones; these were not encounter groups. The psychodynamics that emerged in the interactions and discussions suggested that many of the Black trainees, and the Whites as well, had feelings to be worked through with respect to their role as mental health professionals. Many trainees, Black, White, and Hispanic, verbalized conflicts of having assimilated alien values in the professional role. However, Blacks worried particularly about alienation from their roots, often evoked by their visits to Black neighborhoods reminiscent of their youth. We feel, in sum, that the training had a salutary effect in unearthing unresolved conflicts which inevitably interfere with appropriate countertransference. . ., or with the therapeutic interaction with different SES clients of the same and/or contrast cultures. This interpretation tended to be confirmed in some of the unsolicited "testimonials" received from trainees long after the workshops, describing their CCTI experiences as highly productive of insight and growth. (Lefley, 1981)

Values and World View

Although there are at least a dozen scales that presumably measure the values construct, none was exactly appropriate for our purposes. In conceptualizing how we wanted to operationalize "values" in the present research, Levitan's (1974) discussion and definition seemed closest to our thinking. Functionally, she describes value as "a king of 'meta-attitude' not directly accessible to observation but inferable from verbal statements and other behaviors" (p. 492). More substantively: "The value realm consists of enduring and central clusters of beliefs, thoughts, and feelings which influence or determine important evaluations or choices regarding persons, situations, and ideas (propositions)" (p. 494).

In our evaluation, these "central clusters" were intended to cover a range of stimuli that would cover most of the important aspects of culture as they are perceived by other individuals. Framed as attitudes toward such phenomena as human nature, life and death, social institutions, age and sex roles, familial roles and relations, authority, religion, education, sexuality, and societal handling of deviant behavior, values thus became a culture's world view.

Method

The format and some of the content of a measure that first came to our attention in Pedersen's (1979) **Beyond Tourism** seemed to lend itself admirably to our purposes. Adapted from materials by Janet Bennet, the scale, simply called "Value Survey" had as its objective: "To contrast values of two persons from different cultures on basic world views" (p. 39). The stimulus was framed as "attitude toward. . .man's basic nature. . .life. . .death. . .problem solving. . .etc." with dichotomous instrumental descriptors ("Basically good, basically evil" and the like) as the extremes in a semantic differential format. A five point scale between the extremes permitted a comparison of scores for oneself and another. For our purposes, this instrument was extensively modified and expanded to 42 stimulus items with a total of 53 component responses. As in the case of the other instruments, modification was based on extensive discussion with professionals from Black and Hispanic cultures to include the most salient stimuli.

The items were then ordered in such a way that the trainees were required to give four responses to the same world view item: their own attitudes toward the stimulus event, and their perception of the attitude of most people in their own culture and the two contrast cultures. Since no Hispanic trainees were involved in the evaluation, both Black and White trainees assessed modal attitudes in the Hispanic culture as one of the contrast cultures. They were asked to anchor their responses to the Hispanic group with which they were most familiar, or alternatively, to "Hispanics generally." Most chose "Hispanics generally."

The format of this instrument enabled us to ask a number of basic questions:

(a) How do trainees perceive their own and contrast cultures on various values related to world view? How do the cultures differ?

(b) How does the trainee differ in values from the perceived values of his or her own culture?

(c) How does the trainee differ from the modal values of other cultures?

(d) In what way do these perceptions change over time? Are these perceptions validated by moving closer to the modal perceptions of persons from the contrast culture?

These questions thus refer to (a) value knowledge, and (b) value proximity. Of the two, the former was considered by far the most important issue. In anthropological fieldwork as in cross-cultural training, it is not expected that individuals adopt the emic of another culture as part of their personal armamentarium. In fact, abnegation of one's own value system would be highly counterproductive. Rather, it is the understanding of another's value system that is desired. Thus questions (a) and (d) were considered the most critical. Item (b), however, the perceived value distance between a person and his/her own culture, was viewed as an index of alienation and used in this way for further analyses.

Analysis and Results

Each item on the World View Survey (WVS) has four responses: (1) self attitudes (respondent's own attitudes), (2) perceived modal attitudes of own culture, (3) perceived modal attitudes in other cultures (Black and White), and (4) attitudes in Hispanic culture. Six discrepancy scores are derived for each item by taking all possible differences between the four responses. These scores represent perceived discrepancy between (1) self and own cultures (SO), (2) self and other cultures (SOt), (3) self and Hispanic cultures (SH), (4) Anglo and Black cultures (AB), (5) Anglo and Hispanic cultures (AH), and (6) Black and Hispanic cultures (BH).

Analysis I

For the first analysis these six scores are summed over all 53 items and the six means calculated. The data used for this analysis are these six average discrepancy scores on the pretest and six on the posttest. A 2x6x2 ANOVA was performed with rater ethnicity the grouping variable and the six discrepancy scores and the pretest-posttest factor as repeated measures. Cell means were tested for significance with Tukey's w.

Results

Main effects due to ethnicity were not significant. Effects due to time, however, were significant with discrepancy scores increasing over time ($F(1,122) = 28.22$, $p < .001$). There were also some significant differences among the six discrepancy scores. The Black-Hispanic discrepancy (BH) was significantly smaller than any of the other five scores ($p < .01$). Also, self-own culture (SO) was significantly less discrepant than any of the others except BH previously mentioned ($p < .01$). The other four scores were statistically similar.

Interaction effects were significant ($F(5,610) = 21.64$, $p < 0.001$). Tukey's w analysis indicated AB and AH scores were significantly higher for Blacks than for Whites ($p < 0.01$) and SH was significantly higher for the Whites ($p < 0.01$). A time by ethnicity interaction showed that the differences between Anglos and Hispanics, as perceived both by White and Black trainees, increased significantly more than all other discrepancies from pretest to posttest ($F(5,610) = 9.67$, $p < 0.001$). At this level of analysis, with discrepancy scores significantly increasing over time, it appeared that perceptions of cultural differences were sharpened during the CCTI training and that in the posttest trainees were reporting these perceptions of discrepancies in world view.

Analysis II: Factor Analysis

The WVS consists of 53 items including the component responses under each numbered attitude heading. A factor analysis was performed on the "self attitude" response in order to reduce these items into underlying factors. The principal components method with iteration was used with varimax rotation. The first five factors were used in subsequent analyses since after that the factors consisted of only one highly loading item each. The first five factors accounted for 56.7 percent of the variance on the scale. Post-hoc comparisons were made using Tukey's w.

Analysis of Variance on WVS Factors

ANOVA was done on each factor 2x4x2. The first factor is ethnicity. The second is repeated measures on 4 ratings (S, O, Oth, H), and the last factor is repeated measure pre and post.
Note: All of the following reported differences were significant as $p < 0.01$.

Factor 1 - Traditional Views

The participants, despite their own ethnicity, felt that they were less traditional than their own culture and the other cultures. White participants rated themselves less traditional than Blacks did.

Factors 2 - Government and Authority

White participants felt that they were more positive toward government than the majority in their own culture and the other cultures.
White participants felt that Black culture was more negative about government and authority than Black participants did.
Blacks felt that their culture was more positive about government than White or Hispanic culture.
All participants felt that the other cultures were more negative than themselves and their own cultures toward government/authority.
Participants showed less alienation from government/authority for

themselves and their own culture over time and more alienation for the other (Black or White) culture.

Factors 3 - Parents and Elders

Respect for elders diminished the more one moved away from his own reference group. As a group, the participants felt that both they as individuals and their own culture had more respect for elders than the Hispanic culture. However, Black trainees viewed all reference groups as showing more respect for parents and elders than did the White trainees.

Note: The first item was a surprising finding. It suggested that the Ss may have been responding to the intergenerational conflict emphasized in the discussion of Hispanic acculturation, rather than to stable characteristics of Hispanic culture.

Factor 4 - Status and Materialism

As a group, the participants felt that status was less important for themselves than it was for most people in their own culture or other cultures. The participants felt that status was more important to people in their own culture than in the other two cultures.

Factor 5 - Religion

Blacks felt that religion was more important to the majority in the White culture than Whites did.
Whites felt it was more important to the majority in the Black culture than Blacks did.
Blacks felt it was more important to White culture than the majority in Black culture.
Blacks felt it was more important to themselves than to others in their culture.

Time was significant as a main effect. All trainees thought that religion became more important to every reference group, including themselves, in the posttest, $F(1,120) = 14.28$, $p < .001$. The reference group was also a significant main effect. Both Black and White trainees saw religion as less important in their own culture than in the other culture, $F(3,360) = 33.28$, $p < .001$.

Overall: Perceptions of White trainees moved more toward perception of Black trainees on all discrepancy scores for all reference groups from pretest to posttest, $F(5,610) = 9.67$, $p < .001$.

Reliability and Other Correlations

There was good response stability for both Black and White trainees across time, with almost all pre-post reliabilities significant at the .001 level. An interesting finding emerged, however, in the correlations between self and own/other culture responses among the trainees. For example, in the case of traditional values, in the pretest, White trainees showed significant intercorrelations among all reference group responses, p<.001 for all. They saw all cultures, and themselves as well, as being close in values. In the posttest, while they continued to see a significant correlation between Black and White and Black and Hispanic cultures, p<.001 for both, the correlation between self and own culture dimished to .06, and between self and Black culture, to r = .01. In contrast, Black trainees did not show a correlation between self and own culture either in the pretest (r = .03) or in the posttest (r = .03). Nor did they show a correlation between self and Hispanic culture (r = 05 pretest, .12 posttest). However, the Black participants did show a significant correlation between self and White culture, r = .31 (p<.01) in the pretest, and r = .39 (p<.001) in the posttest.

Summary of Findings Relevant to Clinical Training

1. Initially, trainees tended to be relatively undifferentiated in terms of values, particularly White trainees. They saw all cultures, and themselves as well, as sharing a similar world view. Discrepancy scores among reference groups increased significantly over time, indicating that perceptions of cultural differences were sharpened during the CCTI training. This was particularly true for differences between Anglo and Hispanic cultures, perceived as the most diverse of the cultural pairs.

2. Over time, the discrepancy scores of White trainees moved significantly closer to those of Black trainees. This suggested that with CCTI training on Black culture, Whites' perceptions moved closer to the modal perceptions of persons from the contrast culture.

3. Respect for parents and elders was perceived as diminishing the more one moved away from one's own reference group. Trainees perceived Hispanics as more lacking in such respect—a surprising finding. This was attributed to the emphasis on Hispanic acculturation in the lectures, particularly to the clinical emphasis on intergenerational conflict as a function of the acculturative process, rather than to any stable characteristic of the Hispanic culture. This finding

highlighted the need to differentiate more strongly, in future training, between synchronic and diachronic processes. It also indicated
the need to emphasize in greater detail the traumatic effects of value
disruption and the clinical interpretation of rapid social change.

4. Despite good response stability, Black trainees showed little correlation between their own values and the perceived modal values of
Black culture. The data suggested that Black professionals seem to
perceive their values as closer to those of the dominant culture and to
a lesser extent, Hispanic culture, than to their own culture. This was
another finding considered of great importance for professional
training. It is elaborated on in greater detail in the final recommendations.

Behavioral Measure: The Videotaped Interview

The final pretest-posttest was designed to answer the evaluation
question: Can the trainees demonstrate, behaviorally, greater therapeutic effectiveness after training, as perceived by knowledgeable members of different ethnic groups?

This question involved two evaluation components: (a) demonstration of actual skill development through transfer of training, and
(b) target group satisfaction, a measure of a client's likelihood to continue and benefit from treatment. The demonstration of actual skill development was to be assessed by observations and rating of mental
health professionals; target group satisfaction involved assessment by
members of the ethnic groups who might comprise the potential client
population. Since piloting with clients in a waiting room setting indicated that the task of multiple ratings was too tedious and somewhat
complex for this population, we decided to use community college students who could provide a sufficiently large N for ethnic matching.

In our final design, trainees were videotaped in interaction with a
role-playing "client" (a Black social worker), using a standardized format. The interview was not only prestructured but focused on an empirically derived representative case. The tapes were viewed and rated
by clinicians and also by a large number of community college students
(A.A. candidates) representing Black, Hispanic, and non-Latin White
populations. Most of the Black students, in particular, were from the
neighborhoods served by the community mental health center and
were quite familiar with the type of case presented by the Black social
worker.

In these ratings, time was the major independent variable. The tapes were rated blind, with the raters having no knowledge of whether the interview was before or after the training. The students were not informed that any training had occurred but were simply asked to assess therapists' interviewing skills.

Method

The Videotaped Interaction

A five minute structured vignette was developed by the principal investigator and three Black clinical social workers on the staff of the Community Mental Health Center. The vignette was based on a typical or representative case in a community mental health center serving a low-income minority population. The social workers had seen many such cases and believed it to be one which might cause dilemmas to a therapist who did not have much experience with culturally and socioeconomically diverse groups.

The vignette consisted of six statements, indicated below, which were to be made by a role-playing "client" as her presenting complaint. The statements enbodied a situation in which a mother with two small children whose husband had deserted her and who had no other means of support, had been referred by the local welfare agency to the community mental health center. Apparently the woman had manifested some emotional problems, but she had little idea of why she was referred and kept emphasizing the need to resolve her reality problems. This background material was used as the basis for a five-minute videotaped interaction between a trainee role-playing a therapist and a staff member role-played by only two individuals: both were Black and female, and both were actually clinical social workers.

The vignette was designed to elicit responses that would demonstrate the trainee's skill in dealing with the following issues: client's expectations of therapy; client's expectations of therapist's role; and appeals to the therapists' authority, both as problem solver and as advice giver. These issues are commonly cited in the literature as barriers to effective cross-cultural counseling. Additionally, the videotape was intended to demonstrate the trainee's skill in dealing with both the concrete and symptomatic aspects of a common reality problem.

The role playing staff members were given the above information, as well as the following instructions:

THERAPEUTIC INTERACTION VIGNETTE
FOR VIDEOTAPE

The following six statements are made by the person role-playing the client. Statements are inserted in sequence as appropriate. While the timing will flow with the interaction, each statement should be made within the five minute period. In this setting, the client tends to dominant the interaction by pushing for answers to her questions until she gets a reaction. She does not permit empty space or silence.

1. Mrs. Johnson from County Welfare sent me here.
2. Well, you all can't help me.
3. I need money.
4. I can't sleep at night 'cause I can't pay my bills. Can you help me get some food stamps?
5. Can I get some medication so I can sleep? Can you get the doctor to give me some?
6. You tell me what I'm supposed to do.

Research Design: Control for Practice Effects

During the first Institute all of the trainees received the pre- and posttest on the videotaped interview. In order to control for effects of the pretest on the posttest, a group was needed that attended the Institute, yet only received the posttest. Therefore, for the second, third, and fourth Institutes, half of the trainees were randomly assigned to a pre-post group and half were assigned to a post only group. Videotaping was discontinued after the fourth Institute since a large enough N (102) had been attained.

Selection of Videotaped Sample

After rigorous piloting, the following procedure was followed: (a) selectees' numbers were placed in a box for random drawing including pre-post, and post only; (b) the first five numbers were chosen from the pre-post group; then the order of presentation was determined by random number; (c) an equal number were chosen from the post only group, with random order of presentation; (d) matching was implemented to select for ethnicity and sex from the pool. This was done as randomly as possible. The final selection included: from the pre-post group, 6 Blacks, 9 Whites; 6 males, 9 females. From the post only group: 4 Blacks, 6 Whites; 3 males, 7 females.

The N of 15 pre-post **Ss**, or 30 vignettes in all, proved the highest feasible N for each to be viewed by equal numbers of students from three ethnicities. In all, it took over 1,000 students to produce the needed ratios (see "Rating the Tapes").

The Instrument

The quality of the taped interview session was assessed with the 12-item, 5-point CCTI Interview Rating Scale. These twelve items were chosen from a longer, 20-item form of the questionnaire which had initially been piloted by 15 CMHC clinicians, the majority of them Black. A principal components factor analysis with varimax rotation was performed on the 20 items version. The 12 items on the shorter form all loaded highly on one factor which accounted for 85% of the variance. This factor was perception of the therapist's problem solving abilities. The other two factors were: (a) specific attending skills, and (b) rapport. The rating scale had been developed by the Principal Investigator and several CMHC clinicians from various informal instruments used to assess psychiatric residents and other clinicians in training.

The Raters

The raters were all freshmen or sophomores in social science classes at one of two colleges in Dade County. Tapes were shown to a total of 1,008 students, 362 males and 646 females. The ethnic ratio was 453 White, 350 Black, and 205 Hispanic.

A typical class would see four pretest tapes and the corresponding four posttest tapes in random order. The students were told that they would see mental health professionals interviewing one of two role-playing clients, and that some "therapists" might be seen more than once. They were then given basic instructions about how to fill out the rating scale. Fifteen tapes, in all, were fully rated in the above manner for the pre and post tests. Of these, six tapes were of Black trainees and nine were of White trainees. Since the twelve items on the questionnaire measure the same factor, the mean of these twelve items was used as a summary score. These summary scores were averaged within rater ethnic categories for each tape. Therefore, we had a Black, White, and Hispanic rating for each of the 15 tapes, pre and post.

To determine whether student ratings of these tapes validly assess the skills of the trainee and the quality of the interview, the 15 tapes were also rated by clinicians on our staff; one minority and one non-minority professional.

Interrater rs. A change score was obtained by taking the difference between the pre and post test rating for each tape. The three pairs of scores (pretest, posttest, and difference) for the two clinicians were correlated yielding Pearson r's of .84, .89, and .76 for pretest, posttest, and difference scores, respectively. All of these are significant at $p < .001$. Thus, a high agreement between the two clinicians was established.

The 15 student change scores were correlated with the 15 clinician changes scores. A Pearson r of .98 ($p < .001$) was obtained, indicating a high agreement in the magnitude of perceived change in the interviews and suggest that student ratings are a valid measure of the skill of the trainee and the quality of the interview, if we can assume that two agreeing clinicians validly assess these variables.

Both students and clinicians also showed good reliability. The students' pre-post r ($df = 38$) was .50 ($p < .001$). The clinicians' pre-post r ($df = 14$) was .63 ($p < .01$).

In addition to the 15 tapes fully rated by both the students and clinicians, there were an additional ten tapes of the posttest only control group that were rated by the clinicians. The means of these ten were compared with the means on the other 15 posttests tapes rated by the clinicians to determine whether the pretest had a significant effect on the posttest. The difference between these two means was tested using Student's t. The difference was small and non-significant, thus indicating that the pretest had little, if any, effect on the posttest, and any pre-post differences can be attributable to the Institute.

A note may be added about determining the criteria the raters used in making their judgements. Althought this was not done in any systematic way, informal discussion with a few students and with both clinicians suggested a common pattern; "therapists" were rated high when they took immediate steps to deal with the client's reality problem and thus alleviate her anxiety. Concrete steps, such as telephoning for an immediate referral or to find out how to resolve problems she might face with "Welfare" in obtaining emergency financial aid, were rated most highly. A therapist who sloughed off the reality problem to ask about feelings, or who focused on the client's psychological problems, i.e., her mention of sleeplessness and request for medication, without first addressing her survival needs, received low ratings. Those who competently addressed all needs in the classical Maslovian hierarchy, received highest ratings. It was suggested that in the event this type of evaluation is replicated, a **post hoc** systematic survey might be indicated for assessing the subjective criteria used in the ratings.

Results

A 2x3x2 repeated measures ANOVA was performed on the 15 sets of pre-post scores obtained from the student rates. The first factor was therapist ethnicity (Black, White), the second factor was rater ethnicity (White, Black, Hispanic), and the repeated measure was time (pre, post).

1. The main effects due to rater ethnicity were significant at $p < .01$ ($F = 5.56$, df $= 2.39$). Inspection of the means of the three ethnicities show that the Hispanic raters gave better scores than did the other two ethnicities.
2. Main effects due to time were also significant at $p < .001$ ($F = 12.14$, df $= 1.39$), with scores decreasing significantly in the posttest. This indicated an increase in the quality of the interview.
3. There were no main effects for therapist ethnicity, although inspection of the means indicated that while Black and White therapists were seen to be about equal in the pretest, the Black trainees received more positive ratings in the posttest. This was almost significant at $p < .051$ ($F(1,39) = 4.04$). However, the fact that therapist ethnicity was not significant, given the ethnicity of the "clients" and the problem situation, adds support to the conclusion that the cross-cultural training was instrumental in increasing the perceived therapeutic effectiveness of all trainees.

II. LONG-RANGE EVALUATION: EFFECTS ON INSTITUTIONS AND CLIENTS

Action Plans

Rationale

The development of action plans served a dual purpose within the conceptual framework of the project. First, it was designed as a critical component of the training activities, the logical wrap up session for each Institute. It involved having trainees actually sit down, think about, and operationalize the transfer of training. This four-hour process typically consisted of the joint effort of two or more participants from a particular agency with the assistance of CMHC staff. Even though we recognized the need for the customary overall processing or wrap up session, we wanted to take it a step further and have it result in a concrete mechanism whereby we could increase the odds of changes occurring at the home agencies as effected by the training. Recognizing the need for an instrument or technique that would permit the efficient setting of action goals in operational terms we selected Goal Attainment Scaling, G.A.S., (Kiresuk & Sherman, 1968). The techniques were initially developed for and usually applied to direct services (patient treatment evaluation) but has subsequently been successfully utilized in setting administrative, programmatic goals.

The G.A.S. technique not only served to formalize and synthesize the action planning process, but, also provided us with the means by which we could achieve our second purpose, that is, that of utilizing the implementation of action plans as one of our long-range evaluation measures. The Kiresuk-Sherman technique provided the mechanism for operationalizing goals and measuring their attainment within a specified time frame.

Methodology

Upon completion of the Action Plan Development session each agency team or individual submitted a completed G.A.S. containing the goals negotiated by them and the CCTI staff. Each agency team was asked to review their G.A.S. with the appropriate administrative staff upon returning to their agency. This allowed for fine tuning with overall agency goals, reinforcement of the previously expressed support of executive directors who had sent their staff to CCTI, and the setting of more realistic goals following the period of euphoria generated during the training. Final Plans were due at our offices three weeks after the Institute. Follow up of goals occurred six months after submittal date for the final action plans even though the agencies were asked, for their own monitoring purposes, to do a preliminary follow up after three months. All participants were sent a follow up packet with copies to the executive directors. This packet contained instructions, a sample evaluated G.A.S. and a copy of their original action plan. Written statements were solicited, along with the follow up grid, regarding any obstacles or problems that explained less than expected attainment of goals.

Results

Out of 86 separate action plans developed throughout the various Institutes 52 (61%) were returned with complete follow up information. It is known that a number of key personnel had moved from the agencies at which they had been employed and that information could not be gathered. At any rate, the percent of return was very good, no doubt a result of the ease with which follow up can be performed and reported utilizing the G.A.S. technique.

Goals were categorized and first analyzed. Of the 221 goals contained in the Action Plans, 71 (32%) were attained at the expected level of success, 28 (13%) at the more than expected level, and 24 (11%) at the most favorable outcome possible. Thus, for 56% of all goals, the expectations were met or exceeded.

Overall Goal Attainment scores (unweighted) were then computed according to the Kiresuk-Sherman method. Distributions of Goal Attainment scores commonly have a mean of 50 and a standard deviation of 10. Agencies met or exceeded ($\bar{x} \geq 50$) the goals set within the following categories: Cross-Cultural Training for Other Agencies; Ethnic Representation on Advisory Boards; Public Information and C & E; and Development of Services for Special Populations. Agencies very nearly attained goals at the expected level within the categories of Cross-Cultural Training for Agency Staff; Development of Culturally Sensitive Treatment; Needs Assessment of Ethnic Populations; Community Liaison and Outreach; Recruitment of Minority Staff; and Continuing Education.

Mean Goal Attainment scores were then analyzed for clinicians and administrators, including executive directors as a subgroup. Administrators had significantly higher success levels than clinicians ($t = 3.05$, $p < .01$). Expectedly, agencies sending their executive directors attained the highest level of success.

Other Agency Changes and Spinoff Effects

There were multiple examples of structural changes and spinoff effects that were not included in the original action plans, e.g., development of courses on cross-cultural issues in social services for a local university; at least two state community support program projects focusing on cross-cultural issues in working with the chronically mentally ill; a replication of the CCTI model focusing on providers of human service to refugee populations; and special training projects for police officers, hospital staff, and others working in multiethnic centers.

The most dramatic spinoff effects was a decision by the executive director and key staff of a large community mental health center in Tennessee, to begin decentralization of their center immediately after attending CCTI. The Executive Director and other staff who had participated in the training were impressed with the success of the decentralized community clinic structure of the University of Miami-Jackson Memorial CMHC. Thus, in addition to implementing cross-cultural training, the mental health facility took steps to provide better services to its largely minority catchment area by totally restructuring its service delivery model. The center's technical assistance request extended to our CMHC's needs assessment approach, operating relationships, reporting forms, etc. — i.e., to a number of different parameters that come under the rubric of cross-cultural training which aims at better service provision to minorities. All of the Tennessee center staff who interacted with us during our agency site visit attributed the new organizational change directly to their participation in the CCTI. After two years, the staff brought their decentralization program into full effect with three clinics operating out in the community. From the provision of cross-cultural training for their own staff, they moved on to other agencies. Many other agencies and CCTI trainees have taken less ambitious but no less effective steps to bring about structural changes in services. An example is a CMHC in South Carolina establishing a clinic at a local Baptist church to improve both geographic and psychological accessibility for the local Black population.

Minority Utilization and Client Dropout Rates

Rationale for Study

As an objective indicator of efficacy of training, one of the most critical long-range evaluation measures focused on the hypothesis of (a) an increase in minority utilization and (b) a reduction in client dropout rates. Dropouts are probably the best indicator of inacceptability of services. More than client satisfaction studies and other self-report measures that may be subject to an acquiescence response style, the failure of a client to return, without prior reason or subsequent notification, is the clearest indication that the client feels that he is not benefitting or can benefit no further from the clinical services offered. Research indicates that by far the majority terminate because of negative attitudes toward the therapist or because therapy is perceived as being of no benefit, rather than because of self-perceived improvement (Acosta, 1980).

Our basic hypothesis was that the level of cultural awareness will be increased in the clinicians and administrators who attend CCTI, and that this would be reflected in an observed decrease in client dropout rates in two areas: (1) the clinicians' personal caseload due to a better understanding of the client's culture and needs, and (2) in the overall agency dropout rate due to culturally sensitive procedures initiated by the administrators.

It was predicted that the client dropout rates six months after participants' attendance at CCTI would be significantly less than the dropout rates six months prior to attendance at CCTI. The premise was that these effects would generalize to all clients — minority and non-minority alike — as a result of heightened awareness and sensitivity.

Method: Problematic Aspects of Research Design

Although standard N.I.M.H. criteria were used for defining dropouts, they were applied on a post-hoc basis. In the present research, it was advisable that trainees should have no knowledge of the dropout study in order to avoid confounding the results by differential treatment of patients. For this reason, and because we are dealing with a variety of agencies, it was impossible to develop a preoperationalized procedure for establishing criteria and maintaining a uniform data base across facilities. An additional reason was that the final selection of candidates typically took place within three months of the workshops, rather than six months prior to the workshop, to insure careful adherence to selection criteria needed for training and research, as well as logistics of housing arrangements.

In terms of the research, then, both selection procedures and design requirements militated against preassessment of dropout rates. It would have been extremely difficult if not impossible to develop a separate dropout data collection system with program evaluators or other MIS personnel without knowledge of the CCTI partipants from a particular agency.

One of the major problems was the restrictive range of available data sources. Despite an expressed desire to cooperate in data collection, many participating agencies could not contribute data for the following reasons: (a) they did not compute dropout rates; (b) they used different criteria for computation; (c) they did not keep a separate breakdown by ethnicity for dropout rates; (d) they retained statistics only on an annual basis, with manual systems precluding easy retrieval of data. This MIS heterogeneity also militated against developing an effective control group design. The highly variable MIS and inability to plan observations also precluded the type of control that might have been achieved if a quasi-experimental design using a time series had been possible.

This study used each mental health facility as its own control. The investigation did not use a control group, i.e., a matched group of mental health facilities which did not receive cross-cultural training. Although this would have made for a far more elegant and rigorous design, the logistical problems, as well as the basic problem of contamination discussed earlier, militated against this methodology. However, without this control, it might be argued that a reduction in dropout rates could merely reflect the passage of time, possibly attributable to a general increase in therapeutic sophistication of staff and/or consumer satisfaction with the therapist during the second six month period. Two factors militate against this argument. First, our participants were for the most part trained individuals with years of experience in the field, who would not be expected to show a significant increase in therapeutic sophistication in six months time without an intervention. Second, and more important, is the fact that trends in NIMH Annual Biometry Inventory data do not support this conclusion. Normative data on all federally funded CMHC's indicate remarkable stability in dropout rates across time. The national dropout rates in the last two biometry inventories, for example, deviated by only 0.2%, two-tenths of one percent over a two year period (NIMH, 1980, 1981). This tended to support the assumption that changes in dropout rate, if observed, could not be attributed to time alone.

A difference in proportions test was employed to test the hypothesis that the average drop-out rate would decrease after attendance at CCTI. Additional analysis included (a) determining whether changes in dropout rates could be attributed to changes in ethnic ratios, and (b) a test of the relationship between agency dropout rates and numbers and types of participant administrators. Additionally, percentage dropout rate was assessed in terms of the level of attainment of goals — overall G.A.S. score and G.A.S. score for cross-cultural training of staff.

The caseload and dropout data were broken down by ethnicity. It should be noted that not all of the agencies/clinicians providing caseload data were able to provide dropout data. Therefore, dropout rates were calculated using only those agencies/clinicians with complete data. The changes in dropout rate before and after was calculated and presented as a percent of the dropout rate before.

Table I

AGENCY CASELOAD CHARACTERISTICS AND DROPOUT DATA FOR SIX MONTHS BEFORE AND SIX MONTHS AFTER CCTI ATTENDANCE

	Caseload/Minority Utilization All Reporting Agencies (N = 22)				Dropout Characteristics Agencies with Pre-Post Dropout Data (N = 11)								
	(a) CL Before	(b) CL After	(c) Δ CL (b-a)	(d) %Δ CL (c/a)	(e) # DO Before	(f) CL→DO Before	(g) CL→DO Rate Before (e/f)	(h) # DO After	(i) CL→DO After	(j) CL→DO DO Rate After (h/i)	(k) Δ DO Rate (j-g)	(l) %Δ DO Rate (k/g)	(m) z
All Clients	30373	30899	+526	+2%	2238	10109	.22	1788	9857	.18	−.04	−18%	7.04**
White Clients	20732	20893	+161	+1%	1482	5809	.26	1188	5300	.22	−.04	−15%	3.82**
Black Clients	8886	9149	+263	+3%	464	2040	.23	448	2134	.21	−.02	−9%	n.s.
Hispanic/Other Clients	755	857	+102	+14%	79	396	.20	20	456	.04	−16	−80%	7.07**

** $p < .001$

Note: Row 1 Dropout table includes one agency with no ethnic breakdown: therefore, rows 2, 3, and 4 (White, Black and Hispanic) do not add up to total.

Legend:

CL = Caseload
ΔCL = Change in Caseload
%ΔCL = Percent Change in Caseload
#DO = Number of Dropouts
CL→DO = Caseload Contributing to Number of Dropouts

Results

Agency Data

A total of 22 agencies sent caseload statistics but only 11 agencies could provide standardized dropout data for both time periods required. It can be seen in columns (k) and (l) that the dropout rate decreased in most cases. For the agencies, three differences were significant at $p < .001$. There was a significant decrease in dropout rate in the agency data for (1) Total clients, (2) White clients, and (3) Hispanic/other clients.

In order to determine whether changes in dropout rates reflected changes in the ethnic composition of the total caseload, the percentages for each group were calculated before and after. However, despite increases in minority utilization, the ratio of ethnicities was constant over the two periods.

It should be noted that the significant dropout reduction among Hispanics was largely attributable to a few agencies with large Hispanic caseloads. Other agencies had minimal Hispanic/others, although the findings were in the predicted direction. This suggests that among agencies serving Hispanic populations, training effects were particularly salient, at least in terms of these data.

Since it was hypothesized that CCTI participation would generalize on an agency wide basis, it was important to determine whether a relationship existed between percentage reduction in dropout rate and (a) number and types of administrators participating in CCTI, and (b) G.A.S. scores. Percentage rates were rank-ordered from high to low, together with rankings of a weighted score for administrative participation (number of agency participants x weighted administrative function). This yielded a **rho** of .61 (df = 9), $p < .05$. However, the G.A.S. scores did not show a significant relationship with dropout rate reduction. This may have been because of the considerable variability in goal categories, some of which did not bear a direct relationship to client treatment and characteristics.

Clinician Data

For the total caseload, 26 clinicians responded. However, only 23 clinicians were able to provide caseload plus dropout data for the two time periods. Individual clinician caseload increased dramatically from time period 1 to time period 2. For total caseload, the mean increased from 70 to 84 per clinician. For those providing dropout data, the average increase was commensurate; from 71 in the six months prior to training, to 82 in the six months following training. With this increase, we might expect greater attrition, rather than less, in the six months following training because of an increased workload and commensurate reduction in time and energy allocated to each client. For these reasons, the relative reduction in dropout rate was all the more remarkable. However, there were significant reductions in Hispanic clients only ($p < .05$), paralleling the agency findings.

It was apparent that among both clinician and agency respondents, reduction in the overall number of dropouts reflected a savings in invested time and effort; this could be given a dollar value as well as a human one.

Cost-Benefit Analysis of the Dropout Study Findings

The agency wide reductions in dropouts, which seem to follow a consistent pattern for the agencies that were able to send us the relevant statistics, are important not only in terms of their inferential statement of client satisfaction, but also in terms of mental health costs. Cost-benefit analysis is typically done on three bases: individual, societal, and cost to some other institution. Unfortunately, we simply do not have the data base available for looking at the first two variables. From the literature we would assume that clients who continue in therapy, rather than dropping out, are satisfied with their therapist and feel that they are getting something of value from the experience (see Acosta, 1980, for clients' reasons for dropping out). The cost benefit to individual clients and their families in terms of productivity, improved role functioning, improved interpersonal relations, and subjective well being can not be assessed here; we do not have individual data to undertake this ambitious level of analysis. We also can not assess societal benefit given the limitations of our data base. From the demonstrated fulfillment of action plans and other activities that have resulted in generalization of information, it is quite possible that an increasing number of institutions may have been affected by the CCTI, with commensurate improvement of services and reductions in premature termination of treatment. However, there is no available data base for costing out benefits which remain at the putative rather than demonstrated level.

The present analysis, therefore, is at the level of savings in costs to the mental health agencies which serve multi-ethnic, multi-cultural clienteles. These costs have been computed for agency wide statistics and for individual clinicians' caseloads.

Cost Analysis: Methodology and Results

Agency Data. The cost analysis is based only on caseloads for which full pre and post dropout data were available. Using the pre period (six months prior to training) as a baseline dropout rate, we determined the expected dropout rate for the post period, (columns g x i), and deducted from this the actual or observed number of dropouts. The number of dropouts saved for a 12 months period (760) was multiplied by the mean expenditure per patient care hour ($27) based on reports of 513 community mental health centers reporting to NIMH by June 12, 1981 (NIMH, 1981). For the eleven reporting agencies, this generated a savings of $1,865 per agency per year.

There were 97 agencies represented in the CCTI training; of these, 82 provided direct mental health services to clients. These included psychiatric hospitals, CMHC's, mental health facilities and social service agencies with psychiatric components. The contributory agencies were representative of this spectrum. At an average savings of $1,865, the 82 agencies would have saved $152,930 per annum. This savings, for one visit, is more than the average annual cost of this project.

Because of the considerable variability in caseload and type of agency, it was considered advisable to attempt to determine the reliability of the estimated savings. The 11 agencies were treated as a sample of the universe of 82 mental health facilities participating in the CCTI. With each agency, we used the pre period as a baseline dropout rate and applied the same procedure as above to determine savings in predicted dropouts. This figure, multiplied by $27, yielded a dollar score for each. Using a standard formula for estimating the sampling error and parameter at the 95% confidence level (M ± t05 x SEM), we determined that the agency savings fell within the range of $70,028 to $236,652. This covered a spectrum of mental health facilities with caseloads ranging from 272 to 2,540.

Clinician Data

Because clinicians have much smaller caseloads, the cost savings are not so dramatic as in the case of total agency caseloads. Nevertheless, using the same methodology, we find a savings of $59 per individual clinician per annum. Since there were a total of 113 individual clinicians attending the CCTI, this would be a projected savings per annum of $6,667 based, as in the agency case, on one visit only.

Projected Savings

It should be noted that this costing out is based on only one output unit, i.e., the last scheduled appointment for which therapist time has been made available. In actuality, dropouts affect the return on total investment, i.e., the output value relative to the amount of program resources invested. A comprehensive cost analysis of mental health care by Binner, Halpern, and Potter (1973) demonstrates that "benefits derived from treatment are directly related to treatment extent" (p. 154). An overview of characteristics of treatment dropouts by Rosenberg and Raynes (1973) indicates "There is considerable evidence that the patients who stop coming to treatment often regress—alcoholics return to drink, addicts to their drugs, and those who attempt suicide are more likely to try again" (p. 229). Mental health care is sequential, requiring building toward an objective. Therefore, many cost analysts believe that all costs incurred toward getting there must be reinvested if the process has to be repeated.

Using the mean number of outpatient episodes (3,249) and mean number of outpatient visits per year (16,207) as indicated in the most recent NIMH Provisional Data on Federally Funded CMHC's (NIMH, 1981), we computed an average of 5 visits per outpatient episode. The mean number of persons served during the year, 3,561, is quite close to the number of episodes and suggests minimal duplication. Based on the rationale previously discussed, it might be argued that the agency investment was actually five times the amount indicated, and that the projected savings might be $764,650 for prospective dropouts prevented by CCTI training. For individual clinicians, savings would be $33,335 per annum. While these data are offered tentatively, it should be emphasized that they refer to one year only of patient treatment. There are adequate bases for assuming that training effects are cumulative, and might very well be projected for forthcoming years. Training of nonparticipant staff, in terms of the numerous cross-cultural training workshops administered to other practitioners at home sites, is reflected in the present analysis of agency data but also may be projected in terms of further spinoff effects. Additionally, as we have indicated previously, there was no way of determining the cost benefit to individual clients and their families in terms of productivity, role functioning, and well being. Nevertheless, we suggest that these also enter into the cost analysis in terms of human and dollar savings by reducing the rates of premature termination of treatment.

Discussion and Conclusions: Dropout Study

Although we have attempted to be as rigorous as possible, we are mindful of the fact that the relatively low N, an artifact of the low return rate, has necessitated extrapolations for which the total error variance is unknown. The findings are clear in the case of the 11 agencies; the reduction in dropout rate is unmistakable and highly significant and we have been able to establish an error range for costs at $p < .05$.

With respect to the inferences drawn from the agency data, it should be noted that 73% of the agencies represented in the dropout study sent administrators. Of the 11 agencies, only three sent clinicians alone. This, together with the significant correlation between administrative function and numbers and dropout reduction in agency caseloads, tends to support the inference that agency change was related to administrators' participation in CCTI. It also tends to support extrapolation of cost-benefits to other agencies, 58% of whom had sent administrators to CCTI.

Dropout rates are particularly critical with minority populations. Hertz & Stamps (1977) cite five studies indicating that "members of ethnic minorities, especially Blacks and Spanish-speaking are more likely to break appointments." Wolkon, et al. (1974) have reported drop out rates as high as 74% for Black clients and 75% for Mexican Americans. In the Seattle Project, assessing data on nearly 14,000 CMHC clients, S. Sue (1977) indicated that the failure to return rate after one contact was about 50% for Blacks, native Americans, and Asian Americans, with a 42% rate for Chicanos and Mexicans. This was significantly higher than the 30% rate for Whites, even with income and education controlled. Even for those who did not dropout after one appointment, ethnic minority patients averaged significantly fewer sessions that did White Americans.

Discussions of reasons for dropout have indicated that therapist variables are among the most salient reasons for a client's premature termination of treatment. In a comprehensive overview of twenty years of literature on the subject, Baekland & Lundwall (1975) found that therapist attitudes and behavior, and discrepancies between patient and therapist treatment expectations, were among the major factors predicting patient dropout. Acosta (1980), who conducted the first study to solicit patients' actual reasons for dropping out from three ethnic groups (Mexican Americans, Black Americans, and White Americans), found that "the highest ranking reasons across all ethnic groups were negative attitudes toward therapists and perceiving therapy as of no benefit. These findings support the impression from other studies and investigators that the behaviors, treatment approaches, and attitudes of some therapists may be the most critical variables in explaining high rates of leaving therapy among low-income and minority patients" (p. 441).

This statement, together with all of the confirmatory data in the literature, reinforces the importance of the findings in the current research. While it is evident these findings require replication, they do seem to indicate that just eight days of intensive cultural training may enable therapists and other service providers to significantly reduce premature termination of treatment among some of their minority clientele.

Summary of Evaluation Findings

The following represents an overall summary of all evaluation modalities used in assessing the effects of CCTI on the trainees, their clients, and their institutions.

Participant Feedback

There were highly positive responses on daily ratings of modules, with most given a mean rating of 4.00 or more out of an optimum score of 5.00. Trainees' suggestions were incorporated in current or forthcoming workshops to the greatest extent possible.

Reports of long-range subjective impact, 6-18 months after CCTI training, indicated changes in participants' work, self-concept, views of good mental health care, and assessments of professional education.

Cognitive Distance

Significant rises in learning occurred on both cognitive measures, including identification of important historical or contemporary personages in Black, Hispanic, Haitian and American Indian cultures, and significantly higher knowledge of Black language terms and lifestyle items. This evaluation component tested motivation rather than mere retention of content, since answers were not purposively included in the formal lectures.

Attitudinal Distance

Overall, all trainees tended to show positive attitudes toward minority groups and to disagree with prejudicial or stereotypic statements, such as too rapid progress made by minorities in terms of economic advancement, affirmative action, integration, and political power. Main effects were due to ethnicity rather than time, with Black trainees showing significantly stronger disagreement with the stereotypes than White trainees. However, on one factor there were significant changes over time in both groups. In posttest response, White trainees showed greater acceptance of the need for preferential treatment of minority groups, while Black trainees, although still agreeing, reduced the strength of their affirmation of this need on this dimension.

Social Distance

This test tapped social distance to persons of three socioeconomic levels in three ethnic groups (Black, Anglo, Hispanic) in four interactional contexts (residential, physical, interpersonal, and positional). On almost all dependent variables White trainees showed the predicted decrease in social distance, while Black trainees showed an increase. This was primarily reflected in increased social distance to professionals of all cultures with a significant rise in social distance to their own peers— Black professionals.

Values and World View

Discrepancies between perceived values of self, own culture, other culture (Black or White) and Hispanic culture increased over time, indicating sharpened perceptions of cultural differences from a relatively undifferentiated baseline. Over time, the discrepancy scores of White trainees moved significantly closer to those of Black trainees, suggesting that with CCTI training on Black culture, Whites' perceptions moved closer to the modal perceptions of persons of the contrast culture.

Therapeutic Skill: The Behavioral Measure

A videotaped vignette with a role-playing "client" and trainee "therapist" was rated by 1008 community college students of three ethnicities (Black, Hispanic, Anglo), with time as the major independent variable. Matched numbers of ethnic students rated both pretest and posttest interviews of a sample of 15 trainees with no knowledge of when they were taped. Two mental health professionals, one minority and one nonminority, similarly rated the tapes.

A posttest-only control group was also rated to control for pretest effects on performance. Inter-rater reliabilities between clinicians and between student and clinician rating were highly significant. All ratings showed a significant increase in therapist performance and in the quality of the interview over time. With the control measure, this seemed to be attributable to cultural training rather than to practice effects.

Action Plans

Action plans submitted by 52 agencies (a 61% return rate) included 221 separate goals in the following areas: cross-cultural training for agency staff and for other agencies; development of culturally sensitive treatment approaches; needs assessment of ethnically diverse populations; community liaison and outreach; ethnic representation on advisory boards; affirmative action/minority recruitment; C & E; continuing education for staff; development of services for special populations; utilization review/ethnic client caseload characteristics. Pre-operationalized at five levels of expected attainment, according to the Kiresuk-Sherman GAS method, results indicated that 56% of the goals were attained at the expected level and above, while 44% were attained below the expected level. Scores of action plans developed by agencies that sent at least one trainee whose duties were purely or primarily administrative, were significantly ($p < .01$) higher than those of agencies sending teams or individuals whose duties were purely or primarily clinical.

Agency Changes and Spinoff Effects

Over and above the action plans, agency changes directly attributed by administrative participants to their CCTI experience included: a) total restructuring and decentralization of an urban community mental health center to provide better services to its largely minority catchment area; b) development of a Minority Issues in Mental Health Training package for a state Community Support Project; c) at least four cross-cultural training workshops conducted by the cited CMHC within a one-year period for 40-150 trainees at each workshop; d) a cross-cultural training program for 600 metropolitan police officers; e) cross-cultural training for elementary school teachers and other educators; f) course developed and taught on cross-cultural issues in social services at a major university; g) cultural training for health professionals and other medical staff at a large metropolitan county hospital; h) development of the New Horizons Mental Health Human Services Training Center at University of Miami School of Medicine to respond to the Haitian and

Cuban refugee crisis in Miami, providing cultural training to human service providers serving refugee populations; i) a Mental Health Minority Awareness Training Project, assisting established deinstitutionalization projects in the State of Florida in developing, managing, and enhancing culturally appropriate community support services to minority groups, including conceptualizing and designing all aspects of after-care-community support system operations. More recent spinoffs have included two workshops, by a CCTI trainee, using material learned at CCTI, conducted under the auspices of the Washington State Ethnic Minority Mental Health Consortium in Spokane and Seattle, as well as a two-day workshop on Human Sexuality and Culture conducted by the New Horizons CMHC and the CCTI.

Client Dropout Rates

It was hypothesized that increased cultural awareness in clinicians and administrators would be reflected in an observed decrease in client dropout rates in two areas: a) clinicians' personal caseloads, and b) overall agency dropout rates due to culturally sensitive procedures initiated by administrator-participants. Because of different submissions, there was minimal overlap in the two data sets. Comparison of dropout rates six months before and six months after CCTI participation, using the prior period for baseline percentages, indicated the following: 1) there was an increase in minority utilization, both in clinician and agency caseloads; 2) there was a significant reduction in agency dropout rates for overall caseloads, for White clients, and for Hispanic clients ($p < .001$ for all). For Black clients, the 9% reduction was not significant but in the predicted direction; 3) for individual clinicians, there was a significant reduction in the dropout rate of Hispanic clients; 4) cost-benefit analysis suggested a projected mean annual savings of $152,930 based on only one output unit — the last scheduled appointment. This savings was estimated to be more than the mean annual cost of the CCTI project.

Implications of the Findings

We belief there are three major findings that have important implications for the field. These are (a) the fact that in a mere eight-day training session, mental health professionals can learn and experience enough to generate significant changes in themselves, their clients and their institutions; (b) disclosure of specific needs of minority mental health professionals in applying their training to serving their communities; and

(c) the finding that administrative participation in mental health training facilitates transfer of clinical training skills, as well as ensuring optimal implementation of action plans.

Because we feel these are important findings, these are discussed in considerable detail below. They are discussed under two headings: first, the implications of administrative participation; and second, the implications for professional education.

1. **Administrative Participation.** There are at least two lines of evidence suggesting that involvement of administrative staff in cross-cultural training is critical for effective implementation and spinoff of results. The dropout study indicated that dropout reductions in total agency caseloads are significantly related to administrative participation in cross-cultural training. This includes nonclinical administrators as well as those combining administrative and clinical functions. The G.A.S. study of action plan development indicates that administrators are able to achieve goals at significantly higher attainment levels than clinical staff alone. The implications here are that cross-cultural training efforts that are orientated specifically toward professional education and skill development may produce more sensitive clinicians, but diffusion of knowledge and substantive changes in service delivery requires administrative initiative and input.

2. **Implications for Professional Education**
Mental Health Professionals from the Dominant Culture. In the main, cross-cultural training efforts have been oriented toward the White, middle-class individuals who still comprise the vast majority among mental health professionals. The literature continues to focus on this group with respect to the negative effects of their failures to understand and communicate with clients from contrasting cultural and socioeconomic groups.

With this particular category of mental health professional, represented by the White trainees in the current research, cross-cultural training appears to have significant positive effects in reducing cognitive, social, attitudinal and value distance from other cultural groups. In addition to significant changes in self-report instruments, this learning is manifested behaviorally in several ways: a) an increase in therapeutic skill when interviewing and dealing with the problems of a low-income Black client; b) a 17% decrease in dropout rate of Black clients and a significant 44% decrease in dropout rate of Hispanic clients. These are very important changes and suggest that this target group is easily accessible to knowledge and skill development which, with a short period of training, pays off in highly improved services and considerable cost savings for the mental health service delivery system.

Minority Mental Health Professionals. Almost all of the findings cited above hold true for both minority and non-minority professionals. However, several issues have been raised with respect to reactions of Black professionals which, it is believed, have profound implications for professional education in addition to those omnibus issues that have already been cited.

Several lines of evidence point to identity and role conflict, and perhaps redefinition, among Black trainees. The social distance study gives the clearest indication of this, where the major change was the significant rise in social distance to their own peer group. In effect, it appeared that Black trainees were distancing themselves from themselves. The second line came from the world view study, in which Black trainees showed significant positive correlations between their personal values and the perceived modal values of the White culture, and to a lesser extent the Hispanic culture, but correlations that were mostly in the zero range with the perceived modal values of their own culture. Another line came from the attitude study, where Black trainees, although still affirming the need for preferential treatment of minorities, showed significantly less affirmation in the posttest (while White trainees showed more). If some perceived themselves as receiving preferential treatment, this seemed to be another self-distancing response. Yet, there was such a substantial improvement in therapeutic proficiency with a lower SES Black "client" in the videotaped interview that the differences between Black and White clinicians approached significance at the .05 level.

These "hard" findings were combined with "soft" data of the verbalizations during the group processing periods. At these times, particularly following the street and church experiences, many Black trainees suggested conflicts in two critical areas. One referred to their own self-evaluation and role-conflict as educated middle-class professionals who had moved a great social distance from their own roots. Although some of the Black trainees came from middle-class families, and others from lower SES backgrounds, almost all felt that on some level they had moved away from the majority of Black culture. The other, interrelated conflict referred to the uses of their professional training in providing effective clinical services for the majority of Black clients. Many raised precisely the issues that had been raised earlier in this report regarding basic value assumptions of psychotherapeutic interventions; the sedentary, non-action oriented context of counseling (see Calia, 1966); various inappropriate modes of interaction they have been taught; the culture-bound nature of so many therapeutic goals; and above all, the failure to prioritize and deal with the basic reality and survival problems faced by so many of their clients.

These conflicts are not new to Black professionals. They have been discussed with specific reference to Black mental health professionals by Banks (1980), Jackson (1980), and Jones (1980) among others. Jones specifically states:

> The Black clinician. . .is required to evelute much of this training and much of his thinking about psychology and Black people. . .What is demanded in this kind of personal reevaluation is particularly difficult because it includes social emotional, cognitive, as well as self-image dimensions. . .He knows what effects internal conflicts can have on behavior, and he has conflicts. He is Black and oppressed like his brothers everywhere, but he often enjoys enough environmental comforts to be able to think that he escapes the full effects of oppression some of the time. His effectiveness with community agencies, Black patients, and clients depends on how successful he is in dealing with these conflicts (Jones, 1980, p. 419).

Although this deals specifically with Black trainees, there are indications that the findings might also generalize to other minority groups had there been sufficient numbers to assess in the training. Pedro Ruiz, a psychiatrist who has done much work with Hispanic populations, states categorically: "Suffice it to say that most of what one learns in our classical training programs has little application to this type of program" (services in community mental health centers) (Ruiz, 1982, p. 13).

When the Principal Investigator mentioned some of the preliminary findings to American Indian psychologists, there was instant recognition of the problem and an urging to publish the results. Similarly, among Hispanic professionals, statements were made at some of the institutes — particularly the last workshop where there were relatively more Hispanic professionals — such as "Our training is a million miles away from our communities," "We might just as well not have gone to school. . ." And "What do Freud and Adler have to do with our clients?"

These findings suggest two recommended lines of future training. One requires discrete courses in the special problems of culturally diverse, and acculturating, groups, and interrelated courses in the special behaviors which reflect reactive (or adaptive) responses to minority status and racism. In other words, in addition to attending to the exotic "culture-bound" syndromes clinicians should also be trained to become sensitive to "culture-bound" behavior which comes to professional attention but which may be adaptive rather than pathological. The second line of training refers to a type of self-exploration which probably should be a uniformly systematic component of all professional education, just as psychoanalysis is required for psychoanalytic training. It is apparent that in one way or another, countertransference or its analogue appears in the therapist's interaction with her/his clients. To date, our cross-cultural training efforts have been unidirectional, i.e., we have tried to train White, middle-class Americans, to learn how to be sensitive to the needs of those of culturally contrasting background. There is an apparent need, however, for all therapists to have training in cultural self-awareness. People who have been socialized in a system which has accorded their group second-hand citizenship status, just as those from the dominant culture, need values clarification and identity resolution in order to become optimally effective in helping others.

There are a number of specific recommendations one might draw from these findings: (1) development of culturally appropriate therapeutic modalities for Black, Hispanic, and other ethnic minority clients in which professionals and academicians from these groups take an active leading role, in developing new theoretical as well as empirical approaches to treatment; (2) incorporation of courses in anthropology, sociology, and cultural history as a basic rather than an elective component of professional training of mental health practitioners; (3) internship and practicums in clinical facilities serving low-income, culturally diverse populations, preferably in decentralized neighborhood settings; (4) sensitivity sessions for all graduate students entering a mental health profession, with group processing of issues relating to self-awareness, cultural identity, and perceptions of other cultural groups, and the interrelationships of these perceptions to one's role as a therapist. On the basis of the CCTI experience, it is recommended that such processing take place initially within one's own cultural group, where the climate for self-disclosure and experiential sharing is much more conducive to that type of ego identity which may be essential for optimal effectiveness as a mental health professional.

NOTE

1. A more detailed discussion of research design, comprehensive statistical tables, and copies of instruments may be found in Lefley & Urrutia, 1982. See also Lefley, 1985, for an integrative analysis of the differential impact of training on Black and White mental health professionals.

REFERENCES

Acosta, F. X. (1980). Self-described reasons for premature termination of psychotherapy by Mexican American, Black American, and Anglo American patients. *Psychological Reports, 47,* 435-443.

Alcohol, Drug Abuse, and Mental Health Administration. (1980). *National data book.* Rockville, MD: ADAMHA, Office of Program Planning and Coordination.

American Psychiatric Association Commission on Psychotherapies. (1982). *Psychotherapy research: Methodological and efficacy issues.* Washington, DC: Author.

Baekland, F., & Lundwall, R. (1975). Dropping out of treatment. A critical review. *Psychological Bulletin, 82,* 738-.

Banks, W. M. (1980). The social context and empirical foundations of research on Black clients. In R. L. Jones (Eds.), *Black psychology* (2nd ed., pp. 283-293). New York: Harper & Row.

Binner, P. R., Halpern, J., & Potter, A. (1973). Patients, programs, and results in a comprehensive mental health center. *Journal of Consulting, 41*(1), 148-156.

Calia, V. F. (1966). The culturally deprived client: Reformulation of the counselor's role. *Journal of Counseling Psychology, 13,*(1), 100-105.

Fromkin, H. L., & Sherwood, J. J. (Eds.). (1976). *Intergroup and minority relations: An experimental handbook.* San Diego, CA: University Associates.

Guttentag, M., Kiresuk, T., Oglesby, M., & Cahn, J. (1975). *The evaluation of training in mental health.* New York: Behavioral Publications.

Hertz, P., & Stamps, P. L. (1977). Appointment-keeping behavior re-evaluated. *American Journal of Public Health, 67,* 1033-1036.

Ivey, A., & Authier, J. (1978). *Microcounseling: Innovations in interviewing, counseling, psychotherapy, and psychoeducation* (2nd ed.). Springfield, IL: Charles C Thomas.

Jackson, G. G. (1980). The emergency of a black perspective in counseling. In R. L. Jones (Ed.), *Black psychology* (2nd ed., pp. 294-313). New York: Harper & Row.

Jones, F. (1980). The black psychologist as consultant and therapist. In R. L. Jones (Ed.), *Black psychology* (2nd ed., pp. 418-428). New York: Harper & Row.

Kiresuk, T. J., & Sherman, R. E. (1968). Goal attainment scaling: A general method for evaluating community mental health programs. *Community Mental Health Journal, 4,* 443-453.

Lambert, M. H. (1981). Evaluating outcome variables in cross-cultural counseling and psychotherapy. In A. J. Marsella & P. B. Pedersen (Eds.), *Cross-cultural counseling and psychotherapy* (pp. 126-158). New York: Pergamon.

Lefley, H. P. (1981, June). *Cross-cultural training for mental health professionals in the United States.* Paper presented at the XVIII Interamerican Congress of Psychology, Santo Domingo, Dominican Republic.

Lefley, H. P. (1985). Impact of cross-cultural training on Black and White mental health professionals. *International Journal of Intercultural Relations, 9,* 305-318.

Lefley, H. P., & Urrutia, R. E. (1982). *Cross-cultural training for mental health personnel. Final Report.* Unpublished report. NIMH Training Grant No. 5 T24 MH15429. Miami, FL: University of Miami School of Medicine, Department of Psychiatry.

Levitan, T. (1974). Values. In J. P. Robinson & P. R. Shaver (Eds.), *Measures of social psychological attitudes* (rev. ed.). Ann Arbor, MI: Institute for Social Research.

National Institute of Mental Health. (1980, May). *Provisional data on federally funded community mental health centers, 1977-1978,* Table 11. Unpublished report. Rockville MD: NIMH, Division of Biometry and Epidemiology, Survey and Reports Branch.

National Institute of Mental Health. (1981, September). *Provisional data on federally funded community mental health centers, 1978-1979,* Table 11. Unpublished report. Rockville, MD: NIMH: Division of Biometry and Epidemiology, Survey and Reports Branch.

Pedersen, P. B. (1979). *Beyond Tourism: Alternatives for intercultural awareness.* Preliminary draft, unpublished manuscript, University of Hawaii, Culture Learning Institute, East-West Center.

Renwick, G. (1981). Evaluation: Some practical guidelines. In M. D. Pusch (Ed.), *Multicultural education: A cross-cultural training approach.* Chicago: Intercultural Press.

Rosenberg, C. M., & Raynes, A. E. (1973). Dropouts from treatment. *Canadian Psychiatric Association Journal, 18*(3), 229-233.

Ruiz, P. (1982). Response and critique to L. R. Faulkner, J. S. Eaton, J. D. Bloom, & D. Cutler. The CMHC as a setting for residency education. *Community Mental Health Journal, 8*(1), 13-14.

Spitzer, R. L., & Klein, D. F. (1976). *Evaluation of psychological therapies.* Baltimore: John Hopkins University Press.

Sue, D. W. (1981). Evaluating process variables in cross-cultural counseling and psychotherapy. In A. J. Marsella & P. B. Pedersen. (Eds.), *Cross-cultural counseling and psychotherapy* (pp. 102-125). New York: Pergamon.

Sue, S. (1977). Community mental health services to minority groups. *American Psychologist, 32,* 616-624.

Sundberg, N. D. (1981). Research and research hypotheses about effectiveness in intercultural counseling. In P. B. Pedersen, J. G. Draguns, W. J. Lonner, & J. E. Trimble (Eds.), *Counseling across cultures* (rev. ed., pp. 304-342). Honolulu: University Press of Hawaii.

Triandis, H. C. (1977). Theoretical framework for evaluating cross-cultural training effectiveness. *International Journal of Intercultural Relations, 1*(4), 19-45.

Westie, F. R. (1953). A technique for the measurement of race attitudes. *American Sociological Review, 18,* 73-78.

Wolkon, G. H., Moriwaki, S., Mandel, D., Archuleta, J. Bunje, P., & Zimmerman, S. (1974). Ethnicity and social class in the delivery of services. *American Journal of Public Health, 64,* 709-712.

PART VI

NEW DIRECTIONS FOR PROFESSIONAL EDUCATION

CHAPTER 15

ATTAINING THE TRANSCULTURAL
PERSPECTIVE IN HEALTH CARE:
IMPLICATIONS FOR CLINICAL TRAINING

HAZEL H. WEIDMAN

THIS CHAPTER offers a step-by-step model for attaining the transcultural perspective in health care generally. The schematization that is offered is one the author has used in general medical as well as mental health contexts. It is a model which has been used to order comparative data and cross-cultural training materials in educational, religious, and law enforcement contexts as well. Its value lies in the fact that it provides a framework within which the richness of culture-specific knowledge, the process of achieving self-cultural knowledge, and the details of developing cultural mediating skills may be understood. It allows one to be articulate about the processes and goals of cross-cultural training programs in whatever field they are conducted. The content of such programs may vary; the sequence in which the training materials and experiences are introduced may vary; but, ultimately, in order to attain a transcultural stance, it is necessary to acknowledge the operation of cultural processes and to master the various cognitive stages that support such a posture.

The mental health field is a component of the orthodox health institution. As such, it reflects a range of problems that cannot be restricted to mental health as only one part of the whole. The issues raised in previous chapters of this book apply as well to other components of the total health care delivery system. The schematization to follow can be appropriately elaborated for any specialty area within the orthodox health institution (Weidman, 1982, 1983, 1985). Its contribution in the context of this volume may be that it makes explicit some of the steps in the process of shifting from a unicultural to a transcultural posture in health care generally and mental health care specifically.

Certainly, the evidence is impressive. Culture counts. Ethnicity is a critical factor in the health field but one that is being overlooked or disregarded by many practitioners within the orthodox health care system and by many educators in various professional schools. Despite the fact that a growing cadre of researchers, practitioners, and educators have been working to introduce cultural variables into research protocols, and cultural sensitivity into both service programs and educational processes in health institutions, few have been able to influence the provision of health care in any systematic way. Researchers often are in no position to help plan services which take their findings into consideration. Their impact upon health care is often less direct than that of the practitioner or the educator of health professionals. Nevertheless, even practitioners may incorporate cultural considerations into their own therapeutic efforts without having much impact upon health care generally. And educators may have input into segments of the complex training process without altering the basic paradigm underlying the very structure of that educational system.

Ultimately, in order to better meet the needs of multiethnic patient populations, it will be necessary to convince the majority of our health practitioners, health professional educators, and health system administrators that a transcultural perspective in the provision of health care is more efficacious in achieving health-related goals than is the unicultural (biomedical) perspective now utilized by the majority of health care providers.

Lefley comments in the Introduction to Part II of this volume that the three training programs that are described have in common the goal of bringing participants to a generalizable transcultural perspective. While this may be so, there is little overt acknowledgement of this fact. In the view of this writer, the failure to make adoption of a transcultural posture an explicit goal represents one of the most serious weaknesses in the literature on cross-cultural training. What, precisely, does adoption of a transcultural perspective mean? Why does it make such a difference in outcome for patients and personal satisfaction for health care providers? One of the assumptions regarding the value of such an approach is that it allows health professionals to bridge the gap of social and cognitive distance that may exist between them and some of their patients (and their families).

When health care providers and those who seek care hold different culturally influenced assumptions, they act on the basis of those assumptions. The consequence is that cognitive and social differences create a liminal area between the two that is fraught with ambiguities, misunderstandings, and failures in communication. Liminal or threshold areas are always generative of great confusion; so that anyone attempting to interact across the chasm of cultural difference is, to a certain extent, vulnerable to holding inappropriate expectations, being the recipient of unpredictable types of responses and, therefore, experiencing social and psychological discomfort. This is unacceptable under any circumstances, but particularly so in relation to health care. The ultimate goal of cross-cultural training programs, then, is to improve health care by eliminating the gap (Lefley, this volume) and allowing providers of health care to be more intentional in their attributions and behaviors (Pedersen, this volume). The programs described in this book, and the chapters focusing upon specific cultural groups, certainly, represent efforts in that direction.

As has been pointed out in one way or another through previous chapters, an understanding of cultural differences, alone, will not, in itself, enable health professionals to be responsive to the diverse needs of patients. Learning to individualize care in a culturally sensitive manner is a dynamic process requiring a perceptual shift of a fundamental nature. It literally means defining reality in a new way and enlarging the moral universe within which one works (Weidman, 1976a, 1981). It is a process which begins with cultural awareness, gains momentum with cultural knowledge, including self-cultural knowledge, and is carried forward with the development of skills which allow mediation between separate systems of meaning and behavior (Weidman, 1985). Adoption of a transcultural perspective is required to adequately **assess** significant issues regarding cultural factors in health care. Attempts to **resolve** those issues require adoption of new characteristics in professional roles. These are freeing characteristics rather than limiting ones, however, and may be embraced with enthusiasm.

The step-by-step cognitive model that the author has employed since the early 1970s to help bring colleagues, health professionals, faculty, graduate students, and others to a transcultural posture ordinarily introduces or concludes a series of presentations not unlike those included herein. The transcultural cognitive and perceptual posture is seen as an operational base from which to approach both theoretical and practical problems in the field of health care. It is different from the cognitive and perceptual operational base ordinarily employed. Thus, it represents a new paradigm.

The topic is initiated by describing individuals interacting with others in patterned ways that suggest boundedness:

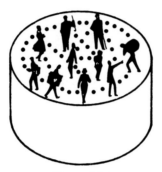

Figure 15-1

Their behavior is guided by certain assumptions they make about the state of their world and the way they should behave within it:

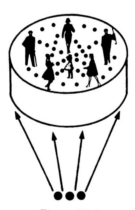

Figure 15-2

Even though such cultural assumptions set the tone and substance for much of what people do, there is always a range of variation in their individual understandings and behaviors:

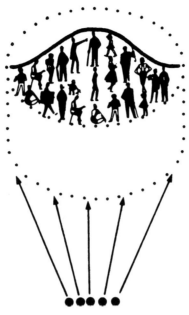

Figure 15-3

It is the dominant patterns of behavior in such a range of variation that leads to stereotyping by others who are not participants in the system. Moreover the individuals in such a system fit into social categories and roles that are hierarchically ordered. Consequently, certain persons in the social system have access to greater resources than others (status/ power/wealth/knowledge, etc.).

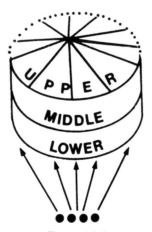

Figure 15-4

Within a social system defined as a nation, there are also groups of individuals whose cultural origins lie outside the boundaries of the nation. These are the resident and immigrant ethnic groups whose members also show a range of variation and are hierarchically ordered in their own right. When such groups accommodate to the host social and cultural system, however, they comprise component parts of the overall structure. Some of their members function within each of the social class levels while maintaining, in varying degrees, both their ethnic affiliation and their representation in the national social and cultural system:

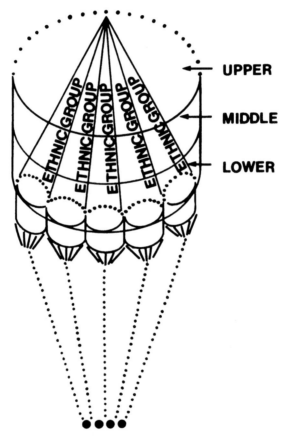

Figure 15-5

Aside from reflecting a range of variation and hierarchical ordering, each cultural system changes through time:

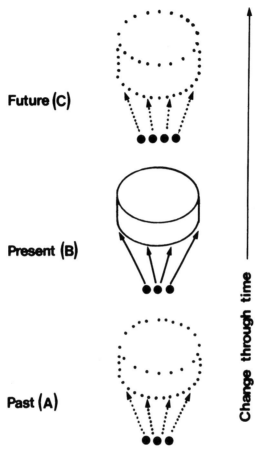

Figure 15-6

While system (a) is not the same as system (b), and system (c) will not be the same as either (a) or (b), there are cultural continuities in basic assumptions and core values that assert their influence through various stages of transformation. These provide orientation and stability in the face of various degrees of social change.

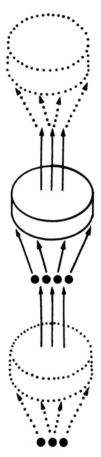

Figure 15-7

Particularly in relation to health and illness do we find tenacity in the retention of beliefs and practices that have security-maintaining functions. Language may change; dwelling types, clothing, modes of transportation, food, and levels of income may change; but the meaning systems which give direction to the manner in which health is maintained and sicknesses are treated change very slowly. They may accumulate new elements, but, ordinarily, these are incorporated peripherally, while the central features are held intact. Even those members of diverse ethnic groups who function in middle and upper socioeconomic statuses may be expected to retain certain understandings and perceptions related to maintaining health and avoiding or treating illness, that have been pervasive in their upbringing. The reason is that these function as elements of a world view that is not always fully transformed along with other behavioral changes that occur through accommodation to or assimilation into the host social and cultural system. Thus, the diagrams introduced to this point (Figures 1-7) may be viewed as representing general cultural systems or they may be seen as representing health cultural systems.

Any number of definitions of the concepts of **culture** and **health culture** might be offered, but the following have been utilized in previous publications and may be introduced here. **Culture** may be understood as "the learned patterns of thought and behavior characteristic of a population or society—a society's repertory of behavioral, cognitive, and emotional patterns" (Harris, 1971). The emphasis upon learning is crucial. When one illustrates the significance of the culture concept by focusing upon the enormous amount of learning that makes it possible to function with ease within a particular society, respect for cultural differences is enhanced (Harris, 1971; Weidman, 1973). There is no way to argue that one process of learning is superior to another. And when we begin to examine systematically the layers upon layers of meaning behind the symbols that organize social life, there is no way to suggest that the complexity of one system is superior to the complexity of another. All have their own logic and integrity. All provide meaning and coherence in support of a way of life that allows survival by meeting both individual and group needs. It is this type of relativity and respect that Matheson stresses in her chapter in this volume. It is this type of relativity that extends as well to an understanding and respect for diverse health cultural traditions.

Health culture is a concept that refers to all of the phenomena associated with the maintenance of well-being and problems of sickness with which people cope in traditional ways within their own social networks and institutions (Weidman & Egeland, 1973). It is a general term that includes both the cognitive and social-system aspects of healing traditions. The cognitive dimension relates to values and beliefs that serve as guidelines for health action. It requires us to understand theories of health maintenance, disease etiology, prevention, diagnosis, treatment and cure. The social system dimension refers to the organization of health care or the health care delivery system. It calls for an understanding of the structure and functioning of an organized set of health-related social roles and behaviors (Weidman & Collaborators, 1978).

Inasmuch as health cultural traditions are integrally linked to general cultural processes, they should command respect as components of the cultural context in which an individual lives and functions. This has not been the case, however, as the chapters in this volume attest and as a now massive cross-cultural literature demonstrates.

In the contemporary world, global migration patterns and cross-cultural research have established two overarching social facts: (1) the populations for which national governments and their human service programs are responsible are now multicultural in character; (2) the orthodox institutions serving these multicultural populations remain unicultural in design, substance, and mission (Weidman, 1981). In the cognitive model under review here, this point is utilized in the effort to help health professionals understand the importance of shifting to a transcultural perspective. The full-blown unicultural paradigm is portrayed as follows:

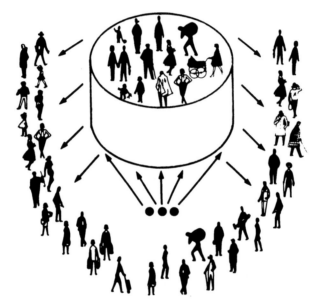

Figure 15-8

The cultural premises which undergird the orthodox health care system in its position of perceived superiority and universal applicability are those that place the highest value upon a rational approach to knowledge, scientific method, professionalism, and technological achievements in the quest for mastery over biological processes and conditions that cause disease (Weidman, 1979, 1985). Those who accept the unicultural health paradigm as the operational base from which they

function, recognize no other social and cultural system as carrying sufficient weight and substance to require their focused attention.

Investigators who have engaged in culture-specific research within
various ethnic groups have established the fact that orthodox health professionals are wrong in their assumption that orthodox health care is
universally applicable in the social sense, i.e., universally understood,
and universally well-received. The data provided by culture-specific re-
seachers have served to bring the concepts of culture, cultural process,
and cultural difference into the awareness of many practitioners of
orthodox health care (Weidman, 1976b).

When professionals within such a system become aware of the concept of culture and cultural differences, social and cultural configurations other than their own begin to be recognized. Cultural awareness
may be portrayed as follows:

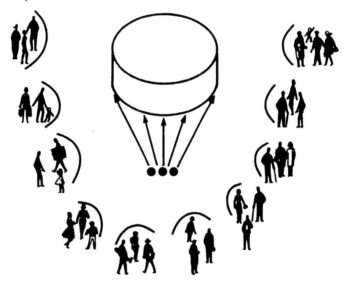

Figure 15-9

Images of those other systems are sketchy and poorly formed, however.
Behavior is seen as fragmented and making little sense, overall. It is only
when cultural knowledge allows a fuller configuration to be drawn that
an appreciation is developed for cultural and health cultural systems as
"sense making wholes" with an integrity of their own. The acquisition of
cultural knowledge may be portrayed as follows:

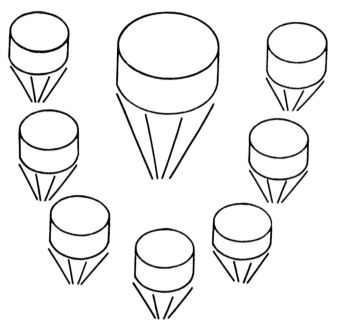

Figure 15-10

Even this recognition does not ensure adoption of a transcultural posture. As suggested by the diagram, the unicultural paradigm may continue to assert its influence through descriptors that contrast "minority" traditions with that of the "majority" (Weidman, 1976b, 1981).

The author has attempted to encourage health professionals to move beyond such asymmetrical assignations by focusing upon equivalence of function, meaning, and worth to participants involved in each of the separate traditions. A fully transcultural posture is portrayed as follows:

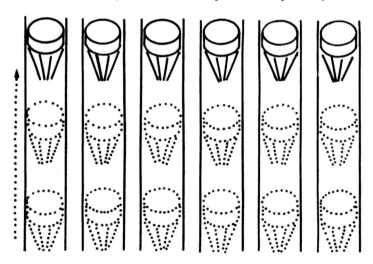

Figure 15-11

True, only one of these — the orthodox health care system — is legally, socially, and politically sanctioned as carrying responsibility for the health of national populations. Nevertheless, in terms of meaning, significance, and worth to participants in the various cultural and health cultural traditions, the systems carry co-equal status. It is for this reason that we have utilized the concept of **co-cultures** in our attempts to help health professionals move from a unicultural to a transcultural posture in providing health care (Weidman, 1973, 1975, 1976a, 1976b).

When health professional and patient meet in clinic settings, they bring meaning and significance of comparable value to each party involved in the interchange. The concept of co-cultures is designed to restructure perceptions from asymmetrical minority/majority distinctions or invalid/valid health knowledge distinctions (Weidman, 1979) toward acknowledgement of co-equal status. This is what Matheson (Chapter 6, this volume) meant when she asked as follows: "Regardless of how honest we are, how can we begin to treat another person with honesty until we are prepared to deal in truths from both points of view?" (p. 7). Co-cultural status is portrayed as follows:

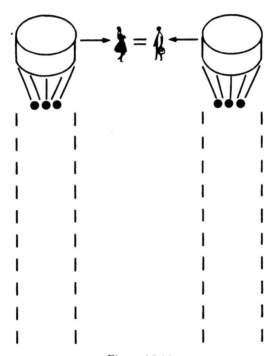

Figure 15-12

In the same way that the concept of co-cultures helps us to attain a transcultural posture; so, also, does the transcultural posture help us to see the need for new terms to both reflect and support that stance. Jackson (this volume), for example, avoids confusion in use of the term, "ethnocentrism," which, in much of the advocacy-type, culture-specific literature has been applied to the orthodox health care system only (this, despite the applicability of the term to all cultural systems). Jackson avoids the lexical complexities that might arise in attempting to use the word to describe a class of behavior applicable to participants in every cultural system while, at the same time, using the term to describe the ethnocentrism of Euro-Americans and the ethnocentrism of Afro-Americans specifically. Instead, he refers to culturalism as a general category, of which Eurocentrism and Afrocentrism are specific examples within the general class. By doing so he asserts unequivocally the transcultural view upon which his discussion is based.

These conceptualizations represent important contributions to a field that is in the process of formalizing a new paradigm for research and practice. The more we can introduce concepts that will hold us to a transcultural posture in our perceptions, in the types of questions we ask and in the strategies of intervention that we develop, the closer we will come to achieving the goals of cross-cultural training that are set forth in this volume.

The transcultural perspective allows clinicians to cognitively, perceptually, and, to a certain extent, affectively, remove themselves from that professional context in which they are ordinarily embedded (Weidman, 1976a, 1976b). From this more "distant" position, they are free to become, initially, more cultural learner than practitioner. The challenge is to move from cultural awareness to cultural knowledge, not only in relation to the patient and the patient's family but in relation to the self as therapist and representative of the orthodox health care system. While the schematization offered here makes this process seem very easy, the Cohen chapter in this volume holds us to the hard realities of clinical assessments in multicultural settings. Despite the complexity of the issues raised by Cohen, however, it may be much easier to fill in the cultural details for the patient than for the self. The contributions of Matheson, Charles, and Sandoval (this volume) are particularly noteworthy in this context.

Once the cultural premises and the contours of the patient's meaning system are understood, however, there is a basis for making explicit comparable premises and value orientations that guide the therapist's behavior and goals. When one juxtaposes the two cultural systems that have come into contact via patient and therapist because of illness, it becomes possible to identify points of congruence or lack of congruence between the two. The Jackson and Sandoval chapters in this book are masterful statements in this regard. The knowledge of similarities and differences in cultural premises, explanatory models (Kleinman, 1980) and co-cultural traditions provides the basis for developing therapeutic strategies that build upon the similarities and mediate between the differences. The acquisition of such skills qualifies one as a **culture broker.** The culture broker position may be portrayed as follows:

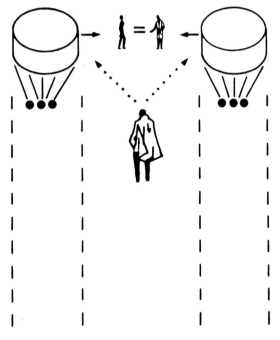

Figure 15-13

Although Szapocznik (Chapter 13, this volume) does not utilize this term in his Bi-Cultural Effectiveness Training, such a training model, incorporated as a therapeutic intervention, builds upon both a transcultural posture and a mediating role that is characteristic of cultural brokerage. Furthermore, the therapeutic technique itself is designed to move the bi-lingual, bi-cultural person to a role more self-consciously like that of culture broker. Also, even though the culture broker concept has not been introduced by authors in this volume who describe their cross-cultural training programs, the skills training they provide requires adoption of some of the characteristics of such a role. When such training is not provided, it constitutes a weakness in the program (Spiegel and Papajohn, Chapter 3, this volume). Cultural brokerage or cultural mediation becomes a central feature of therapeutic intervention in programs serving multiethnic client populations. The brokerage tasks may cover a wide range, indeed (Bestman, Chapter 11, this volume; Lefley & Bestman, 1984; Root, Ho, & Sue, Chapter 10, this volume; Sussex & Weidman, 1975; Weidman, 1975, 1983; Weidman & Collaborators, 1978).

At times, when comparisons are made of separate culture/health cultural traditions, many areas of congruence may be found and only a few of conflict. On the other hand, there will be instances in which the areas of difference are so great that there may be no ground on which negotiation might occur. If one's strategies do pay off, and the patient/family/community benefit from them, there will be considerable personal and professional reward in what has been achieved (see Lefley, Chapter 2, this volume). If there is no basis for negotiation, and the patient is withdrawn (or withdraws) from care, there may be disappointment, but there should be no sense of failure. The choice will have been made within the social context and meaning structure of the patient and his/her family. The attempt to force a culturally dystonic cure upon them would be intrusive, indeed. This is a very different situation from that in which a patient withdraws because of confrontation with a unicultural approach which does **not** take into consideration his own cultural framework and value system.

Let us focus, for a moment, specifically upon mental health care. We have been fortunate in Miami in that we were able during the early 1970s to design a community mental health program on the basis of extensive research into the health beliefs and practices of the five dominant ethnic groups in the inner city area (Weidman & Collaborators, 1978). The program of which I speak, incorporated a negotiating model based upon an explicit transcultural perspective (Lefley, 1975; Sussex & Weidman, 1975; Weidman, 1973, 1975). This proved to be a very successful program which led, subsequently, to the training of mental health professionals from throughout the nation. Cross-cultural training was initiated with the intent to bring care givers to a transcultural posture and provide them with skills to serve clients from varying cultural backgrounds (Lefley, 1982a, 1982b). Evaluation procedures were built into both of these endeavors, one a service program; the other an educational one.

On the basis of this integrated approach to research, service, and training, it has been demonstrated that a transculturally-oriented model of **mental health care** is more efficacious than a standard, biomedical or unicultural model of care (Lefley & Bestman, 1984). Also, it has been established that a transcultural model of **training** serves to enhance knowledge of other cultures, increase self-cultural knowledge, improve clinical skills and performance, and that this is manifested in improved patient care (see Lefley, Chapter 14, this volume).

Perhaps the time has come to move these integrated models of research, service, and training more broadly into the mental health arena but, also, into other medical specialities as well. Can the same positive results be expected in the fields of internal medicine, pediatrics, or family medicine, for example?

At the heart of most cross-cultural training programs is the assumption that, at the clinical level, the sequence of action between patient and practitioner will require dealing with the following basic issues (among a host of others, of course):

Patient enters clinic setting with patient-recognized problem "x" and begins treatment for clinician recognized problem "y."

Issue No. 1: Is problem "x" recognized by health team?

Issue No. 2: Does problem "x" impinge on patient anxiety and solution to "y"?

Issue No. 3: Can problem "y" be cured without resolving problem "x"?

Issue No. 4: Does health care team have the means (skills, knowledge, resources) to resolve "x"?

Issue No. 5: Does health care team take the time/make the effort to resolve "x"?

Issue No. 6: Does patient return home improved or with the potential of being cured of both "x" and "y"?

Issue No. 7: In order to restore the patient to an acceptable level of functioning, is it necessary to modify or even abandon treatment of "y" in favor of treating "x"?

As simple as this schematization may be, it captures the essence of the problem of providing orthodox health care to patients from multiethnic backgrounds. Similarly, it captures the meaning of the phrase, "the social and cognitive gap" between health care provider and client from contrasting cultural background. Significantly, such a sketch may be drafted only from a transcultural posture. Similarly, resolution of the issues raised may be approached only from a transcultural posture.

There is no way to either recognize or deal with them from a unicultural position.

Cross-cultural training programs attempt to illustrate the value of the transcultural perspective by bringing health professionals to the point that mediation between disparate meaning and behavioral systems is possible. The hope is that the knowledge, principles, experiences, and affects derived from such training will contribute to a shift from a unicultural to a transcultural stance. The intent is that the perspective and the assumptions supporting it will be internalized. The premise is that the transcultural paradigm, by enlarging the moral universe within which practitioners function, both allows and encourages the development of new therapeutic skills and strategies to better serve multiethnic client populations. Skills training is designed to both show the way and reinforce the negotiating posture that accompanies adoption of the transcultural approach to health care.

Even if a patient population should be monocultural, however, the personal realms of meaning and behavior of therapist and client may be approached with the same model. Instead of being transcultural in the broader sense, it becomes trans-personal in this more limited sense (Weidman, 1982, 1985). And here, Kleinman's concept of individual explanatory models (Kleinman, 1980) or Pedersen's concept of "salient culture" held by individuals who are members of "cultural" clusters determined by age, gender, social class, occupational group, etc. are pertinent (Pedersen, Chapter 4, this volume).

While a transcultural approach is by no means a panacea, we do have evidence now that the acquisition of mediating skills within the transcultural framework does, indeed, allow for more individualized and culturally sensitive care while alleviating some of the stresses experienced when health care is provided to multiethnic patient populations from a single perspective in which culture is not taken into account.

Evaluation data presented in this volume suggest that a transcultural approach to both mental health care and the training of mental health professionals is of value in meeting the needs of individuals and families of diverse ethnic background. If evaluation data from other medical specialities were to demonstrate similarly beneficial results following adoption of such an approach, a point would be made that would be very difficult to refute. This is the type of "hard data" that may eventually convince the majority of our medical practitioners, medical educators, and administrators that a shift from a unicultural to a transcultural paradigm is justified. If that should occur, we might be well on the way toward closing the gap of social and cognitive distance between health service providers and clients of contrasting cultural background. In the happy event that the transcultural posture is generalized to all patients as a trans-person approach, the orthodox health care system will have been transformed, and there will be no further need for specialized cross-cultural training programs. They will have become integral parts of all health professional training programs. It will be a major breakthrough if this book contributes significantly toward that end.

REFERENCES

Harris, M. (1971). *Culture, man, and nature.* New York: Thomas Y. Crowell.

Kleinman, A. (1980). *Patients and healers in the context of culture.* Berkeley, CA: University of California Press.

Lefley, H. P. (1975). Approaches to community mental health: The Miami model. *Psychiatric Annals, 5*(8), 26-32.

Lefley, H. P. (1982a). *Cross-cultural training for mental health personnel* (Final Report). Miami: University of Miami School of Medicine, Department of Psychiatry.

Lefley, H. P. (1982b). *Cross-cultural training for mental health personnel* (Final Report Executive Summary). Miami: University of Miami School of Medicine, Department of Psychiatry.

Lefley, H. P., & Bestman, E. W. (1984). Community mental health and minorities: A multiethnic approach. In S. Sue & T. Moore (Eds.), *The pluralistic society* (pp. 116-148). New York: Human Sciences Press.

Sussex, J. N., & Weidman, H. H. (1975). Toward responsiveness in mental health care. *Psychiatric Annals, 5*(8), 8-16.

Weidman, H. H. (1973, March). *Implications of the culture-broker concept for the delivery of health care.* Paper presented at the annual meeting of the Southern Anthropological Society, Wrightsville Beach, NC.

Weidman, H. H. (1975). Concepts as strategies for change. *Psychiatric Annals, 5*(8), 17-19.

Weidman, H. H. (1976a). The constructive potential of alienation: A transcultural perspective. In R. S. Bryce-Laport & C. Thomas (Eds.), *Contemporary perspectives on alienation* (pp. 335-357). New York: Praeger.

Weidman, H. H. (1976b). On getting from "here" to "there" (Guest Editorial). *Medical Anthropology Newsletter, 8*(1), 2-7.

Weidman, H. H. (1979). The transcultural view: Prerequisite to interethnic (intercultural) communication in medicine. *Social Science and Medicine, 13B*(2), 85-87.

Weidman, H. H. (1981). Dominance and domination in health care: A transcultural perspective. In M. S. Staum & D. E. Larson (Eds.), *Doctors, patients, and society: Power and authority in medical care* (pp. 133-143). Waterloo, Ontario: Wilfrid Laurier University Press.

Weidman, H. H. (1982). Research strategies, structural alterations and clinically applied anthropology. In N. Chrisman & T. W. Maretzki (Eds.), *Clinically applied anthropology* (pp. 201-241). Boston: D. Reidel.

Weidman, H. H. (1983). Research, service and training aspects of clinical anthropology: An institutional overview. In D. B. Shimkin & P. Golde (Eds.), *Clinical anthropology: A new approach to American health problems?* (pp. 119-153). Lanham, MD: University Press of America.

Weidman, H. H. (1985, October). *Transcultural issues in pediatric oncology.* Keynote address presented during the ninth annual conference of the Association of Pediatric Oncology Nurses, Key Biscayne, FL. To appear in the *Journal of the Association of Pediatric Oncology Nurses.*

Weidman, H. H. & Collaborators. (1978). *The miami health ecology project report* (Vol. 1). Miami: University of Miami School of Medicine.

Weidman, H. H., & Egeland, J. A. (1973). A behavioral science perspective in the comparative approach to the delivery of health care. *Social Science and Medicine, 7*(11), 854-860.

NAME INDEX

A

Abad, M., 24, 27, 37n, 38n
Abbott, W. L., 24, 37n
Abel, T. M., 23, 24, 37n
Acosta, F. X., 27, 28, 37n, 161, 180n, 289, 294, 297, 306n
Adebimpe, V. R., 16, 19, 24, 26, 30, 37n
Alcohol, Drug Abuse, and Mental Health Administration, 306n
Al-Issa, I., 11, 37n
Alpert, M., 27, 41n, 160, 161, 180n
Alvarex, R., 11, 42n, 135, 146n, 160, 180n
American Academy of Child Psychiatry, 225, 242n
American Psychiatric Association, 266, 306n
Anderson, R., 143, 146n
Annis, R., 247, 261n
Aranalde, M. A., 175, 181n, 247, 261n
Archuleta, J., 307n
Arieti, S., 41n
Arredondo-Dowd, P., 7, 10n
Ashe, P., 133, 149n
Atkinson, D. R., 28, 37n
Attneave, C., 42n
Authier, J., 83, 85n, 265, 306n

B

Baekland, F., 27, 37n, 297, 306n
Bailey, F. M., 82, 85n
Banks, G., 133, 146n, 304, 306n
Barnlund, D. C., 85n
Bass, B. A., 31, 37n
Bateson, G., 117, 120, 130n, 146n
Batts, V., 145, 148n
Bazzoui, W., 22, 37n
Beaton, S. R., 27, 37n

Becerra, R. M., 12, 26, 37n, 38n, 160, 180n, 241, 242n
Beiser, M., 42n
Bell, C. C., 12, 17, 18, 33, 37n, 38n
Bell, R. A., 43n, 131, 146n
Belmaker, R. H., 22, 38n
Benjamin, L., 28, 44n
Bennett, A. B., 12, 39n
Bennet, J., 276
Bergman, R., 129
Bernal, G., 26, 38n, 203, 205, 209n
Bernier, J. E., 87n
Berry, J. W., 247, 261n
Bertelsen, A. D., 23, 38n
Bestman, E. W., 9, 92, 110n, 111n, 161, 180n, 209, 209n, 213, 214, 224n, 326, 327, 329
Better, S., 133, 146n
Biggs, J. T., 30, 44n
Bingham, R. P., 83, 86n
Binner, P. R., 296, 306n
Bjorck, J., 42n
Blazer, D. G., 15, 38n, 42n
Bloom, J. D., 307n
Blum, J. D., 26, 42n
Boyce, E., 27, 37n
Braswell, L., 23, 38n
Brislin, R., 10n, 39n, 86n
Britain, S. D., 24, 38n
Brodie, H. K. H., 41n
Brooks, G., 133, 149n
Brough, J., 77, 78, 85n
Brown, B. S., 40n, 134, 149n
Brussel, C. B., 229, 242n
Bryson, S., 7, 10n
Buck, M., 133, 146n
Buhl-Auth, J., 16, 35, 44n
Bunje, P., 307n

SUBJECT INDEX

A

Acculturation
 acculturation stress 58, 247; Bicultural Effectiveness Training 255-260; and coping mechanisms 34-35; Cubans 34-35, 255-260; Haitians, 35, 193-195; Hispanics, 165, 228-235, 247-248; structural aspects of 316
Adaptive strengths/coping mechanisms 12, 31-35, 37, 196-198
Administrators,' training 96-98, 107-108, 286-297, 302
Affective disorders (*See also* Depressive disorders) 19-22, 25, 29
 Bipolar-unipolar ratio 22
Africans 24, 32, 227
Afro-Americans (*See* Black Americans/Afro-Americans)
Afro-Caribbeans (*See* Black-Caribbeans)
Agency characteristics
 CCTI trainees 97-98; and effects of training 286-296
Alternative healing systems (*See also* Supernatural belief systems; Root medicine; *Espiritismo; Santeria; Vodou*) 32, 99, 104, 143, 161, 175, 187-191, 199, 222-223, 237
American Indians 8, 14, 18, 49, 97, 105, 205, 269
 alcoholism 122; depression 18; and diagnosis 23, 124; drop-out rates 26, 297; mental health professionals 304; mental health services 107, 115-130; world view/values 121-127
American Psychological Association 6, 73-74, 79, 200, 207-208, 266
Amish, Old Order 20, 22

Anglo Americans/White Americans 49, 91, 97, 178, 205, 213, 215, 222, 230
comparative statistics 179-180; and diagnostic tests 23-24; drop-out rates 297-298; and epidemiology 15-16; and Eurocentrism 132; mental health professionals 132-134, 302-303, 305; and psychotherapy 164, 166, 175-178; responses to cross-cultural training 270-306; value orientations 54-56, 157-160, 175-178; world view 275-281
Anthropology 48, 276, 305
Asian-Americans-Pacific-Americans (*See also* specific ethnic groups) 9, 14, 49, 97, 199-209
 and alternative healing 199; chemotherapy response 29-30; drop-out rates 26, 200, 297; family and family therapy 28, 201-202; mental illness rates 18; National Asian-American Training Center 205-208; psychotherapy with 201-202; utilization of services 199-200

B

Bahamians, 48, 91, 99, 180, 215, 222
 Bahamian mental health team 217, 223
Behavioral measures 281-286
Beliefs; Belief systems (*See* World view and Values; *also* Supernatural Belief Systems)
Bicultural Effectiveness Training 35, 104, 255-260, 325
Biological-cultural interaction 36, 29-31, 242
Black-Americans/Afro-Americans (*See also* Africans; Black-Caribbeans) 8, 13, 48, 49, 60, 91-92, 96-97, 99, 102-103, 104, 131-149, 178, 180, 227, 269

339

Refugees (*See* Cubans, Haitians, Indochinese, etc.)
refugee experience 171, 183-186, 229-223; Cuban 171, 183-184, 223, 232, 235; Haitian 183-186, 223, 230; Vietnamese 230; Nicaraguan 231
Religion (*See also* Alternative healing systems; Supernatural belief systems)
in Black and White cultures 137-138; as cultural strength 31-32, 102; in Haitian culture 187-191; in Hispanic culture 175-176
Research
action-oriented 92; cross-cultural 77, 90-92, 203; on training programs 265-307; on training techniques 82-83
Root Medicine 104

S

Santeria 32, 104, 175, 237
Schizophrenia
comparative rates 15, 18; diagnosis, cultural differences 19-22; International Pilot Study of Schizophrenia 24, 33-34
Self-cultural awareness 13, 108-109, 305
Sex differences
and epidemiology 16-17; in Haitian culture 193-195; in Hispanic culture 155-156; sex role definition 136-137
Socioeconomic status/social class
and cultural immersion 102; and epidemiology 16-17; and mental health services 89-93; and symptomatology 18
Social distance scale 272-275
Social support system 12, 32-34, 37, 108, 196-198
Spanish Family Guidance Center, University of Miami 247, 255
Strengths (*See* Adaptive strengths; Social support systems)
Stress
buffering mechanisms 33, 196-198
Subjective culture 12
Substance abuse (*See also* Family therapy; Family Effectiveness Training) 17, 246-255, 258-260
Suicide 18-19
Supernatural belief systems (*See also* Alterna-

tive healing systems; *Espiritsmo;* Root medicine; *Santeria; Vodou*) 104
American Indian 123-127; Hispanic 175; Haitian 187-191
Symptomatology
and behavioral norms 20-21, 236-237; and diagnosis 18; and epidemiology 18
Syracuse University

T

Trainee characteristics 47-48, 50, 78-79, 96-98
ethnic differences in response to training 270-306
Training, cross-cultural (*See also* individual program names)
goals and objectives 5, 11, 58-59, 92-94, 286-288, 291, 300; in clinical psychology programs 203; effects on agencies and clients 286-296; effects on Hispanic clients 293-294; effects on trainees 105-110, 269-286; evaluation of 64-65, 77-78, 105-110, 265-307; for mental health administrators 96-98, 107-108, 297; methods 52-58, 61-62, 76-83, 100-104, 203-208; minimal competencies 6, 79-80; training approaches 6, 74-77
Training Program in Ethnicity and Mental Health 47, 49-72
Trance possession 190-191
Transactional Systems Theory; also Transactional Field Theory 8, 49, 52-53
Transcultural perspective 47, 104, 257, 311-330
Transference, countertransference 13, 193, 275, 305
Triad Model for Cross-Cultural Counseling (Pedersen) 81-83, 103

U

United Kingdom 21-22, 33
University of Hawaii (*See* Developing Interculturally Skilled Counselors—DISC)
University of Miami (*See also* Cross-Cultural Training Institute for Mental Health Professionals) 48, 74
University of Miami-Jackson Memorial Hos-